k

Budgeting and Financial Management for Nurse Managers

—— The Jones and Bartlett Series in Nursing ——

Budgeting and Financial Management for Nurse Managers

Russell C. Swansburg, Ph.D., R.N.

Jones and Bartlett Publishers
Sudbury, Massachusetts

Boston • London • Singapore

Editorial, Sales, and Customer Service Offices

Jones and Bartlett Publishers
40 Tall Pine Drive
Sudbury, MA 01776
(508) 443-5000
info@jbpub.com
http://www.jbpub.com

Jones and Bartlett Publishers International
Barb House, Barb Mews
London W6 7PA
UK

Library of Congress Cataloging-in-Publication Data

Swansburg, Russell C.
    Budgeting and financial management for nurse managers / by Russell C. Swansburg.
        p.   cm.   —   (The Jones and Bartlett series in nursing)
    Includes bibliographical references and index.
    ISBN 0-7637-0232-3
    1. Nursing services—Business management. 2. Budget. I. Title. II. Series.
    [DNLM: 1. Budgets—nurses' instruction. 2. Nursing, Supervisory—organization & administration.   WY 105 S972b 1997]
    RT86.7.S92   1997
    362.1'73'0681—dc21
    DNLM/DLC
    for Library of Congress   96-50949
                                                                                        CIP

Production Editor: Marilyn E. Rash
Manufacturing Manager: Dana L. Cerrito
Editorial Production Service: Joan M. Flaherty
Typesetting/Design: UltraGraphics
Cover Design: Hannus Design Associates
Printing and Binding: Hamilton Printing Company
Cover Printing: Coral Graphics, Inc.

Printed in the United States of America

01 00 99 98 97   10 9 8 7 6 5 4 3 2 1

To my wife,
Laurel C. Swansburg, R.N.

Contents

9   Personal Financial Management for Nurses   **291**

Russell C. Swansburg
Philip W. Swansburg
Richard J. Swansburg

Preface

This book is based on the premise that the nursing budget should be decentralized to cost-center managers. In nursing such managers were frequently titled *head nurses*; they are now more accurately titled *nurse managers*. Teaching nurse managers the basic concepts of budgeting empowers them, stimulates their motivation to increase productivity, and builds a healthy financial foundation for the organization.

All nurse managers have three main elements of the budget for which to plan: personnel, supplies and equipment, and capital budgets. The basic theory underlying budgets and the concepts involved in planning and managing them are the same for all organizations, although budgeting procedures vary by organization. This text provides examples of actual nursing budgets.

The model for costing and pricing nursing services is based on the *Medicare Cost Report*. Although seldom used, it could be the basis for modeling and forecasting health-care budgets. A nursing price index could be a similarly useful tool. Because financial forecasting should include identification of new products and services, a chapter is devoted to writing a business plan. The actual plan was developed by doctoral students in a health-care economics course taught by the author.

A short chapter on personal financial planning completes this book. Because jobs as we know them are fast disappearing to temporary workers, outsourcing, and other changes in the workforce, personal financial planning is important to every nurse manager, as well as to every clinical nurse.

Budgeting and Financial Management for Nurse Managers

1

Principles of Budgeting

Because the amount and quality of nursing services depend on budgetary plans, nurse managers should become proficient in related procedures. This proficiency will provide the resources necessary for safe and effective nursing care. With limited resources and a competitive market, personnel and material resources need to be used wisely and efficiently. The enlightened nurse manager knows that the person who controls the budget is the person who controls nursing services. The costs of nursing services have been identified for many years, but the income earned from nursing services has been included in "bed and board" on the budget sheets. This practice will cease when, through the efforts of nurse managers, it becomes possible not only to justify the price put on this service but also to institute programs and procedures for charging for direct nursing care. To achieve reimbursement for nursing services will mean that many government regulations and third-party payer policies will need to be changed to allow for direct payment to nursing providers, based on the amount of care given and the skills of the persons giving it.

Budgeting is an ongoing activity in which revenues and expenses are managed to maintain fiscal responsibility and fiscal health. The nurse manager has financial responsibility and is accountable for managing the nursing budget. The nurse manager makes all of the decisions about how to adjust the nursing budget to manage programs and costs. These include adding and dropping programs, expanding and contracting programs, and all modifications of revenues and expenses within the nursing unit.

Basic Planning for Budgeting

Planning yields forecasts for one year and for several years. The budget is an annual plan intended to guide effective use of human and material resources, of products or services, and of managing the environment to improve productivity. Budgetary planning ensures that the best methods are used to achieve financial objectives. It should be based on valid objectives to provide a product or service that the community needs and for which it will pay. In nursing, budgetary planning helps assure that clients or patients receive the nursing services

they want and need from satisfied nursing workers. A good budget is based on objectives, is simple, has standards, is flexible, is balanced, and uses available resources first to avoid increasing cost.

Planning frequently distinguishes business success from business failure. By encouraging managers to think ahead in a coordinated fashion, the budget process is useful during all phases of business operations. Not only do budgets enable management to anticipate problems, they serve also as standards for performance as the business moves forward.

There is no formula for the form, detail, or periods covered by budgets. Each budget system is designed for the situation at hand, bearing in mind the character of the company, its position, and the nature of the plans involved. Ordinarily the budget system is most detailed in aspects of operations most important to the firm's success. Furthermore, the period covered by the budget varies with the nature of the plans and with the degree of accuracy possible in the preparation of estimates.[1]

A nursing budget is a systematic plan that is an informed best estimate by nurse administrators of nursing revenues and expenses. It projects how revenues will meet expenses and projects a return on equity, or profit. It should be stated in terms of attainable objectives so as to maintain motivation of nurse managers at unit or cost-center levels. The nursing budget serves three purposes: (1) to plan the objectives, programs, and activities of nursing services and the fiscal resources to accomplish them; (2) to motivate nurse managers and nursing workers through analysis of actual experiences; and (3) as a standard to evaluate the performance of nurse administrators and managers and increase awareness of costs. These objectives should include the mission, strategic plans, new programs or projects, and goals. Managing the financial end of nursing through an operational budget obviously can create a new dimension for nurse managers. The budget can be a strong support for developing written objectives for the nursing division and for each of its units. It can provide strong motivation for effective planning and it can certainly provide standards by which to evaluate the performance of nurse managers.[2] Effective planning provides for contingencies by indicating which programs or activities can be reduced or eliminated if budget goals are not met. This is best taken care of with a reserve or contingency (rainy-day) fund.

Revenues and costs, or expenses, and operating and capital budgets should all be projected for the long term. Possible problems in future years should be flagged. Every planning decision, whether long- or short-term, should be accounted for in the budget.[3]

Budgeting Procedures

Decentralized budgeting involves the nursing unit managers and their staffs in the process. Nursing service is labor-intensive, which is reflected in the fact that the first six budget-planning steps pertain to that area. Note that only steps 7 and 8 are concerned with nonlabor expenses. The steps are:

1. *Determine the productivity goal.* The director of nursing services and the nurse manager determine the unit's productivity goal for the coming fiscal year.

2. *Forecast workload.* The number of patient days expected on each nursing unit for the coming fiscal year are calculated.
3. *Budget patient-care hours.* The expected number of hours devoted to patient care for the forecasted patient days are calculated.
4. *Budget patient-care hours and staffing schedules.* The budgeted patient-care hours are reflected in recommended staffing schedules by shift and by day of the week.
5. *Plan nonproductive hours.* Vacation, holiday, education leave, sick leave, and similar hours are budgeted for the coming year.
6. *Chart productive and nonproductive time.* To aid in the planning process, a graph is used to show head and assistant head nurses how the level of forecasted patient days, and therefore the staffing requirements, are expected to increase and decrease during the year. Productive time is the time spent on the job in patient care, administration of the unit, conferences, educational activities, and orientation.
7. *Estimate costs of supplies and services.* The supplies and services to be purchased for the year are budgeted.
8. *Anticipate capital expenses.* The expected capital investments for the coming year are figured into the budget.

These eight steps result in a proposed budget that goes to the nursing administrator for review. After preliminary acceptance, this budget is sent to the accounting department, where the forecasted patient days are turned into expected revenue. The budgeted productive and nonproductive time is converted to dollars, as are the costs for supplies, services, and other operating expenses that will be allocated to a given nursing unit for the coming year. A pro forma operating statement is then returned to the director of nursing for review with the head nurse. When the director of nursing and the head nurse accept the budget, it is returned to the accounting department and forwarded with the rest of the hospital managers' budgets to administration and the board of directors.[4]

People who pay high prices for health care want accountability of both costs and quality of service. The nursing budget can be a shared responsibility, with unit budgets being prepared with staff involvement at the clinical level. The planning and controlling processes are ongoing. Through their participation, clinical nurses enhance their professional stature. A budget prepared and executed as a shared experience becomes an object of ownership to a staff who will put forth effort to work within its framework.

According to Osborne and Gaebler, budgets should be developed without line items, based on the idea that funds can be moved around to fit shifting needs. Many health-care organizations follow this rule. In one instance a new cardiac rehabilitation program was developed and budgeted based on this rule. Cost-center managers agreed to shift funds because they could see the advantages of the program and had been led to believe that they owned their budgets. All unused funds should be carried over into the new budget. This policy reduces the wasteful practice of spending money to keep budgets constant or to prevent reduction.[5]

Managing Cost Centers

A cost center is a given area of assigned accountability for both direct and indirect expenditures. A department of nursing is a cost center, as are each of its

units, each clinic, in-service education, surgical suites, and any other section with a nursing mission in which nurses provide services to clients. Each cost center is assigned a code. A reference (Seawell) is available for a uniform accounting and reporting system for hospitals. An organization may use this coding system, which is usually referred to as the patient-care system. It requires workload measurements, sometimes referred to as performance classifications or units of measure. The unit of measure for each cost center is identified as a specific, quantitative statistic, such as inpatient days or relative value units (RVUs). The number of RVUs defines the tangible things done as evidence of production and to measure quantity, quality, and cost.

Each cost center is an internal department dealing with distribution of services and products. The cost-center manager is responsible for determining the cost of each service or product and how these services or products are distributed within the organization. Two types of cost centers are mission, or revenue-producing, and service cost centers. Examples of mission, or revenue-producing, centers are radiology and laboratory departments. They have monetary income relating to the purpose of the organization. Service centers are support centers that provide a service to other units and charge for that service; there is no exchange of revenue. The unit served adds the costs of these support services to its costs of output.[6] Examples of these centers are communication, purchasing, and laundry.

Each cost center has a manager, called the cost-center manager or the responsibility-center manager, who is responsible for identifying needs for equipment and programs to maintain progress at the current level of technology in the unit.

Budgeted costs within the cost center are broken down into subcodes. This promotes better budgetary planning and control, because items are specifically identified during the budget planning process. Also, each item purchased is charged to (debited from) the balance shown for that specific subcode.

Many hospitals do not credit nursing units as income-producing (mission or revenue) centers; it is time they did so. The same codes can be used for income-producing centers as for cost centers; in fact, in some organizations they are known as "activity centers." Nurse managers establish systems for (1) determining that work is being performed by the appropriately skilled person and (2) determining the charges for each hour of care a patient receives. Controlling processes determine that a registered nurse (RN) does not often perform activities that can be performed by nursing assistants. Although shifting performance of activities that require less skill should be expected as practical and necessary, nursing workers should not be expected to perform activities for which they are not educated, skilled, or licensed.

Teaching patients can be charged for and paid by third-party payers when it is planned with initiative. Nordberg and King recognized the need to educate patients and took action to accomplish third-party payment. They emphasize low-key approaches to financial reimbursement for teaching patients and acknowledged the assistance of their organization's controller. They recommend a thoroughly prepared and documented proposal covering the program's history, behavioral objectives, operational objectives, chart forms, teaching methods, evaluation tools, follow-up procedures, evidence of cost effectiveness such as decreased admissions or hospital stays, and teachers' qualifications. Such a

thorough approach to professional nursing services is often successful in obtaining third-party reimbursement, and will help to move these services out of the arena of "room and board" or "staff nursing care services."[7]

Relationship of Budget and Objectives

One of the chief planning activities is to identify the objectives of the nursing division and each of its units. This includes developing a management plan with a budget for each objective. One of the first sources of budgetary information is the statement of nursing objectives. By using these objectives nurse managers see the benefit of developing pertinent, specific, practical budgetary objectives.

Stages of the Budget

For practical purposes there are three stages of development of the nursing budget: (1) the formulation stage, (2) the review and enactment stage, and (3) the execution stage. These are sometimes labelled forecasting, preparation, and control.[8]

Formulation Stage

The formulation stage is usually a set number of months (six or seven) prior to the beginning of the fiscal year for the budget. During this period procedures are used to obtain an estimate of the funds needed, funds available, expenses, and revenues. These procedures, and the instructions for performing them, should be communicated by the budget officer to nursing administrators and unit or cost-center managers.

Financial reports of expenses and revenues of the previous fiscal year and year-to-date will be analyzed by the chief nurse executive, department heads, and cost-center managers.

One of the first steps in writing a budget is gathering data for accurate prediction of expenses (costs) and revenues (income). This task can be developed into a system. Primary sources of data are the objectives for the division of nursing and for each cost center. Each program and activity needs to have an estimated cost placed on it. If in-service educators want new audiovisual equipment, they should not walk into the nurse administrator's office and expect to have it next week or even next year. It should be planned for six to seven months before the next fiscal year begins, and it may be budgeted for any quarter or month within that fiscal year. In surveying the objectives, nurse administrators and managers evaluate the previous year, review the philosophy, and rewrite the objectives for the future.

Other data include programs from other departments that will require use or expansion of nursing resources, expansion of nursing clinics and client-teaching programs, travel costs for attendance at professional and educational meetings, incentive awards, library requirements, clinical and office supplies and equipment, investment equipment and facilities modification on a five-year plan, and contracts for such items as intravenous pumps and oxygen equipment. Data can be obtained from historical financial records of the organization.

Budgeting is described in terms of programs and activities that are planned to accomplish specified nursing objectives. That is why the writing of objectives is so important and why unit or cost-center budgeting is important. Productivity and accomplishments can be related directly to the unit's programs and activities. This allows financial managers to provide costing and pricing for packages of care. Such a method is referred to as *performance and program budgeting* and requires nurse managers to evaluate deliberately the purposes for which money and resources are expended. It relates productivity and costs to objectives, making nurse administrators and managers cost conscious.

Among the cost-center reports that assist the nurse manager are the following:

daily staffing reports
monthly staffing reports
payroll summaries
daily lists of financial categories of patients
biometric reports of occupancy
biometric reports of workload
monthly financial summaries of revenues and expenses

Review and Enactment Stage

Review and enactment are budget development processes that put together all the pieces for approval of a final budget. After the cost-center managers have presented their budgets to the budget council, the chief nurse executive consolidates the nursing budget. It is then further consolidated into an organizational budget by the budget officer. Approval is made by the chief executive officer of the organization and the governing board. During this entire process there are conferences at which budgets are adjusted.

Nurse managers should be prepared to sell their budgets during budget meetings and other management meetings where products and services are discussed. These are five steps that help:

1. *Be prepared to defend the budget.* Every program must be carefully thought through. Although each budget committee member will have figures at hand, each nurse administrator and cost-center manager needs a detailed plan. This plan includes justification of need, objectives, cost of additional resources (personnel, supplies, equipment, space), and sources of funding.

2. *Initiate a marketing strategy.* This can include selling programs to committee members before meetings to review your budget. For example, to get approval for costs of joint appointments of nursing faculty as nursing staff in a university medical center, a carefully made plan, supported by nursing service and nursing college administrators, could be sold to the vice president for academic affairs. Secure the support of interested parties beforehand and decide how to use that support successfully.

3. *Anticipate challenges.* Who might oppose your program? Why will they be against it? Prepare a sound defense for each anticipated challenge. When nurses are plentiful, finance personnel are prone to want to cut salaries and

fringe benefits. Be prepared to defend call pay, shift differentials, pay for clinical ladders, overtime pay versus compensatory time off, weekends-only shifts, flextime, and other gains made to reduce nursing turnover and boost morale.

4. *Be persuasive without being emotional.* If the clinical ladder is under attack, present the different performance requirements for each level and relate them to productivity.

5. *Work for win/win situations.* Plan fallback positions in the management plan. These could range from optimally to minimally acceptable. Begin with the optimum and if the committee and executives want cuts, negotiate so that they win concessions and the nurse manager wins a program.[9]

Preparation of a sound budget by nurse administrators and cost-center managers will promote favorable action by the budget committee. The nurse administrator can defend the budget alone or jointly with each cost-center manager. Whichever strategy is used, it should be well planned. When these meetings occur, budget committees are interested in and favorably impressed by well-prepared plans. The objectives should be clearly stated, the costs should be accurate, and the revenues should be defensible. Although some budget requests can be disallowed, there are generally few setbacks when a reasonable and well-prepared budget is ably defended by informed cost-center managers.

Execution Stage

Both the formulation and the review and enactment stages of the budget are planning activities. Execution of the budget involves directing and evaluating activities. The budget is executed by the nurse administrators and managers who planned it. Revisions in execution of the budget are scheduled at stated intervals, frequently once or twice during the fiscal year. There are procedures for evaluating the budget at cost-center levels. Budgets are prepared for either fiscal years or calendar years, depending on the policy of the organization.

The entire budgeting process is given a specific time frame with target dates assigned for each step (see Exhibit 1.1). During the fiscal year of the execution stage of budgeting, the formulation and review and enactment stages for the next fiscal year are being carried out.

Cost Accounting

Objectives

Like all other aspects of financial management, cost accounting is part of the total management plan for all levels of hospital personnel and is used by hospital administrators and regulators or third-party payers. Nurse managers, with the hospital administrator and associate administrators, develop clear financial objectives, which are used in all strategic plans and subsequent operational plans. They become an integral part of many management strategies, of communication, of budget negotiations and revisions, of staffing, of cost/price projections, and of cost management.

EXHIBIT 1.1   The Budget Calendar

Formulation Stage (July–December, current fiscal year)
1. Develop objectives and management plans.
2. Gather all financial, historical, and statistical data and distribute to cost-center managers.
3. Analyze data.

Review and Enactment Stage (January–June, current fiscal year)
4. Prepare unit budgets.
5. Present unit budgets for approval.
6. Revise and combine into organizational budget.
7. Present to budget council.
8. Revise and present to governing board.
9. Revise and distribute to cost-center managers.

Execution Stage (July–June, succeeding fiscal year)
10. Direct and evaluate expenses and receipts.
11. Revise budget if indicated.

Nurse managers use various objectives and methodologies of cost accounting to measure the intensity or severity of illness, as well as case mix of patients. Nurses have done more in this area than other operational hospital administrators. It is also important to have objectives and methods for measuring performance or outcome against standards, including those for short-term expenses for all resources. Information is relayed to all managers, particularly cost-center managers.

Nurse managers also have objectives and methods to control variable costs, which fluctuate with volume. They can be controlled most easily through staffing, inventory control, and pricing practices. All objectives for cost accounting should be coordinated with accounting, data processing, plant management, and other affected departments if they are to be effective in controlling costs. Cost accounting is important to cost management because it describes spending behavior.

Cost Factors

Cost is money expended for all resources used, including personnel, supplies, and equipment. The volume of service provided is the greatest factor affecting costs. Others include length of patients' stays, salaries, prices of material, case mix, seasonal factors, and efficiencies such as simplification of procedures and quality management to prevent errors that increase patient complications (morbidities and mortalities) and increase costs. Other factors that have an impact on cost are regulation and competition, third-party payers, the age and size of the hospital, type and amount of services provided, the hospital's mission, and relationships among nurses, physicians, and other personnel.

Accrual accounting counts any future obligation incurred as an expense. Cash accounting, on the other hand, counts expenses only as they occur.[10]

Fixed, Variable, and Sunk Costs

Fixed costs are not related to volume. They remain constant as volume increases and decreases over a period of time. Among fixed costs are depreciation of equipment and buildings, salaries, fringe benefits, utilities, interest on loans or bonds, and taxes.

Variable costs do relate to volume and census. They include such items as meals and linen. Supplies are usually volume responsive, meaning that total costs increase or decrease according to use. For example, supplies vary by patient census, physicians' orders, and diagnosis. Surgical dressings increase in cost when a patient's wound has drainage and dressings must be changed frequently. As census (patient days) vary, the costs of supplies also vary, increasing or decreasing with the census. For this reason, there should be an established unit of measure for productivity in every cost center. This unit may be numbers of tests, procedures, patients of a specific acuity type, hours or minutes of service, discharges, or RVUs. Most activities include elements of both fixed and variable costs. For example, personnel costs and utility costs can be both fixed and variable, since there is a minimum number or amount that is required.

Sunk costs are fixed expenses that cannot be recovered even if a program is cancelled. Advertising is a good example.[11]

Direct and Indirect Costs

Direct costs are the costs of providing the product or service and are often considered to be those directly related to patient care. These include personnel costs and the variable costs of supplies. The definition of direct costs varies by department. In areas removed from direct patient care, each department incurs its own category of direct costs.

Indirect costs are those incurred in supporting the provision of the product or service. These costs are not directly related to patient care, and include utilities, administration, housekeeping, and building maintenance. However, as mentioned above, they are direct costs for the source department. Some indirect costs are fixed, such as depreciation and administration. Others, such as laundry and accounting, are variable. All indirect costs are allocated or transferred by a specific method to the departments that use the services.

Every hospital has a method of establishing costs, including the *Hospital Health Care Complex Cost Report Certification and Settlement Summary*, commonly known as the *Medicare Cost Report*. In a few hospitals, the method is more refined. Nurse administrators should become informed about this activity.

Cost Accounting

A cost-accounting system assigns all costs to cost centers. Periodic, usually monthly, reports of costs are provided to cost-center managers, but they do not reflect all costs. There are many indirect costs that are allocated only once a year in the Medicare Cost Report. These include the costs of utilities, accounting, administration, data processing, admitting, and other items. Informed and influential nurse managers use these cost allocations when preparing budgets. Such allocations are usually hidden in the operational budget under the category of "room costs."

There are two systems of cost accounting, process costing and job-order costing. Process costing is a system whereby costs for an item are accumulated and averaged as unit costs within a cost center. They are then added to the product or service. Supply costs, which are calculated on the basis of cost per patient day, are an example.

Job-order costing accumulates the costs related to a product or service for each order. Although it is done by averaging, resources are more specifically identified for each unit of product or job lot. Better job-order costing is done in hospitals now that a diagnosis-related–group (DRG) system exists. It will become more job- and product-specific as a severity-of-illness index is used and the room rate is unbundled. Costs will then become patient-specific instead of charge-specific. As this occurs, nurse managers will be able to evaluate and compare performance and productivity among cost centers.

Cost assignments to cost centers are made on the basis of direct costing if they are direct costs of patient care. Otherwise they are made by transfer costing from a patient-care support department, or by cost allocation if not related to direct patient care or support. Job-order sheets are used to account for all services to patients. If direct overhead costs cannot be identified with specific services rendered, they are allocated based on some other measurement such as square feet of floor space.

The present cost-accounting system for manufacturing is being modified, with time replacing labor costs as the measurement unit. Quicker customer service reduces inventory time (Drucker uses sunk cost as the term for inventory of finished goods); and reduced inventory time reduces sunk costs. This change in cost accounting can be applied to nursing. Charges for the surgical suite are already partly time based. Also, although hospital accountants say that the Medicare Cost Report is not the best cost-accounting system, an alternative has not been forthcoming. Certainly nurse managers should advocate the unbundling of the hospital income and expense system to account for direct nursing costs by individual cost centers. A time-based cost system could then be developed.[12]

Service Units

Service units are measurable units of productivity or volume that are used to identify and count costs. They must be measurable, known to managers, and affected by volume. Productivity is measured by service units produced.

With the increased sophistication of hospital information systems, it is easier for nurse managers to become involved in identifying and costing service units. It can be done by hours of nursing care per category of acuity of illness. To make this an RVU, all other direct and indirect costs must be allocated on the basis of hours of nursing care per category of acuity of illness.

Chart of Accounts

A chart of accounts that includes a number and table for each cost center is available (see Seawell in references section of this chapter). The chart is subdivided into major classifications and subcodes, such as salaries and wages, employee benefits, medical and surgical supplies, professional fees, nonmedical and nonsurgical supplies, purchased services, utilities, other direct expenses, depreciation, and rent. These classifications are further subclassified.

All movement of labor and materials between cost centers must be recorded in order to be assigned to the correct cost center. All fringe benefits must be charged to the appropriate cost center by some established method. So must all purchases, including those shared. This is usually done using allocated shares of service units.

Amortized expenses are deferred charges allocated to units over a specific period of time. These include depreciation charges for hospital plant and equipment, in addition to prepaid items. Usually the prepaid items are charged monthly as service units. Other deferred expenses include unamortized borrowing costs and costs incurred for capital expansion or renovation programs.

Inventory and Cost Transfer

Identifying actual costs of any service unit is improved through an accurate system of inventory control. Based on the number of orders or requisitions for any item, the appropriate proportion of its costs can be transferred to the cost center that ordered it.

Performance Reporting

Cost-center managers measure performance on the basis of the costs under their control. They cannot control building depreciation, the salaries and fringe benefits of administrators and support personnel, or plant and grounds management.

When actual service-unit costs vary from budgeted costs, cost-center managers should be able to determine the cause. There obviously needs to be a good system of recording activity to identify and control such costs.

Financial Standards and Responsibility Accounting

In an era of retrenchment in the hospital industry, professional nurses will be asked to reduce waste. While they will be expected to maintain high standards of care, they will also be expected to compare treatment expenses with clinical benefits. This will mean making objective, economic choices in use of supplies, equipment, and services. One way nurses can do this is through a system of responsibility accounting.

According to McCullers and Schroeder, a responsibility accounting system for making efficient decisions has these characteristics:

1. *Decision usefulness*. Information is relevant and reliable.
2. *Timeliness*. The information is available before the decision maker loses the capacity to economize on expenditures.
3. *Favorable cost/benefit ratio*. The benefit desired from the information exceeds the cost of collecting, maintaining, and processing it.
4. *Understandability*. Information content is intelligible to those who must handle it and is presented in a form they can grasp.
5. *Relevance*. The information collected actually makes a difference in decisions to be made.
6. *Reliability*. Information faithfully represents what it purports to represent.
7. *Verifiability*. Agreements among independent measures using the same measurement methods can demonstrate content validity to referents.
8. *Materiality*. Information magnitude has a significant impact on the resources of the unit or the organization as a whole. However, magnitude by itself is not sufficient for a decision. The nature of the item and the circumstances in which the decision is made must also be considered.

9. *Comparability and consistency.* Currently collected information can be compared with similar information about the same unit for some other time period.
10. *Neutrality.* Accounting methods are free from bias towards a predetermined result.
11. *Predictive value and feedback value.* The information helps predict or confirm expectations.[13]

Like all other characteristics of quality control, a system of responsibility accounting needs pertinent standards against which accurate amounts can be measured. Financial standards can be developed by using historical data from the accounting division. These will include standards for staffing, medical supplies, equipment, and services. Nurse managers should be sure they obtain input for these standards from practicing nurses. Responsibility accounting can be a motivational factor in making clinical nursing decisions.

In being assigned and accepting financial accountability, nurses have a first duty to their patients, who have given them their trust. They should be accountable to themselves for their work, to their professional peers, to their employers, and in publicly funded institutions, to taxpayers.

One way or another patients pay the costs of health care. It may be through insurance premiums, taxes, fringe benefits, or from their own pockets. Financial accountability means that nurses and others can account for the efficient spending of the money paid for health care.

Nurse managers need information on the costs of all services provided by their institutions and competing institutions. This knowledge will, in turn, be provided to clinical nurses who should know what it costs to do their work. Cost consciousness leads to reduction of waste and to effective cost management.

Some managers believe that overspending can be controlled by controlling nursing labor power and expenditure. This misconception can be rectified by holding nurses accountable for their budgets, both revenues and expenses.

Nurse managers have to justify the cost/benefit ratio of services provided and devise new methods to increase cost effectiveness. They should learn to use computers to their advantage. Increasingly, information-processing technology is covered in nursing curricula. As continuing education becomes more important, a stronger link between academics and clinical practitioners should be formed.

The Cost of Nursing Care

To determine the cost of nursing care, several factors should be considered. Nursing charges should be quantifiable. A patient-acuity system would serve this purpose. The patient-acuity system usually separates patients into four or five levels of nursing care, and enumerates nursing requirements for each level. Charges could be set by level and negotiated with third-party payers. These costs could be separated from the cost of non-nursing requirements. Non-nursing tasks would be reassigned to ensure that the charges for nursing care reflect the actual costs of providing such care.

A second method of costing nursing is determining what share of total hospital costs is attributable to nursing. This would vary by DRG. An industrywide effort for each region could produce standards for nursing costs and charges. Otherwise a majority of the approximately 6,500 acute-care hospitals in the

United States would need to undertake research to determine nursing costs and charges on a hospital-specific basis. Multinational corporations, of course, could apply research studies across member institutions.

Definitions

Budget

According to *Webster's New Twentieth Century Dictionary, Unabridged, Second Edition,* a budget is "a plan or schedule adjusting expenses during a certain period to the estimated or fixed income for that period."

Herkimer has stated that "an effective budget is the systematic documentation of one or more carefully developed plans for all individually supervised activities, programs, or sections. . . . The budget is a tool which can aid decision makers in evaluating operating performance and projecting what future operations might produce."[14]

A budget is an operational management plan, stated in terms of income and expense, covering all phases of activity for a future division of time. It is a financial document that expresses an operation's plan of action. In the division of nursing it sets the limits of financial support, thereby controlling the extent and quality of nursing programs. The budget will determine the number of kinds of personnel, material, and financial resources available to care for patients and to achieve the stated nursing objectives. It is a financial statement of policy. Budgeting is the process whereby objectives and plans are translated into financial terms and evaluated by financial and statistical criteria.

Unit of Service

The unit of service is a measurement of the output of hospital services consumed by the patient. In the surgical suite and recovery room, it is minutes or hours; in the emergency room, it is visits or time and procedures; and in the nursing units, it is the acuity category of patients and hours per day expressed in RVUs. Types of measurement include procedures, patient days, patient visits, and cases.

Revenue

Revenue is the income from sale of products and services. Traditionally, nursing revenue has been included with room charges. Increasingly it is being unbundled from the room rate as a separate charge per patient acuity category and per visit, day, or procedure.

Revenue can include assets such as accounts receivable and income-producing endowments. The latter can be restricted to specific purposes. Buildings, land, and other items can be assets if they produce income or are capable of producing income. Total income is frequently termed *gross income*, with the excess of revenues over expenses being known as *net income* or *profit*.

Revenues also come from research grants, gift shops, donations, gifts, rentals of cots and televisions, parking fees, telephone charges, and vending machines, among other sources. Many may be elements of product lines such as

orthopedic services that include orthopedic nursing, traction equipment, and prostheses, among others.

Revenue Budgeting

Revenue budgeting, or rate setting, is the process by which a hospital determines revenues required to cover anticipated costs and to establish prices sufficient to generate that revenue. Complicating the process is the fact that all patients (purchasers) don't pay an equal, fair share of a hospital's costs.

To remain viable, any business, including a hospital, must generate sufficient revenue to cover operating costs and make a profit. These include increases in working capital, capital replacements, and inflation adjustments. "Nonprofit" hospitals are identified as such for tax status only! Nonprofits use profits to improve plants and services; profits do not go to stockholders or owners. Profits appear as positive balances on account ledgers.

Fundamental to the rate-setting process are adequate statistical data, historical and projected, for implementing the rate-setting method to be employed. This includes, on a departmental basis, volume of services, current rate, allocated costs, and rate increase constraints. The goal is to obtain the greatest impact from a minimum cumulative rate increase in today's cost-management environment. This is done by increasing rates in high-profit departments while instituting rate reductions in low-profit departments so that they offset each other.

In today's reimbursement milieu, revenues are often budgeted before expenses. This is necessary to determine how much revenue will be available.

Expenses

Expenses are the costs of providing services to patients. They are frequently called *overhead*, and include wages and salaries, fringe benefits, supplies, food service, utilities, and office and medical supplies. As part of the budget they are a collection or summary of forecasts for each cost center's account.

Full costs include both direct and indirect expenses. While direct costs such as nursing can be traced to the source, indirect costs such as utilities, telephones, or purchasing services are allocated to the source department by a standard formula. Accountants use a process called *cost-finding* to determine full cost by allocating indirect costs. Revenue and expense budgets are also called *sales budgets* because sales of products and services are the principal income for paying operating expenses and producing profits.[15]

Expense Budgeting

Expense budgeting is the "process of forecasting, recording, and monitoring the manpower, materials and supplies, and monetary needs of an organization in such a manner that the operation of the various components of the organization can be controlled."[16] The components of expense budgeting are cost centers. Purposes of expense budgeting include

- to predict labor hours, material, supplies, and cash flow needs for future time periods;
- to establish procedures for making comparative studies, and

- to provide a mechanism for determining when changes in procedures need to be made, providing gross information on the kinds of changes needed, and providing evidence that control has been established or reestablished.

Historical trends are the single best inexpensive indicator of expenses available to the institution. They are valid for prediction of present and future trends most of the time.

Patient Days

Patient days are used to project revenues. They are commonly used as units of service to compute staffing. Patient-day statistics are usually derived from census reports that are done daily at midnight, and summarized monthly for the year to date and annually. A patient admitted on May 2 and discharged May 10 is charged for nine patient days. See Exhibit 1.2 for an illustration of patient days per unit for one month (July and June columns).

Fiscal Year

The fiscal year (FY) is the budgetary or financial year. It may be the calendar year in some organizations, beginning on January 1 and ending on December 31. Many organizations use October 1 to September 30 as the fiscal year; some use July 1 to June 30. This is done to coincide with budget decisions of state legislatures and the U. S. Congress. In the latter examples, the fiscal year obviously overlaps two calendar years.

Year to Date

The term *year to date* (YTD) describes the accumulated units of service at a particular point in the fiscal year. If the fiscal year begins October 1, the year-to-date patient days for December 31 would be the summary for 92 days. See Exhibit 1.2 for an illustration of year-to-date statistics.

Average Daily Census

The census is summarized for a specific number of days and divided by that number of days. As an example, the average daily census (ADC) for the month of June would be the total patient days for June divided by 30. From Exhibit 1.2 the number of patient days for June was 7436. When this is divided by 30, the average daily census is 248.

Hours of Care

From the nursing viewpoint, hours of care have traditionally been the number of hours of care allocated per patient per day (24 hours) on a unit. With the use of patient-acuity rating systems, hours of care can be determined to the hour or even parts of an hour. Usually patients fall into one of four or five patient-acuity categories, each of which is assigned a specific number of hours of care per patient day.

EXHIBIT 1.2   A Patient-Day Census

	Current Year			Year to Date		
	July	OCC (%)	June	Current Year	OCC (%)	Previous Year
Nursing Station						
3rd Floor	1,014	79.8	833	9,792	78.6	8,650
4th Floor	811	76.9	718	7,834	75.8	7,255
5th Floor North	526	65.3	524	5,300	67.1	4,838
5th Floor South	622	77.2	592	5,587	70.7	5,603
6th Floor	792	71.0	866	8,730	79.8	8,176
7th Floor	850	68.5	895	9,086	74.7	8,885
8th Floor	0	0.0	0	0	0.0	4,403
8th Floor North	376	60.6	383	4,624	76.1	2,393
8th Floor South	303	69.8	274	3,253	76.4	1,729
9th Floor	0	0.0	0	0	0.0	5,138
9th Floor North	526	84.8	501	5,332	87.7	2,690
9th Floor South	481	77.6	506	5,118	84.2	2,617
MINU	104	83.9	89	1,041	85.6	432
SINU	73	58.9	84	964	79.3	471
Burn Unit	173	79.7	188	1,723	81.0	1,912
Labor and Delivery	138	37.1	99	1,228	33.7	1,258
CCU	206	83.1	148	1,848	76.0	1,937
Clinical Research Unit	137	73.7	132	1,342	73.6	1,361
EAU	23	0.0	7	390	0.0	634
MICU	213	85.9	191	2,099	86.3	2,291
PICU	169	54.5	112	1,612	53.0	1,834
SICU	229	92.3	207	2,175	89.4	2,302
NTICU	209	84.3	87	1,891	77.8	2,277
Totals	7,975	73.1	7,436	80,969	75.7	79,086
Nursery						
Newborn	832	103.2	632	7,666	97.0	7,307
Intermediate	577	103.4	457	4,761	87.0	3,991
Intensive Care	955	110.0	716	8,526	100.2	7,022
Totals	2,364	105.9	1,805	20,953	95.7	18,320

Source: Courtesy of the University of South Alabama Medical Center, Mobile, Alabama.

Caregiver

Each nurse who works with patients is labelled a *caregiver*. In nursing the three common types of caregivers are registered nurses, licensed practical nurses, and nurse aides or extenders. Most personnel budgets have a ratio of registered nurses to other caregivers. There is considerable research supporting an all-RN caregiver staff. The current cost-management environment will alter this goal.

Operating Budget

The overall plan identifying expected revenues and expenses, both fixed and variable, for the forthcoming fiscal year is termed the *operating budget*. It is an annual budget that includes the cash budget and the capital budget. In addition, the operating budget identifies the source and nature of expected revenues and

EXHIBIT 1.3   Cost-to-Charge Ratios

Cost Center	Cost-to-Charge Ratio	Cost Center	Cost-to-Charge Ratio
Operating Room	1.072993	Cast Room	0.238285
Recovery Room	0.731813	Emergency Room	1.131543
Delivery Room	0.920547	Routine Inpatient	1.321196
Radiology	0.846045	Surgical ICU	1.044988
Laboratory	0.502010	Coronary Care	0.892522
Respiratory Therapy	0.288370	Burn Unit	2.054106
Physical Therapy	1.261435	Pediatric ICU	1.153027
EKG-EEG-CVL	0.698327	Medical ICU	1.038597
Fiberoptic Lab	0.815626	Nursery ICU	0.756198
Medical Supplies	0.303416	Nursery	1.138131
Drugs	0.275234		

Source: Courtesy of the University of South Alabama Medical Center, Mobile, Alabama.

expenses. The operating budget determines the per diem and other charges to be made to the patient. A cost-to-charge ratio is used.

Cost-to-Charge Ratios

Cost-to-charge ratios are convenient tools for computing the cost of providing a service. For example, if the charge to a patient for fiberoptic laboratory services were $1,000, and the cost-to-charge ratio 0.815626, one would know that the cost to the hospital for these services was approximately $815.63 (see Exhibit 1.3). This cost includes the expense of running the fiberoptic laboratory and a portion of the hospital's overhead cost. In some instances the cost-to-charge ratios are greater than one, which means the cost of operating these cost centers is greater than the charges.

The hospital has two types of cost centers. The first are revenue-producing cost centers, such as the fiberoptic laboratory, which bill patients for services provided. The second type are overhead cost centers, such as the accounting department, which exist to support the revenue-producing centers. The cost of the overhead cost centers is allocated to the revenue-producing centers by various statistical methods. For example, utility costs are allocated to the revenue-producing departments based on the square feet of space they occupy. However, the accounting department costs are allocated based on the size of the operating budget of each revenue-producing cost center. The cost-to-charge ratio is computed by dividing the total cost of the cost center, direct and overhead, by the total charges for the same department.

Product Lines

Hospitals are reorganizing on the basis of product lines. These can include outpatient or ambulatory surgery, home health care, a burn center, a comprehensive cancer center, or other "products." As in business or industry, each functions as a profit center within the overall accounting system. Even a single DRG can

be a product. A product must pay for itself, be paid for through cost shifting, or be eliminated and deleted from the budget.

Financial Management Triad

The financial management triad includes planning, budgeting, and evaluation. Planning is essential to development and to survival. It considers philosophy, type of hospital, type of patient, size of units, projected occupancy, physical plant, modality of nursing, availability of ancillary services, staffing, variable costs for office supplies and medical supplies, food, and repair and maintenance of equipment. Planning projects the institution of new programs and expenses as well as curtailment or discontinuance of old programs. Through the operating and capital budgeting process a price tag is put on plans. When they are implemented they are evaluated for effect and efficiency. People involved in the financial management triad put forth an effort to make it work. For this reason, broad participation is preferred over narrow participation by employees.

Cost/Benefit Analysis

Cost/benefit analysis is a planning technique.[17] What are the costs of pursuing a goal, an objective, a program, or a specific nursing intervention? How do costs compare with the benefits? Is the project worthwhile? Comparison of different nursing interventions for the same nursing diagnosis or problem results in using the least costly one to achieve similar or better results. The intervention used is then cost-effective.

Vertical Integration

Purchase or establishment of freestanding diagnostic centers, nursing homes, chronic care facilities, and other organizations by hospitals is termed *vertical integration*. This technique is used to increase financial stability and profit. A hospital may move backward in vertical integration and buy or acquire a medical supply business. Thus the hospital sells products it previously bought, an entirely new service of the hospital. It may move forward and acquire a health maintenance organization (HMO). In horizontal integration, hospitals merge.

Variance Analysis

Variance indicates the difference between the budget and the actual results. It can be positive (a profit or return on investment) or negative (a loss). Cost-center managers investigate variances to determine why they occur. This is called *variance analysis*.

Flexible Budgeting

A flexible budget is designed to allow for evaluation of variable costs and demand, rather than evaluating variances based on a predetermined, fixed level of demand. The flexible budget is adjusted to reflect actual activity levels. It shows meaningful variance analysis.

In preparing a flexible budget, the manager may select 50 percent (or 60 percent or 70 percent or more) of current workload as a baseline. Assuming a linear relationship between expenses and baseline, the appropriate amount of variable costs may be added to a total of 100 percent of actual costs. This flexibility may be applied to depreciation, maintenance, supplies, quality control, labor, and other specific costs.[18]

Contribution Margin

The contribution margin, or percentage, is a mathematical computation that relates charges to variable costs to show the break-even point. A break-even point is the point at which costs and revenues are equal. A positive contribution margin means that each productivity unit makes the organization more profitable. The margin of safety is the point to which charges can be dropped without incurring losses. See the section titled Program Budgeting.

Zero-Base Budgeting

Zero-base budgeting is a method of budgeting used to control cost. It is not derived from the previous budget or historical data. In a zero-base budget the budgeting process starts from zero and everything must be justified by each new budget cycle. A previous activity can be included in the budget, but funding for it must be justified by its relation to the current organizational objectives. In theory, each and every function in a zero-base budget must stand on its own merits, and the merits of each function are reviewed annually. All labor power and costs are recalculated and decisions are made as to whether to continue the function and at what levels.

Zero-base budgeting collects information regarding a program into a *decision package*, an approach that focuses greater attention on the alternative ways in which a program can be offered. A decision package consists of the program purposes, costs and benefits, alternative ways to produce it, alternative levels of quantity, and alternative levels of quality. This provides a mechanism to ensure a formal, systematic review of each budget.[19]

Zero-base budgets are cumbersome, time consuming, and can be manipulated. In actual practice, zero-base budgeting seldom reviews all costs; much of the previous budget is accepted because complete analysis can cost more than it saves. Nevertheless, with cost studies becoming more prevalent in nursing, the application of zero-base budgeting techniques may increase.

Program Budgeting

Program budgeting is a part of budget planning. Such items as continuing education programs, employee benefits fairs, health promotion programs, and other programs should be budgeted with the annual budget. The budget for each program should enumerate fixed expenses, such as rent, advertising, fixed speaker fees, and department overhead; and variable expenses such as food, handouts, and per-person honorarium speaker fees. Some fees, such as advertising, are unrecoverable even if the program is cancelled. They are referred to as *sunk fees* and should be in the cost center's budget as operating expense, and should be included as well in the individual program's budget.

Program budgets should include a break-even analysis. If the cost of the program is $2,000 and the reasonable charge is $50 per participant, the break-even point is 40 paid participants. A break-even chart may be made for each program (see Exhibit 1.4). Income above the break-even point is profit, below is loss.

The point at which the cost to carry out the program is equal to the cost to cancel it is called the *least-loss point*. If enough people have registered to pay the sunk costs, the net loss will be the same whether the program is cancelled or held. It may be good public relations to carry out a program at the least-loss point.[20]

Operating or Cash Budgets

The cash budget is the actual operating budget in detail, usually excluding the capital budget. A cash budget indicates whether cash flow will be adequate to meet anticipated payments such as debt obligations, including replacement and expansion of facilities, unanticipated requirements, the payroll, payment for supplies and services, and a prudent investment program. Cash receipts come from third-party payers, tuition, endowment fund earnings, and sales of food, gifts, and services.

The cash budget is the day-to-day budget and represents money coming in and going out. It is advisable to have cash reserves so that cash flow, the money coming in, will pay the bills. Otherwise, revenues must be speeded up or payment of bills slowed down. Cash reserves should not be excessive; they may represent money that should be working elsewhere for the organization. Cash budgets show revenues and expenses while operating budgets show plans. They are usually considered integrated entities.[21]

Negative Cash Flow

The major factors influencing negative cash flow are

- time lag between delivery of services and collection of payments,
- the difference in cycles between the timing of net income and flow of cash,
- lag created by the large up-and-down cycles of volume during different periods (cash deficit during a high-census cycle or surplus during a low-census cycle), and
- labor expense (60 to 70 percent of operating expense) paid out in salary and wages does not cycle concurrently with collections.

To maintain solvency, cash flow must be managed carefully and cycles of cash shortage planned for appropriately. The cash budget should plan for borrowing cash during shortfalls, investment of excess cash, and *strict* monitoring and reporting of lost charges and of the billing and collecting process. The cash budget is a part of the total budget and is apportioned to departments based on individual cost-center activity.

Developing the Operating Budget

Operating budget information supplied to the chief nurse executive (CNE), department heads, and cost-center managers includes a budget worksheet

EXHIBIT 1.4 Break-Even Analysis

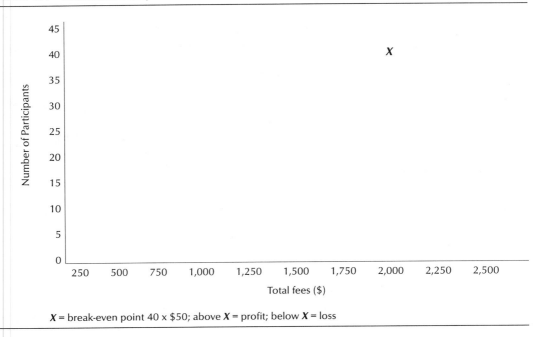

X = break-even point 40 x $50; above X = profit; below X = loss

(Exhibit 1.5) and an adjustment explanation worksheet (Exhibit 1.6). The budget worksheet depicts information by each cost center's account number and subcode. It lists prior-year expense, original budget, and annualized expense. Usually this form is provided during the budget formulation stage for a new fiscal year and the annualized expense is the projected total expense if current rates continue to the end of the fiscal year. The columns headed Budget Detail and Budget Pool are empty so that the cost-center manager can fill in the budget expenses for the projected fiscal year. Note in Exhibit 1.5 that the cost-center manager had projected an increased budget of $10,780 for subcode 211, medical and surgical supplies. This was reduced to an annualized projection of $8,790 at the budget council hearings when hospital administration decided *not* to project inflation.

Also in Exhibit 1.5, note that subcode 232, office supplies, was increased by $138. This was justified on the adjustment explanation worksheet. However, information available to the administrator indicated that $320 had been budgeted and expended in the current year for new chart-backs. Because this was a one-time expense, it was backed out of the budget. A similar transaction for $53 was backed out of subcode 501, minor equipment. Zero-base budgeting would have avoided this cumulative effect. Overall, increases were approved for subcodes 501, and 372, books. The total budget for supplies and minor equipment for this cost center was approved for $14,595.

In the formulation stage described here, the assistant administrator for finance distributes the worksheets to the other assistant administrators and department heads. They develop budgets with their cost-center managers and defend them before the budget council.

EXHIBIT 1.5   Budget Worksheet

Subcode	Description	ABR	Prior Year Expense	Original Budget	Annualized Expense	Budget Detail	Budget Pool
200	Pool-Med/Surg Supply	0	$ .00	$10,975.00		$10,780	$ 8,985
211	Med & Surg Supplies	4	10,893.80	.00	$ 8,790	$ 8,790	
213	Drugs	4	129.59	.00	195	$ 195	
Pool Total			11,023.39	10,975.00	8,985		
220	Pool-General Supply	0	.00	2,705.00			$ 2,848
232	Office Supplies	4	303.34	.00	672	$ 810	−320
234	Printing	4	37.75	.00	3	$ 3	
240	Housekeeping Supply	4	1,404.06	.00	1,482	$ 1,482	
270	Food Expense	4	913.73	.00	523	$ 523	
Pool Total			2,658.88	2,705.00	2,680		
300	Pool-Travel/Entertain	0	.00	110.00			$ 50
314	Local Travel	4	13.80	.00	18	$ 50	
Pool Total			13.80	110.00	18		
320	Pool-Other Expenses	0	.00	130.00			$ 660
336	Equip Maint & Repair	4	66.60	.00	123	$ 610	
372	Books & Subscription	4	25.00	.00		$ 50	
Pool Total			91.60	130.00	123		
501	Minor Equipment	0	.00	.00	72	−53	$ 465
Pool Total			.00	.00	72		
Acct Total			$13,787.67	$13,920.00	$11,878		
						Total	$14,968
							− 373
							$14,595

Source: Courtesy of the University of South Alabama Medical Center, Mobile, Alabama.

Osborne and Gaebler refer to the operational budget as the *expenditure control budget*. It sets up accounts for various major expenditures. These authors recommend shifting among accounts as needed, with departments being allowed to carry over into the new budget what they do not spend. A recommended formula for establishing an expenditure control budget is to take the figure for the previous year plus inflation and growth or decline, plus any carryover funds. Managers should apply additional money for the new initiatives. The strengths of such a mission-driven budget are the following:

- Every employee has an incentive to save money.
- Resources are freed up to test new ideas.
- Managers have the autonomy to respond to changing circumstances.
- A predictable environment is created.
- The budget process is enormously simplified.
- Much money can be saved on auditors and a budget office.
- Managers can focus on other important issues.[22]

Performance Budgeting

Performance budgeting focuses on the activities of a cost center, such as indirect care, direct care, and quality monitoring. Each activity has objectives with specific financial resources; performance budgeting focuses on what is expected

EXHIBIT 1.6 Adjustment Explanation, for calendar year _____

DEPARTMENT NAME ___9th floor_____

DEPARTMENT NUMBER ___60686_____

Subcode Number	Subcode Description	Adjustment Amount	Adjustment Explanation
		$ 30.00	2 lg blue policy binders $15.00 ea
		6.00	1 sm blue policy binder
		32.00	2 large red 4" (8½" × 11") 3-ring binders—normal wear and tear, 2 yrs old
232	Office Supplies	$ 25.00	4 black 3-ring binders (MAR & Kardex)—normal wear and tear
		28.00	48" × 36" cork and wood-frame bulletin boards—↑ appearance ↓ clutter
		17.00	25" × 25" ¼" thick Plexiglas—↑ appearance
		$138.00	
		$ 30.00	*Taber's Medical Dictionary*—ref. book needed to ↑ professionalism
372	Books	$ 20.00	*Webster's Tenth New Collegiate Dictionary*—↑ learning
		$ 50.00	

Source: Courtesy of the University of South Alabama Medical Center, Mobile, Alabama.

to be accomplished. Performance is evaluated based on a variety of outputs. Flexible budgeting that evaluates actual costs based on actual workload is an improvement over traditional budgeting, but is a limited evaluation of nursing performance. Performance budgeting is an improvement over flexible budgeting because it ties performance to consumption of financial resources.[23] The steps in performance budgeting are:

1. Define the performance activities or areas of accomplishment for the cost center. These may include providing direct care, improving quality of care, nursing staff satisfaction, patient satisfaction, productivity, and innovation (see Exhibit 1.7).
2. Identify the line-item operating budget for the cost center being evaluated. These expenses will be for salaries, education, supplies, and overhead (see Exhibit 1.8)
3. Define how much of the resources represented by each line item are to be devoted to each of the performance areas. Exhibit 1.7 shows percentages and Exhibit 1.8 the dollar allocations.
4. Choose measures of performance for each performance area, budget an amount of work for each area, and determine the budgeted cost-per-unit of work based on these measures. For an example of an actual performance budget see Exhibit 1.9.[24]

EXHIBIT 1.7 Summary of Percentage Allocation to Performance Areas

	Quality	Staffing	Cost Control	Productivity	Patient Satisfaction	Staff Satisfaction	Innovation	Direct Care	Indirect Care	Other	Totals
Cost Item											
Nurse Manager	15%	15%	20%	20%	10%	5%	15%	0%	0%	0%	100%
Staff Salary	5	0	5	2	5	0	0	30	30	23	100
Education	20	2	20	20	10	10	20	0	0	0	100
Supplies	0	2	2	0	0	0	0	90	5	1	100
Overhead	0	0	0	0	0	0	0	100	0	0	100

Source: S. A. Finkler. "Performance Budgeting." Reprinted from *Nursing Economic$*, 1991, No. 6, p. 405. Reprinted with permission of the publisher, Jannetti Publications, Inc., Pitman, New Jersey.

EXHIBIT 1.8 Allocation of Expenditures to Performance Areas

	Total	Quality	Staffing	Cost Control	Productivity	Patient Satisfaction	Staff Satisfaction	Innovation	Direct Care	Indirect Care	Other
Cost Item											
Nurse Manager	$50,000	$7,500	$7,500	$10,000	$10,000	$5,000	$2,500	$7,500	$0	$0	$0
Staff Salary	800,000	40,000	0	40,000	16,000	40,000	0	0	240,000	240,000	184,000
Education	20,000	4,000	0	4,000	4,000	2,000	2,000	4,000	0	0	0
Supplies	40,000	0	800	800	0	0	0	0	36,000	2,000	400
Overhead	90,000	0	0	0	0	0	0	0	90,000	0	0
Totals	$1,000,000	$51,500	$8,300	$54,800	$30,000	$47,000	$4,500	$11,500	$366,000	$242,000	$184,400

Source: S. A. Finkler. "Performance Budgeting." Reprinted from *Nursing Economic$*, 1991, No. 6, p. 405. Reprinted with permission of the publisher, Jannetti Publications, Inc., Pitman, New Jersey.

EXHIBIT 1.9   Performance Budget

	Type of Activity	Description of Output Measure	Amount of Output Budgeted	Total Cost of Activity	Average Cost
Quality Improvement	Patient care planning	Patient-care plan compliance	10% reduction in failure rate	$ 51,500	$5,150/Percent drop in failure rate
Staffing	Daily staff calculations	Number of daily calculations	365 daily calculations	8,300	$22.74/Daily calculation
		Reduction in paid hours per patient day over staff guide minimum	0.2 paid hours per patient day		$4,150/0.1 Hour reduction
Cost Control	Reduce	Reduction in cost/patient day	$8/patient day	54,800	$6,850/ $ reduction
Increase Productivity	Revise procedures Work more efficiently	Reduction in total unit cost per direct care hour	$3 reduction per direct care hour	30,000	$10,000/ $ reduction
Increase Patient Satisfaction	Respond to needs	Complaints	10% reduction in complaints	47,000	$4,700/1% reduction in complaints
Increase Staff Satisfaction	Respond to needs	Turnover	25% reduction in staff turn-over	4,500	$180/1% reduction in turnover
Innovation & Planning	Planning sessions	Number of meetings	12 meetings	11,500	$958.33/ meeting
Direct Care	Direct patient care	Hours of care	10,000 hours	366,000	$36.66/direct care hour
Indirect Care	Patient charting	Number of patient days	7,300 patient days	242,000	$33.15/patient day
Other				184,400	
Total				$1,000,000	

Source: S. A. Finkler. "Performance Budgeting." Reprinted from *Nursing Economic$*, 1991, No. 6, p. 405. Reprinted with permission of the publisher, Jannetti Publications, Inc., Pitman, New Jersey.

The performance budget evolves or is converted from the operating budget. Measurements of potential output are proxies and measure both process and outcome. These output measures may include

- compliance with patient-care plan procedures with the goal of a percentage reduction in errors
- improved compliance to reduce errors and achieve goals costs money to fix the problem, which usually requires additional resources of some kind
- staffing decisions take less management time
- cost reduction
- increased productivity
- increased patient and staff satisfaction
- innovation and planning
- direct care
- indirect care

Multiple measures can be developed for each performance area.[25]

Revenues

What are the sources of nursing revenue or for securing a financial base for nursing? They include grants, continuing education, private practice, community visibility, health care for students and staff, HMOs, city health departments, industry, unions, third-party payments, professional corporations, and nurse-managed centers.

Operating room nursing is an example of a cost that can be billed as a source of revenue. This can be done by determining the level of care needed for different procedures and the room charges, based on use of supplies and equipment, and billing the services separately. In computing the nursing charges, the cost of nursing personnel per case can be determined from the records. To this can be added cost for preparation time for assembling supplies and equipment and setting up the room, visiting the patient preoperatively and postoperatively, nursing administration, and staff development. Room costs would include environmental services and maintenance.[26]

Maryland and Maine have passed legislation requiring hospitals to list nursing as a separate item on patients' bills. As the hospital bill is unbundled, all nursing cost centers will become major revenue-producing centers. Then all payers will be paying for nursing services based on business procedures. This will include allocated return on equity (profit) and proportionate losses due to bad debts.[27] (See note.)

Using product-line strategy, nursing divisions can sell staff development programs, consultation services, home health care, wellness programs, computer software, and many other product lines.

Many items and services have been used to generate revenues for hospitals. These include drugs, supplies, respiratory therapy, physical therapy, and others. In most instances, the charges have been excessive and there have been areas where cost shifting accounted for revenues (and profits) to cover services delivered and charged at a price below costs. As the hospital bill is unbundled, charges will eventually reduce to costs at a 1:1 ratio. Not-for-profit hospitals are not allowed a return on equity or credit for bad debts as a cost of doing business; they carry these items as cash or ledger balances.

Budgeting is a competency of nursing managers, indicating responsibility and accountability. A well-prepared unit budget indicates that the best nurse manager has been delegated and has accepted the responsibility for this facet of the job. Management of the budget to keep expenditures and revenues in balance indicates that the nurse manager accepts responsibility for it. Within the budgetary plan, the nurse manager should be allowed some flexibility in making decisions about the mix of expenditures. This would mean that monies for staff, supplies, education, and other budgeted expenses could be interchanged so long as costs do not exceed revenues and the objectives of the unit are being met.

A concept related to budgeting is "value for money." Is the unit or the organization getting full value for the money expended? This question relates to such areas as turnover of personnel, waste of supplies, ineffective use of clinical skills, and inaccurate staffing standards.[28]

Relationship of Patient Acuity Rating Systems to Budgets

Historically, nursing staffing has been based on subjective formulas. The nurse administrator with the most persuasive list of personnel needs was most successful in obtaining greater budgetary allocation. Such a list might include formulas based on research, standards of professional and government agencies, and a number of facts and statements related to average daily census, number of admissions and discharges, number of surgeries, and complaints of stress by nurses and about nurses by physicians and nurse managers. Seldom were all budgeted positions filled, and requests for increased staffing did not usually affect the bottom line—costs. A CEO could respond positively to personnel requests that would probably not be filled.

During the 1980s we saw the disappearance and reemergence of nurse shortages, the advent of prospective payment, and a more scientific, quantitative approach to nurse staffing and personnel budgeting—the Patient Classification System (PCS). A PCS is actually mandated by the Joint Commission on Accreditation of Healthcare Organizations (JCAHO).

During the 1990s we see the potential for nurse surpluses, at least on a geographic basis, and the struggle for health-care reform. Productivity measurements are becoming a necessary element of budgeting.

Among the benefits of a PCS is the reduction of tensions among nursing staff. Managers predict budgetary needs for personnel using objective data. Staffing based on needs becomes predictable to managers and subsequently to the staff.

Some hospitals are using the PCS to bill for actual nursing services. They are using patient classification billing systems composed of

- an accurate patient classification system
- staffing based on patient classification
- patients rated by nurses
- defined units of care
- a rate per unit

The advantages of this system include elimination of the inequities of flat-rate billing systems, which shift costs from patients requiring few units of nursing care to subsidize the nursing care of those requiring many units of nursing care. A PCS also ensures adequate reimbursement for nursing expenses. Professional nurses see value placed upon their work, and their morale is boosted. To bill for nursing services the hospital bill must be unbundled. An example of this is given in chapter 7.

The following are early examples of patient classification billing systems:

1. *St. Luke's Hospital Medical Center, Phoenix (1974).* Points were assigned per nursing task based on time and skills and points per support or education of patient's family or friends; five categories for general units and two for intensive care; 24-hour billing rates.

2. *Montana Deaconess Medical Center (1971).* Patients rated twice daily by nurses by type of service provided; hourly charges; four categories for general

units, four for intensive care, three for intensive care nursery, and five for critical care.

3. *Massachusetts Eye and Ear Infirmary, Boston (1975).* Clinical care units; dollar rate per unit; applied to specific diagnosis; bills varied by length of stay; one-time administrative charge; daily room-and-board fee.

Herzog attributes 50 percent of hospital expense budget to nursing. Since nursing costs are buried within other categories of financial data, including room rates, laboratory charges, radiology charges, and so on, the true costs of nursing must be identified. The patient classification system is one important source for identifying hours of care per category of care given per patient. Nursing research can test nursing treatment modes. These would include selection of a procedure, selection of supplies, selection of category of personnel to perform it, and comparison of outcomes.[29]

While in business and industry technology is used to reduce cost by increasing output, the opposite has been encouraged in the health-care industry by charge-based reimbursement schemes. Increases in equipment costs and types and numbers of procedures were paid for by third-party payers. That has changed somewhat with the prospective payment system (PPS). With control of reimbursement, less expense is best. The old revenue producers such as drugs, respiratory therapies, laboratory tests, X rays, and others are being reimbursed at their true costs. Nursing care is the source of revenue for the future. Nurses must identify the relative value units of care by which they will be reimbursed. They must learn to use information systems to process data, and to select and use the supply item that does the best job for the least money. They must standardize procedures and practices and review and revise jobs.

Their relatively high fixed costs require that hospitals maintain high productivity. If productivity declines, costs must be decreased. This is done by decreasing staff and the use of supplies, and making other reductions in use of resources.

The Controlling Process

Now that the nursing budget has been viewed from its planning and directing aspects, it will be looked at from its controlling or evaluating aspects. The budget establishes financial standards for the division of nursing and through its cost center for each nursing unit. Feedback, on a daily, weekly, monthly, and quarterly basis supplies information to compare managerial performance with the established standards. The results are used to make adjustments. What kind of feedback is needed by nurse managers relative to their budgets and cost control? They need information to tell whether their goals are being met. Are they exceeding the budget? Is the excess both for cost and revenues? Are the supplies and expenses of the quantity and quality planned? Is the equipment being purchased and installed as scheduled? Are employees being recruited and utilized effectively to produce the expected quality and quantity of nursing services? Is employee morale good? What adjustments need to be made? Where are the problems and who is responsible for them?

Budget processes should be flexible to allow for increased and decreased volume of business. The business office provides cost-center managers with biometric information to make adjustments in staffing and in use of supplies.

A planning-programming-budgeting system (PPBS), developed by the RAND Corporation for the Department of Defense in the 1950s and 1960s, has found application in health-care management. Using this concept the nurse administrator prepares a total budgetary package containing:

- definition of the objectives (*planning*),
- analysis of the contributions (outcome) the proposal will make toward accomplishing organizational objectives, including all pertinent costs and benefits that are part of the proposed program (*programming*),
- *budgets* of resources including all future costs and benefits,
- completion of authorized programs (*working*), and
- the analysis employed to *evaluate* alternative approaches for reaching the same goals.[30]

The last criterion is considered a key one. Again, having specific, current, practical, written objectives for the division of nursing and each of its units is imperative to planning, budgeting, and effective cost management.

It should be remembered that a budget is a plan based on the best estimates of the costs of running an organization. It cannot be inflexible, but neither can it hide waste and inefficiency.

The nurse administrator should be sure that nurse managers will not be penalized when budgetary objectives are not met due to events beyond their control. They are working within the confines of an organizational environment that is affected by both internal and external constraints. One of the external constraints facing them is federally mandated cost control or cost containment, which is seen by some administrators as reimbursement control.

The colossal mistakes of budgeting are made in the control area. Top management should view variations in budget as a tool for decision making, not an instance to make arbitrary cuts resulting in unrealistic operating budgets for line managers. One way to overcome this problem is through employee education about the budget process. Such knowledge helps employees view the budget as an aid rather than an obstacle.[31]

Decentralization of the Budget

Cost-center managers, usually head nurses and supervisors of units, are capable of planning and controlling their own budgets. The nurse administrator, assisted by financial managers, should prepare them to do so. Through decentralized budgeting, cost-center managers propose innovative objectives. They gather data to defend their objectives and operating plans. The unit budget becomes their responsibility and they zealously guard its integrity. They sense when adaptations have to be made because of increased costs or decreased revenues, and they make or recommend immediate remedies. Decentralized budgeting provides for internal controls.

Monitoring the Budget

Various techniques have been described and defined for monitoring the budget, however, all budgetary objectives should contain procedures for quality

review including identification of a team to perform such a review. If a program is not successful—is not meeting objectives or is running above predicted costs and below predicted revenues—a decision should be made whether to rework or cancel it. This is very difficult, but it is essential to good control. The technique of cancelling budgeted programs is sometimes referred to as *sunsetting*. A nurse manager should accept the responsibility for sunsetting programs that are costly and unprofitable.

In developing the nursing budget it is necessary that the unit structures for nursing administration are comparable. This can be ensured by developing and providing financial policies and guidelines. This is most successful when the top administrative team works with the budget monitor to develop such financial policies. The nurse administrator is part of this team and brings to its meetings standards of service that are defensible, such as data on workload, including numbers and types of procedures, patients, surgical operations, and visits. These policies should reflect the long-range plans of the governing board.

Part of the information furnished to nurse administrators and managers is in the form of reports. These include statistical reports of revenues and expenditures for the current year. Exhibit 1.10 illustrates financial information that is needed by the cost-center manager and the nursing service administrator.

Note that the account number at the head of the table is 4-60680. The prefix 4 denotes that the account balance does *not* turn over at the end of the fiscal year. The cost center or department is 60680. Financial transactions, including purchase orders for supplies and minor equipment, as well as the payroll, are identified with this cost center number and are charged by the purchasing and accounting departments to this number and to the appropriate subcodes, 100 through 501. Horizontal columns indicate the operational budget, the actual expenditures for the current month and for the fiscal year, open encumbrances, and the balance available. Because 83 percent of the fiscal year (which begins October 1) has elapsed, this has some relationship to the Percent Used column. Although 103 percent of the budgeted salary has been used indicating a variance of 20 percent, only 78 percent of employee benefits have been used, which indicates a use of overtime plus part-time employees working less than the 0.5 FTE required to qualify for fringe benefits. Zero percent of the budgeted money for minor equipment has been spent to date. Total budget expenses were 96 percent indicating a variance of 13 percent overspending. While this report serves as a control for nurse managers, the expenditure of budgeted money for any one subcode could cause the total expenses to date to be greater than the percentage of fiscal year elapsed without creating an alarm. In this instance overspending should be related to increased census and revenue.

Exhibit 1.11 informs the nurse managers of the specific financial transactions that took place during the month of July. They can be checked against Exhibit 1.10.

Information on revenues is reported similarly. Exhibit 1.12 illustrates the inpatient revenue for the Medical Intensive Care Unit, which includes nursing and hotel services. It is all credited to nursing. The revenue account is 4-30815, while the cost center is the same as for expenses, 60680. The budgeted revenues for the year are listed, as are the revenues for the month and for the fiscal year. Note that although 83 percent of the fiscal year has elapsed, only 76 percent of the budgeted revenues have been charged, a variance of –7 percent.

Also, Exhibit 1.13 indicates that 76 percent of budgeted equipment revenues have been billed.

Since the amount billed (that is, the unit's revenues), 76 percent, is less than the 83 percent of fiscal year elapsed, the nurse managers can note that revenues are less than expenses, a negative financial report. The manager's goal is to maintain or improve this financial status to the end of the fiscal year.

Additional financial information can be furnished to each nurse manager. This includes summary reports in whole dollars and for all cost centers supervised. This can be done by subcode (see Exhibit 1.14), by subcode and cost center (see Exhibit 1.15), and by unit or department (see Exhibits 1.16 and 1.17).

"Rollover" funds designated by prefix 3, are also included in the financial reports that can be provided to the chief nurse executive. Balances in these funds are carried over into the next fiscal year to be spent at any future date. An example of a rollover fund is account 3-64155, the maternal child health education fund. Exhibit 1.18 shows activities for this fund for the month, and Exhibit 1.19 shows how the debits were spent.

Rollover funds can be managed by the chief nurse executive, a department head, or a cost-center manager.

Motivational Aspects of Budgeting

Budgeting can be a motivating force for personnel—if current programs must increase in effectiveness and efficiency to remain; if decentralization and staff involvement provides an increased sense of responsibility and satisfaction; and if merit increases, promotions, and bonuses are tied or linked to budgetary performance.

Budgeting facilitates communication among interdependent departments, thus increasing knowledge and understanding of other areas. It provides learning opportunities for future nurse managers.

The budget can be dysfunctional and fail to facilitate attainment of organizational objectives when it is viewed as an end rather than a means. This happens in the following circumstances:

- It is inflexible and permits no deviation from the established plan.
- It is viewed as externally imposed by administrators who do not understand patient care.
- Health-care providers feel left out of budget decisions.
- There is overemphasis on staying within the budget, thus leading to a decrease in interdepartmental communication and cooperation.
- Managers are held accountable without being given authority.[32]

Using the Budget for Innovation

In many hospitals nurse managers manage from 25 to 30 full-time and part-time staff members, with operating budgets exceeding $1 million. This is as much as other major department heads manage, and more than some. The nurse executive encourages and supports nurse managers to develop simulated budgets for proposed expansion and changes in utilization of facilities, or modification of unit schedules. Well-qualified nurse managers do not need to be overseen by

EXHIBIT 1.10 Accounting System Report

Computer Date _____
Time of Day _____
Acct: 460680
Dept: 60680

Account statement in whole dollars for fiscal year ending _____
83% of fiscal year elapsed
Distribution code = 700
Medical Intensive Care Unit–Expense

Subcode	Description	Budgets Original	Budgets Revised	Actual Current Month	Actual Fiscal Year	Open Encumbrances	Balance Available	Percent Used
100	Pool–Salary & Wages	$ 948,742	$ 901,053				$901,053	0%
130	Professional Salary			$ 72,533	$ 775,790		775,790–	***
135	Tech Salary & Wages			4,085	50,947		50,947–	***
140	Office Salaries			4,347	53,168		53,168–	***
155	Service Empl Wages			3,936	52,195		52,195–	***
160	Student Wages	14,898	14,898	1,518	14,898			100
166	Accrued Salaries	32,791	32,791	11,462	32,791			100
	Salaries	948,742	948,742	97,880	979,789		31,047–	103
170	Pool–Empl Benefits	254,683	55,722				55,722	0
182	Employers FICA		112		112			100
183	Group Life Ins		2,569	264	2,569			100
184	Disability Ins		4,869	526	4,869			100
185	Teachers Retirement		134		134			100
188	Group Health Ins		59,973	5,887	59,973			100
198	State Paid Retiremnt		62,158	5,591	62,158			100
199	State Paid FICA		69,146	6,313	69,146			100
	Employee Benefits	254,683	254,683	18,581	198,961		55,722	78
200	Pool–Med/Surg Supply	75,000	23,920				23,920	0
211	Med & Surg Supplies		128,235	14,846	128,235			100
213	Drugs		1,317	140	1,317			100
214	Solutions		36,091	4,389	36,091			100

						Adjustments	Current Enc	
Med/Surg Supplies		75,000	189,563	19,375	165,643		23,920	87
220	Pool–General Supply	5,789	2,553–				2,553–	0
232	Office Supplies		1,070	19	1,069	1		100
233	Copying & Binding		36	30	36			100
234	Printing		1,494	115	1,494			100
235	Printing Paper		633	83	633			100
240	Housekeeping Supply		1,880	323	1880			100
243	Housekeeping Furnish		1,395		1,395			100
244	Linen Replacement		214		214			100
250	Maintenance Supplies		1,001		1,001			100
270	Food Expense		619	49	619			100
General Supplies		5,789	5,789	620	8,341	1	2,553–	144
300	Pool–Travel/Entertain	1,430	1,005		425		1,005	0
316	Workshop & Training		425					100
Travel/Entertainment		1,430	1,430		425		1,005	30
320	Pool–Other Expenses	157,000	12,624				12,624	0
324	Contract Service		140,390	16,720	140,390			100
336	Equip Maint & Repair		3,700		2,950	750		100
372	Books & Subscription		286		286			100
Other Expenses		157,000	157,000	16,720	143,626	750	12,624	92
501	Minor Equipment	4,000	4,000				4,000	0
	Total Expenses	1,446,644	1,561,207	153,176	1,496,785	751	63,671	96
Account Total		$1,446,644	$1,561,207	$153,176	$1,496,785	751	$63,671	96%

Open Encumbrance Status

Account	P.O Number	P.O Date	Description	Original Enc	Liquidating Expenditures	Adjustments	Current Enc	Last Act Date
4-60680-232	H01764	10/06/xx	Waller Brothers	.85			.85	10/18
4-60680-336	H07584	07/24/xx	Scaletronix Inc	750.00			750.00	08/01
			Account Total	750.85			750.85	

Source: Courtesy of the University of South Alabama Medical Center, Mobile, Alabama.

EXHIBIT 1.11 Accounting System Report

Computer Date _____
Time of Day _____
PGM = AM091

Acct: 4-60680
Dept: 60680

Report of transactions for fiscal year ending _____
Distribution code = 700
Medical Intensive Care Unit–Expense

Subcode	Description	Date	EC	Ref.	2nd Ref.	J.E. Offset Account	Budget Entries	Current Rev/Exp	Encumbrances	Batch Ref.	Date
130	Payroll Expense	07/07	64	900001		0-10080-118CR		$ 35,017.03		PPS584	07/07
130	Payroll Expense	07/21	64	900001		0-10080-118CR		37,516.33		PPS588	07/21
130	CM Total Professional Salary							72,533.36			
135	Payroll Expense	07/07	64	900001		0-10080-118CR		1,630.89		PPS584	07/07
135	Payroll Expense	07/21	64	900001		0-10080-118CR		2,454.11		PPS588	07/21
135	CM Total Tech Salary & Wages							4,085.00			
140	Payroll Expense	07/07	64	900001		0-10080-118CR		2,082.44		PPS584	07/07
140	Payroll Expense	07/21	64	900001		0-10080-118CR		2,264.26		PPS588	07/21
140	CM Total Office Salaries							4,346.70			
155	Payroll Expense	07/07	64	900001		0-10080-118CR		1,884.26		PPS584	07/07
155	Payroll Expense	07/21	64	900001		0-10080-118CR		2,051.29		PPS588	07/21
155	CM Total Service Empl Wages							3,935.55			
160	Payroll Expense	07/07	64	900001		0-10080-118CR		494.83		PPS584	07/07
160	Payroll Expense	07/21	64	900001		0-10080-118CR		1,022.81		PPS588	07/21
160	CM Total Student Wages							1,517.64			
166	Susp Corr/Accr Sal	06/30	60		S01544	0-13000-160CR		65.00		HJV002	07/10
	Susp Corr/Accr Sal	06/30	60		S01543	0-13000-160CR		45.00		HJV002	07/10
	RVS Accrd Sal & Wage	07/01	60		075101	0-15300-220DR		40,318.00-		HJV001	07/10
	RVS Accrd Sal & Wage	07/01	60		075101	0-15300-220DR		65.00-		HJV001	07/10
	RVS Accrd Sal & Wage	07/01	60		075101	0-15300-220DR		45.00-		HJV001	07/10
	Accrued Sal & Wages	07/31	60		075100	0-15300-220CR		51,780.00		HJV019	07/31
166	CM Total Accrued Salaries							11,462.00			
183	Payroll Expense	07/21	64	900001		2-77000-180CR		264.04		PPS588	07/21
183	CM Total Group Life Ins							264.04			

184	Payroll Expense	07/21	64	900001		2-77000-180CR	526.48	PPS588	07/21
184	CM Total Disability Ins						526.48		
188	Payroll Expense	07/07	64	900001		2-77000-180CR	65.81	PPS584	07/07
188	Payroll Expense	07/21	64	900001		2-77000-180CR	5,821.12	PPS588	07/21
188	CM Total Group Health Ins						5,886.93		
198	Payroll Expense	07/07	64	900001		2-77000-180CR	2,659.96	PPS584	07/07
198	Payroll Expense	07/21	64	900001		2-77000-180CR	2,930.66	PPS588	07/21
198	CM Total State Paid Retiremnt						5,590.62		
199	Payroll Expense	07/07	64	900001		2-77000-180CR	3,019.55	PPS584	07/07
199	Payroll Expense	07/21	64	900001		2-77000-180CR	3,293.55	PPS588	07/21
199	CM Total State Paid FICA						6,313.10		
211	Inventory Exp Alloc	07/31	60		075264	0-12100-140CR	14,845.75	HJV027	07/31
211	CM Total Med & Surg Supplies						14,845.75		
213	Pharmacy Distrib—Jul	07/31	60		075006	4-60730-213CR	140.34	HJV033	07/31
213	CM Total Drugs						140.34		
214	Inventory Exp Alloc	07/31	60		075264	0-12100-140CR	4,389.27	HJV027	07/31
214	CM Total Solutions						4,389.27		
232	Inventory Exp Alloc	07/31	60		075264	0-12100-140CR	19.49	HJV027	07/31
232	CM Total Office Supplies						19.49		
233	Xerox Expense-J/J 89	07/31	60		075008	4-60960-965CR	30.21	HJV026	07/31
233	CM Total Copying & Binding						30.21		
234	Print Shop Chrgs—Jul	07/26	60		075011	4-60960-960CR	115.20	HJV013	07/27
234	CM Total Printing						115.20		
235	Inventory Exp Alloc	07/31	60		075264	0-12100-140CR	82.69	HJV027	07/31
235	CM Total Printing Paper						82.69		
240	Inventory Exp Alloc	07/31	60		075264	0-12100-140CR	323.42	HJV027	07/31
240	CM Total Housekeeping Supply						323.42		
270	Inventory Exp Alloc	07/31	60		075264	0-12100-140CR	48.61	HJV027	07/31
270	CM Total Food Expense						48.61		
324	Nephrology Applicati	07/26	68		563631	0-15030-211CR	3,520.00	HPD850	07/26
324	Accrue Jly	07/31	60		075259	0-15030-210CR	13,200.00	HJV024	07/31
324	CM Total Contract Service						16,720.00		
336	Scaletronix Inc	07/24	50	H07584			$750.00	HEN010	07/31
336	CM Total Equip Maint & Repair						750.00		
	Account Total						$153,176.40		

Source: Courtesy of the University of South Alabama Medical Center, Mobile, Alabama.

EXHIBIT 1.12 Accounting System Report

Account statement in whole dollars for fiscal year ending _____

83% of fiscal year elapsed
Distribution code = 700
Medical Intensive Care Unit–Revenue

Computer Date _____
Time of Day _____
PGM = AM090-B1

Acct: 4-30815
Dept: 60680

Tab Code	Description	Budgets		Actual		Open Encumbrances	Balance Available	Percent Used
		Original	Revised	Current Month	Fiscal Year			
040	Inpatient Revenue	$1,511,400–	$1,511,400–	$115,500–	$1,146,600–		$364,800–	76%
	Total Revenues	1,511,400–	1,511,400–	115,500–	1,146,600–		364,800–	76
	Account Totals	1,511,400–	1,511,400–	115,500–	1,146,600–		364,800–	76

Source: Courtesy of the University of South Alabama Medical Center, Mobile, Alabama.

EXHIBIT 1.13 Accounting System Report

Account statement in whole dollars for fiscal year ending _____

83% of fiscal year elapsed
Distribution code = 700
Medical Intensive Care Unit–SP&D–Revenue

Computer Date _____
Time of Day _____
PGM = AM090-B1

Acct: 4-30818
Dept: 60680

Subcode	Description	Budgets		Actual		Open Encumbrances	Balance Available	Percent Used
		Original	Revised	Current Month	Fiscal Year			
040	Inpatient Revenue	$1,080,088–	$1,080,088–	$101,637–	$818,031–		$262,057–	76%
	Total Revenues	1,080,088–	1,080,088–	101,637–	818,031–		262,057–	76
	Account Totals	1,080,088–	1,080,088–	101,637–	818,031–		262,057–	76

Source: Courtesy of the University of South Alabama Medical Center, Mobile, Alabama.

EXHIBIT 1.14 Accounting System Report

Summary report in whole dollars for fiscal year ending _____

Distribution code = 750

Computer Date _____
Time of Day _____
PGM = AM095-B1

Subcode	Description	Budgets		Actual			Open Commitments	Balance Available	Percent Used
		Original	Revised	Current Month	Fiscal Year	Project Year			
001	Prior Year Balance		$ 302,976					$ 302,978	0%
002	Transfers								0
010	Income	$16,419,272-	16,419,272-	$1,342,529-	$13,782,618-	$13,782,618-		2,636,654-	84
020	Income			13,078-	127,981-	127,981-		127,981	0
023	Interest Income			1,353-	11,022-	11,022-		11,022	0
025	Original Budget	600,000-	600,000-	77,740-	1,236,565-	1,236,565-		636,565	206
026				191-	210-	210-		210	0
028	Bad Debt Recovery				169,932	169,932		169,932-	0
030									0
040	Inpatient Revenue			1,852-	29,682-	29,682-		29,682	0
041	Outpatient RF								0
042	Outpatient ED								0
050	Ded/Gross Revenue	75,009,000	75,009,000	8,904,127	72,586,402	72,586,402		2,422,598	97
099	State Paid Benefits								0
	Total Revenues	57,989,728	58,292,706	7,467,383	57,568,256	57,568,256		724,450	99
100	Pool–Salary & Wages	1,416,748	82,157					82,157	0
110	Exec & Adm Salaries		170,518	23,443	170,518	170,518			100
120	Instruction Salaries								0
130	Professional Salary		210,392	15,839	210,592	210,592		200-	100
131	Interns Salaries								0
135	Tech Salary & Wages		11,906	1,195	11,906	11,906			100
140	Office Salaries		840,893	79,028	840,893	843,866		2,973-	100
150	Craft/Trade Wages				143	808		808-	0
155	Service Empl Wages					154		154-	0
159	Temp Craft/Trade Wage					2,431		2,431-	0

(Continued)

37

EXHIBIT 1.14 Accounting System Report (*Continued*)

Summary report in whole dollars for fiscal year ending _____

Distribution code = 750

Computer Date _____
Time of Day _____
PGM = AM095-B1

Subcode	Description	Budgets		Actual			Open Commitments	Balance Available	Percent Used
		Original	Revised	Current Month	Fiscal Year	Project Year			
160	Student Wages	$1,416,748		$ 2,678	$ 20,975	$ 20,975		$ 75,591	100%
164									0
166	Accrued Salaries		41,158	10,264	41,158	41,158			100
167									0
168	Tuition Reimbursement		6,971	2,756	6,971	6,971			100
169	Budget Correction								0
	Salaries	$1,416,748	1,384,969	135,202	1,303,156	1,309,378		$ 75,591	95
170	Pool–Empl Benefits	340,007	116,982					116,982	0
180	Employee Benefits	187,747	205,413	3,318	421,300	421,300		215,888-	205
181	Unemployment Ins	41,307	41,307	7,722	22,717	22,717		18,590	55
182	Employers FICA		266	54	266	1,871		1,605-	703
183	Group Life Ins		91,969-	435	91,969-	91,967-		3-	100
184	Disability Ins		9,090	1,015	9,106	9,110		20-	100
185	Teachers Retirement		4		4	4			100
186	Meal Books								0
187	TIAA-CREF Retirement		2,068	259	2,068	2,068			100
188	Group Health Ins		96,262	12,650	116,322	116,342		20,080-	121
190	Tuition Reimbursement	56,911	56,911	7,955	49,916	49,916		6,996	88

Source: Courtesy of the University of South Alabama Medical Center, Mobile, Alabama.

EXHIBIT 1.15 Accounting System Report

Computer Date _____
Time of Day _____
PGM = AM095-B1

Subcode summary audit report for fiscal year ending _____

Distribution code = 750

Subcode	Subcode Description	Original Budget	Revised Budget	Current Month	Year to Date	Project to Date	Open Commitments	Balance Available
001								
364100	General Hospital Fnd	0.00	$ 30,653.57	0.00	0.00	0.00	0.00	$ 30,653.57
364105	Burn Unit	0.00	22,495.81	0.00	0.00	0.00	0.00	22,495.81
364110	Intensv Care Nursery	0.00	4,438.37	0.00	0.00	0.00	0.00	4,438.37
364120	J Erwin Ped Surgery	0.00	942.96–	0.00	0.00	0.00	0.00	942.96–
364127	Heart Statn–Holters	0.00	14,205.00	0.00	0.00	0.00	0.00	14,205.00
364173	Helping Hands/3&4 Fl	0.00	3,618.70	0.00	0.00	0.00	0.00	3,618.70
364174	Telethon–C&W USAMC	0.00	32,797.51	0.00	0.00	0.00	0.00	32,797.51
364175	Heart Fund Donations	0.00	864.10	0.00	0.00	0.00	0.00	864.10
364176	Telethon–C&W	0.00	71,327.96	0.00	0.00	0.00	0.00	71,827.96
364178	WOCD/Palmer Mem Fund	0.00	1,403.81	0.00	0.00	0.00	0.00	1,403.81
364179	Telethon–C&W	0.00	122,923.92	0.00	0.00	0.00	0.00	122,923.92
364197	Payroll Inserter	0.00	1,308.00–	0.00	0.00	0.00	0.00	1,308.00–
	Subcode Totals	0.00	302,977.79	0.00	0.00	0.00	0.00	302,977.79

Source: Courtesy of the University of South Alabama Medical Center, Mobile, Alabama.

EXHIBIT 1.16 Accounting System Report

Time of Day _____
PGM = AM047-H1

Cost-Center 9-82301
Reports to: 9-81000

Responsibility roll-up report as of fiscal year ending _____

Revenue

| | Budgets | | Actual | | | Open Commitments | Balance Available | Percent Used |
Responsibility Units	Original	Revised A	Current Month	Fiscal Year	Project Year B	C	A – B – C	(B + C)/A
Responsibility Units								
Cardiovas Rehab	$ 790–	$ 790–		$ 869–	$ 869–		$ 79	110%
Revenue-Enter Thpy	3,968–	3,968–	$ 2,960–	39,582–	39,582–		35,614	997
Chemothrapy-O/P Revn	90,729–	90,729–	15,107–	110,452–	110,452–		19,723	121
Clinical Research Un	268,800–	482,051–	34,340–	346,521–	346,521–		135,530–	71
Cardiac ICU	1,524,600–	3,254,816–	252,996–	2,426,084–	2,426,084–		828,732–	74
Orthopedic Cast Room	108,459–	108,459–	8,128–	91,765–	91,765–		16,696–	84
5th Floor North/Reve	31,592–	31,592–	4,013–	39,076–	39,076–		7,484	123
5th Floor South/Reve	2,054,000–	2,977,320–	236,359–	2,331,656–	2,331,656–		645,664–	78
Psychiatric Unit/Rev	1,701,300–	1,725,507–	137,906–	1,463,792–	1,463,792–		261,715–	84
8th Flr Medical/Reve	2,315,220–	2,959,584–	216,324–	2,456,181–	2,456,181–		503,403–	82
Medical ICU/Revenue	1,773,840–	2,853,928–	244,778–	2,232,035–	2,232,035–		621,893–	78
Coronary Care/Revenu	2,148,888–	2,148,888–	167,130–	1,801,879–	1,801,879–		347,010–	83
6th Flr Surgical/Rev	1,787,100–	2,409,563–	172,079–	1,930,916–	1,930,916–		478,648–	80
Burn Center/Revenue	1,254,000–	3,090,809–	193,436–	2,155,646–	2,155,646–		935,163–	69
9th Flr Surgical/Rev	2,029,260–	3,122,028–	230,728–	2,446,790–	2,446,790–		675,238–	78
Neuro/Trauma ICU/Rev	1,504,800–	1,504,800–	111,100–	1,035,650–	1,035,650–		469,150–	68

Newborn Nursery/Reve	804,600–	896,817–	87,603–	794,535–	794,535–	102,282–	88
Premature Nursy/Reve	615,672–	615,672–	71,803–	596,432–	596,432–	19,240–	96
Neonatal Nursy/Reven	4,692,600–	5,468,373–	580,112–	5,178,067–	5,178,067–	290,306–	94
Obstetric Unit/Reven	1,930,440–	2,379,997–	217,489–	2,091,217–	2,091,217–	288,781–	87
Pediatric Unit/Reven	1,438,080–	2,013,282–	171,673–	1,658,513–	1,658,513–	354,769–	82
Pediatric ICU/Revenu	1,141,800–	1,915,268–	115,489–	1,208,778–	1,208,778–	706,490–	63
Delivery Room/Reven	3,396,552–	3,396,552–	410,192–	3,553,291–	3,553,291–	156,738	104
Emergency Room	4,922,867–	4,922,867–	446,310–	4,716,353–	4,716,353–	206,514–	95
Totals	37,539,957–	48,373,660–	4,128,055–	40,706,080–	40,706,080–	7,667,586–	84
Rev/Exp by Fund Operating Revenues	37,539,957–	48,373,660–	4,128,055–	40,706,080–	40,706,080–	7,667,586–	84
Totals	$37,539,957–	$48,373,660–	$4,128,055–	$40,706,080–	$40,706,080–	$7,667,586–	84%
Rev/Exp by Type Revenues	37,539,957	48,373,660	4,128,055	40,706,080	40,706,080	7,667,586	84

Expenses
Salaries
Employee Benefits
Med/Sur Supply
Office/Other Suply
Travel/Entertain
Other Expenses
Minor Equipment
Cost Offsets

Total Expenses

Source: Courtesy of the University of South Alabama Medical Center, Mobile, Alabama.

EXHIBIT 1.17 Accounting System Report

Responsibility roll-up report as of fiscal year ending _____

Expense

Responsibility Units	Budgets		Actual			Open Commitments	Balance Available	Percent Used
	Original	Revised A	Current Month	Fiscal Year	Project Year B	C	A – B – C	(B + C)/A
Medical Nursing	$ 1,446,644	$ 1,561,207	$ 153,176	$ 1,496,785	$ 1,496,785	$ 751	$ 63,671	95%
Psychiatric Nursing	659,186	661,552	63,520	590,664	590,664	566	70,323	89
Staff Development	274,449	274,748	17,680	295,828	295,828	2	21,082–	107
Nursing Svcs-Admin	869,036	880,078	91,347	779,791	779,791	6,242	94,044	89
Clinical Resch Unit	211,846	222,854	17,962	250,545	250,545	16	27,707–	112
Cardiac ICU	429,808	429,807	3,424	53,440	53,440		376,367	12
Float Nurses Pool			110	2,589	2,589		2,589–	
Orthopedic Cast Room	27,195	27,196		12,461	12,461	1,172	13,563	50
Employee Health Nurs	155,423	155,423	18,779	149,601	149,601	5	5,817	96
9th Floor-North	527,221	527,222	46,442	496,133	496,133	98	30,991	94
9th Floor-South	521,411	521,412	40,785	461,240	461,240	2	60,170	88
8th Floor-Medical	810,508	894,965	109,696	1,131,504	1,131,504	1,557	238,095–	126
5th Floor-Shrd Supp	66,529	157,455	25,770	185,295	185,295	862	28,702–	118
Burn Center	546,449	940,030	77,567	836,022	836,022	3,353	100,656	89
6th Floor-Surgical	1,222,187	1,363,087	117,908	1,278,709	1,278,709	2,101	82,276	93
Surgical ICU	1,074,332	1,332,394	138,564	1,309,157	1,309,157	338	22,899	98
7th Floor-Shrd Supp	626,522	696,032	72,802	833,026	833,026	787	137,781–	119
Newborn Nursery	667,925	939,9,10	81,197	892,992	892,992	868	46,051	95
Intermediate Nursery	236,612							
Intensive Care Nursy	1,810,927	1,944,960	202,179	1,749,864	1,749,864	1,241	193,856	90

Obstetric Unit	628,047	668,254	64,748	632,055	632,055	226	35,974	94
Pediatric Unit	923,577	998,643	91,105	895,375	895,375	263	103,005	89
Pediatric ICU	560,288	645,410	48,874	568,314	568,314	50	77,045	88
Delivery Room	1,113,286	1,208,604	134,770	1,107,944	1,107,944	20,154	80,506	93
Emergency Room	1,613,253	1,691,149	160,935	1,524,713	1,524,713	13,885	152,550	90
Patient Transport	220,377	220,377	18,889	186,146	186,146	40	34,191	84
Totals	17,243,038	18,962,769	1,798,229	17,720,193	17,720,193	54,579	1,187,999	93
Rev/Exp by Fund								
Nursing Division	17,060,420	18,750,317	1,771,862	17,527,171	17,527,171	53,402	1,169,746	93
Professional Division	27,195	57,029	7,588	43,421	43,421	1,172	12,436	78
Administrative Divis	155,423	155,423	18,779	149,601	149,601	5	5,817	96
Totals	17,243,038	18,962,769	1,798,229	17,720,193	17,720,193	54,579	1,187,999	93
Rev/Exp by Type								
Revenues								
Expenses								
Salaries	12,382,495	12,461,654	1,256,095	12,391,869	12,391,869		69,785	99
Employee Benefits	3,031,241	3,033,250	239,363	2,487,863	2,487,863		545,387	82
Med/Sur Supply	1,502,492	3,020,154	262,420	2,447,985	2,447,985	30,781	541,387	82
Office/Other Suply	109,306	109,306	9,788	107,656	107,656	1,652		100
Travel/Entertain	43,989	45,788	2,209	27,555	27,555		18,233	60
Other Expenses	212,976	211,676	19,555	196,765	196,765	4,019	10,891	94
Minor Equipment	55,585	66,681	7,590	21,443	21,443	18,127	27,113	59
Cost Offsets	14,060	14,060	1,209	39,057	39,057		24,797–	273
Total Expenses	17,243,038	18,962,769	1,798,229	17,720,193	17,720,193	54,579	1,187,999	93
Net Revenue/Expense	17,243,038	18,962,769	1,798,229	17,720,193	17,720,193	54,579	1,187,999	93
Totals	$17,243,038	$18,962,769	$1,798,229	$17,720,193	$17,720,193	$54,579	$1,187,999	93%

Source: Courtesy of the University of South Alabama Medical Center, Mobile, Alabama.

EXHIBIT 1.18 Accounting System Report

Computer Date ____
Time of Day ____
PGM = AM090-B1

Acct: 3-64155
Dept: 64155

Account statement in whole dollars for fiscal year ending
83% of fiscal year elapsed
Distribution code = 700
Maternal Child Health Education Fund

Subcode	Description	Budgets		Actual		Open Encumbrances	Balance Available	Percent Used
		Original	Revised	Current Month	Fiscal Year			
001	Prior Year Balance		$3,624				$3,624	0 %
020	Income				$5,285–		5,285–	***
021	Refunds				55–		55–	***
	Total Revenues		3,624		5,230–		8,854	144–
224	Recreation Supplies				60		60–	***
231	Postage				60		60–	***
234	Printing				257		257–	***
	General Supplies				377		377–	***
311	Travel			459	1,463		1,463–	***
314	Local Travel				27		27–	***
316	Workshop & Training			3,338	3,498	2,500	5,998–	***
	Travel/Entertainment			3,796	4,989	2,500	7,489–	***
422	Honorarium				425		425–	***
450	Expense Offset				1,000–		1,000	***
	Total Expenses			3,796	4,790	2,500	7,290–	***
	Account Totals		3,624	3,796	440–	2,500	1,563	57

Open Encumbrance Status

Account	P.O Number	P.O Date	Description	Original Enc	Liquidating Expenditures	Adjustments	Current Enc	Last Act Date
3-64155-316	HO4118	01/26/xx	Perdido Hilton Hotel	2,500			2,500	03/22/xx
			*** Account Total ***	2,500			2,500	

EXHIBIT 1.19 Accounting System Report

Computer Date _____
Time of Day _____
PGM = AM090

Report of transactions for fiscal year ending _____

Distribution code = 700
Maternal Child Health Education Fund

Acct: 3-64155
Dept: 64155

Subcode	Description	Date	EC	Ref.	2nd Ref.	J.E. Offset Account	Budget Entries	Current Rev/Exp	Encumbrances	Batch Ref.	Date
311	Dorothy May	07/11	48		218418			$ 458.65		HPC804	07/11
311	CM Total Travel							458.65			
316	Perdido Beach Hilton	07/19	48		220893			3,337.73		HPC832	07/19
316	CM Total Workshop & Training							3,337.73			
	Account Total							3,796.38			

Source: Courtesy of the University of South Alabama Medical Center, Mobile, Alabama.

45

directors of nursing so closely that their creativity is stifled. When such excessive oversight occurs, the nurse managers often spend time doing the work of directors rather than their own. In a decentralized organization, nurse managers are department heads who develop their own objectives, programs, and budgets. They are assisted by staff experts in such tasks as staffing and scheduling.

Proposals originated in this way present a variety of options and are subject to cost/benefit analysis, a process with which nurse managers then become familiar. They are provided with staff service in this area by the chief nurse executive or a staff expert.

New Programs

Complete management plans should be made if new programs are to be implemented. The plans should include objectives; actions that identify procedures, supplies, equipment, and personnel; target dates for implementing each action; and accomplishments noted as they occur. Exhibit 1.20 lists programs that would require such management plans. Exhibit 1.21 shows such a plan for a social services department.

Cutting the Budget

When the budget has to be cut, planning is a vital aspect of the process. This is happening today as hospital admissions and stays decrease and reimbursement takes on a new character. The form and the process of nursing management can determine the course of events when the budget has to be cut.

A nursing administration that delegates decision making to the lowest level and encourages participative management is an effective administration. When clinical nurses are informed at the unit level and invited to give their input, they can help with suggestions for cutting costs. They will gladly implement and support the activities they recognize as resulting partly from their input. A nursing organization that promotes self-direction at the clinical nurse level, nurse manager level, clinical consultant level, and executive nurse level will support direction to reduce cost and to increase productivity and profit. As an example, when a hospital CEO discovered that self-pay patient care was the only category not reviewed for use of resources, a review process was established by a clinical nurse. This process was supported by physicians and other health-care professionals.

Nursing budgets are enormous, with budgets for a single unit running into hundreds of thousands of dollars per year. Pay awards or increases have to be met by budget cuts (personnel cutbacks), use of less expensive supplies and techniques, or increased productivity. The latter requires more paying patients, shorter stays, and increased sales of all paying services. When personnel cuts are to be made, numbers make nursing vulnerable. Some cuts can come from all services but nursing has greater numbers. The nurse manager who controls these numbers daily, weekly, and yearly has greater credibility. Many sources indicate that turnover is costly. The cost of turnover of personnel low on the salary scale is sometimes weighed against the higher cost of employees who are

---

EXHIBIT 1.20   New Programs

1. Expand the intensive care bed capacity.
2. Establish a helicopter aeromedical evacuation service.
3. Replace monitoring equipment in MICU.
4. Update defibrillators.
5. Expand clinical ladder levels II and III.
6. Reorganize nursing administration.

---

at the top of the salary scale. An assumption is made that long-time employees are better satisfied with their jobs and do better work, an assumption that needs to be validated through research.

As workload data indicates shifts from one unit to another, resources must be shifted. This can be done by asking for volunteers, moving vacated positions, and using PRN pools. There is a shift today from inpatient procedures in hospitals to outpatient procedures, either in hospitals or at ambulatory surgery centers. Also, many more diagnostic procedures are done on an outpatient basis. As a result inpatients are often a sicker group, requiring more nursing care.

Because nurse administrators control multimillion dollar budgets, they are powerful people. They are also vulnerable for personnel cuts. Much of this vulnerability stems from external controls imposed by the state and federal governments and health insurance companies. Power comes from the ability of nurse administrators to use knowledge and skills in defending their budgets and in directing and controlling them. They learn to hold the line on staffing, on overtime, and on appropriate use of supplies and equipment.

EXHIBIT 1.21   Management Plan

UNIVERSITY OF SOUTH ALABAMA MEDICAL CENTER
MANAGEMENT ACTION PROGRAM
FISCAL YEAR _____
TO: Russell C. Swansburg, Administrator
FROM: G. C., Director of Social Services
SUBJECT: Objectives for Social Service Department

		Resources		Interim Review
Objective	As Measured by	Admin. Cost	Other Cost	Jan./June
4.3 Active membership on hospital committees by all professional staff	A. Participation on one committee by each social worker			
4.4 Increased involvement in patient education	A. Lectures given by professional staff for families and patients			
	B. Staff involvement in support groups			
	C. Distribution of literature to patients and families	$50/yr		
4.5 Involvement in staff development	A. Lectures for hospital staff in such areas as coping with stress, understanding hostility, etc.			

Source: Courtesy of the University of South Alabama Medical Center, Mobile, Alabama.

Legitimate Budget Activities

It is the contention of the author that hospitals should be managed like other businesses. Charges should be determined from costs and should include allowance for profits or return on equity and for bad debts. The practice of cost shifting to make certain services revenue producers should be stopped.

Oszustowizc suggests the following seven-step system by which total financial requirements eventually determine the gross patient revenue equal to meet the financial needs of a department:

1. Detail demand for nursing services and equipment needs.
2. Detail direct expenses.
3. Detail indirect expenses.
4. Detail working capital requirements.
5. Detail capital requirements.
6. Detail earnings (profit) requirements.
7. Detail deductions from patient revenues.[33]

Director of Nursing Planning and Finance

Some health-care organizations have established a director of nursing planning and finance within the nursing division. This role is often filled with a person with a master's degree in either business administration, health-care administration, or nursing administration, and relevant work experience. The person may be either a nurse or a non-nurse. Duties of this role include forecasting productivity goals and workload, budgeting patient-care hours and nonproductive time, forecasting staffing fluctuations, costs of supplies and other expenses, and budgeting capital investments. In addition, the person in this role creates computer models, controls variances from budget, approves expenditures, educates personnel on financial matters, oversees policy developments and implementation on financial matters, and provides data for all areas of financial planning.[34]

While the goal of this role may be financial control or cost management of all nursing activities, the conventional wisdom is that budgeting, both of revenues and expenditures, should be decentralized. Decentralized budgeting is motivating because it empowers first-line managers and clinical nurses. It provides them ownership. Front-line managers and clinical nurses should be able to shift funds from one account to another. They should be able to expend their budgets without authorized approvals of top managers. With these principles in mind, a director of nursing planning and finance role may assist front-line managers and clinical nurses to be more productive and effective.[35]

Summary

It is important for nurse managers to have a working knowledge of the objectives of a cost-accounting system and of component costs such as fixed costs, variable costs, direct costs, indirect costs, service units, costing standards, chart

of accounts, inventory, cost transfer, and performance reporting. Every activity that takes place in a hospital costs money. There must be a standard for assigning costs to user departments. The nursing department should pay its user share and no more. Knowledge of the cost-accounting system will provide accurate information for budgeting and for cost management.

Efficient nurse managers use a budget calendar that covers formulation, review and enactment, and execution stages of the total budget process.

Evaluation is an administrative aspect of budgeting that, in itself, serves as a controlling process. Decentralization vests control at the lowest competent level of decision making. Good budget feedback is essential if the budget is to be an effective controlling process. This includes information about revenues and expenses, and internal comparisons of projected and actual budgets. The budget can motivate professional nurses and facilitate their development of innovations.

The belief of nurse managers that budgets are beyond comprehension can effectively sabotage their effectiveness in a managerial position. Spiraling health-care costs, hospital cost-management efforts, and increasing accountability from individual cost centers should serve as an impetus to learn at least the fundamentals of budgets and the budget process. To assume the responsibility of budget work increases the nurse manager's potential realm of planning, predicting, and reviewing programs within his or her jurisdiction.

Similar to a nursing care plan, the budget is an activity guidance tool. It is a plan expressed in monetary terms, carried out within a time frame. To be effective as a caregiver, the nurse knows how to develop and use a nursing care plan; similarly, to be effective as a manager, the nurse manager knows how to develop and use a budget.

Experiential Exercises

1. Develop a performance budget for a cost center to be used as a model for a health-care organization.
2. Every hospital prepares the *Hospital and Hospital Health Care Complex Cost Report Certification and Settlement Summary,* commonly known as the *Medicare Cost Report.* Obtain the latest one for your employing or clinical experience hospital. Select a nursing cost center and complete the form to prepare a budget for a unit or project.

Unit _____ Revenue Center Number _____

Direct Expenses (Directly Assigned)
    Salaries (attach position questionnaire for new ones) $ _____ . _____
    Employee benefits $ _____ . _____
    Personnel services $ _____ . _____
    Supplies $ _____ . _____
    Other $ _____ . _____

Total Direct $ _____ . _____

Indirect Expenses
    Depreciation of capital buildings and fixtures $ _____ . _____
    Capital equipment (movable) $ _____ . _____
      (attach requests for new items) $ _____ . _____
    Worker's compensation $ _____ . _____
    Life insurance $ _____ . _____
    Communications $ _____ . _____
    Data processing $ _____ . _____
    Purchasing $ _____ . _____
    Admitting $ _____ . _____
    Patient accounts $ _____ . _____
    General administration $ _____ . _____
    Plant operations $ _____ . _____
    Biomedical $ _____ . _____
    Laundry $ _____ . _____
    Housekeeping $ _____ . _____
    Nursing administration $ _____ . _____
    Patient transport $ _____ . _____
    Preparation $ _____ . _____
    Central supply $ _____ . _____
    Pharmacy $ _____ . _____
    College of nursing (or other college) $ _____ . _____
    Interns and residents $ _____ . _____
    Other $ _____ . _____

Total Indirect $ _____ . _____

Total Costs (Direct + Indirect) $ _____ . _____
Total Charges or Revenues $ _____ . _____
Cost-to-Charge Ratio (Divide total costs by
    total charges or revenues.) $ _____ . _____
                            divided by $ _____ . _____
                            minus $ _____ . _____
                                    or _____%

This exercise has acquainted you with the Medicare Cost Report. You can use projected medical inflation rates to prepare a budget for the following year. If they are projected to be 8 percent, multiply all costs by 1.08 to project and budget costs. You will note that intensive care units are budgeted separately. All other inpatient units are grouped as "Adults and Pediatrics (General and Routine Care)." To separate these units for revenue and expenditures, do the following calculations.

2.1 Select a unit.
2.2 Determine the number of patient days of occupancy for this unit (from the biometric records): _____
2.3 From the Medicare Cost Report determine:
 2.3.1 Total direct and indirect costs $ _____
 2.3.2 Total patient days _____
 2.3.3 Divide total direct and indirect costs $ _____ by total patient days _____ = $ _____ cost per patient day.
 2.3.4 Patient days for unit (from 2.3.2) _____ × cost per patient day (from 2.3.2) _____ = $ _____ or approximate expenses for the nursing unit for this year.
3. Using the management plan format in Exhibit 1.21, construct a prime source document that budgets an objective for a nursing division, department, service, or unit.

Notes

1. R. W. Johnson and R. W. Melicher. *Financial Planning* (Boston: Allyn & Bacon, 1982).
2. J. D. Baker. "The Operating Expense Budget, One Part of a Manager's Arsenal." *AORN Journal* 54, no. 4 (1991):837-841; S. Klann. "Mastering the OR Budgeting Process Is Key to Success." *OR Manager* (Oct. 1989):10-11.
3. D. Osborne and T. Gaebler. *Reinventing Government* (New York: Plume, 1992):237, 241.
4. J. N. Althaus, N. M. Hardyck, P. B. Pierce, and M. S. Rodgers. *Nursing Decentralization: The El Camino Experience* (Gaithersburg, Md: Aspen, 1981); G. R. Whitman. "Analyzing and Forecasting Budgets." In *Management Issues in Critical Care*, ed. C. Birdsall (St Louis, Mo: Mosley, 1991):287-307.
5. D. Osborne and T. Gaebler, op. cit., 3.
6. R. N. Anthony and D. W. Young. *Management Control in Nonprofit Organizations* 4th. ed. (Chicago: Irwin, 1988).
7. B. Nordberg and L. King. "Third Party Payment for Patient Education." *American Journal of Nursing* (Aug. 1976):1269-1271.
8. S. Klann, op. cit.
9. B. Huttman. "Taking Charge: Selling Your Budget." *RN* (Apr. 1964):25-26.
10. D. Osborne and T. Gaebler, op. cit., 243.
11. G. J. Talbot. "Key for Successful Program Budgeting." *The Journal of Continuing Education in Nursing* 14, 3 (1983):8-10.
12. P. F. Drucker. "The Emerging Theory of Manufacturing." *Harvard Business Review* (May-June 1990):94-100.
13. L. D. McCullers and R. G. Schroeder. *Accounting Theory Text and Readings* (New York: John Wiley & Sons, 1982):18–23.
14. A. G. Herkimer, Jr. *Understanding Hospital Financial Management* (Rockville, Md: Aspen, 1978):132.
15. H. Koontz and H. Weihrich. *Essentials of Management* 5th. ed. (New York: McGraw-Hill, 1990):414.
16. R. P. Covert. "Expense Budgeting." In *Handbook of Health Care Accounting and Finance*, ed. William O. Cleverly (Rockville, Md: Aspen, 1982):261-278.

17. J. Buchan. "Cost-Effective Caring." *International Nursing Review* 39(4)1992:117-120.
18. B. E. Statlard and C. Roby. "Flexible Budgeting: A Tool for Better Forecasting." *Medical Laboratory Observer* (Jan. 1985):34-41.
19. S. A. Finkler. *Budgeting Concepts for Nurse Managers* 2d. ed. (Philadelphia: W. B. Saunders Co., 1992).
20. G. J. Talbot, op. cit.
21. R. K. Campbell. "Understanding the Management Process and Financial and Managerial Accounting Part IV. Cash Flow Analysis and Budgeting." *Diabetes Educator* (Feb.-Mar. 1989):126-127, 129.
22. D. Osborne and T. Gaebler, op. cit., 119-124.
23. S. A. Finkler. "Performance Budgeting." *Nursing Economics* (Nov.-Dec. 1991):404-408.
24. Ibid.
25. Ibid.
26. P. N. Palmer. "Why Hide the Revenue Produced by Perioperative Nursing Care?" *AORN Journal* (June 1984):1122-1123.
27. In business and industry bad debts are considered an expense of doing business. In hospitals bad debt is subtracted from revenue. It becomes a reduction of revenue rather than a cost of doing business. Profit or return on equity is not allowed by Medicare or Medicaid except in "for profit" hospitals. A few third-party payers allow a return on equity.
28. C. Hancock. "Value for Money." *Nursing Focus* (Sept. 1981):447-449.
29. T. P. Herzog. "Productivity: Fighting the Battle of the Budget." *Nursing Management* (Jan. 1985):30-34.
30. R. M. Hodgetts. *Management: Theory, Process and Practice* (Philadelphia: W. B. Saunders, 1975):208-209; L. C. Megginson, D. C. Mosely, and P. H. Pietri, Jr. *Management: Concepts and Applications* 3d. ed. (New York: Harper and Row, 1989):453-454.
31. G. R. McGrail. "Budgets: An Underused Resource." *Journal of Nursing Administration* (Nov. 1988):25-31.
32. A. E. Hillestad. "Budgeting: Functional or Dysfunctional?" *Nursing Economics* (Nov.-Dec. 1983):199-201.
33. R. J. Oszustowizc. "Financial Management of Department of Nursing Services." NLN Publ. 20–1798, National League for Nursing, 1979, 1-10.
34. B. R. Zachry and R. L. Gilbert. "Director of Nursing Planning and Finance: A New Role." *Nursing Management* (Feb. 1992):50-52.
35. Ibid.

References

Applegeet, C. J. "AORN's Budget—Planning and Forecasting Uncover Future Needs." *AORN Journal* (Aug. 1989):212, 214.

American Hospital Association. *Managerial Cost Accounting for Hospitals* (Chicago: American Hospital Publishing, 1980).

Cochran, Sr., Jeanette. "Refining a Patient-Acuity System Over Four Years." *Hospital Progress* (Feb. 1979):56-60.

Esmond, T. H., Jr. *Budgeting Procedures for Hospitals 1982 Edition* (Chicago: American Hospital Publishing, 1982).

Esterhuysen, P. "Budgeting—A Serious Matter." *Nursing News* (May 1993):8.

Goetz, J. F., and Smith, H. L. "Zero-Base Budgeting for Nursing Services: An Opportunity for Cost Containment." *Nursing Forum* (Feb. 1980):122-137.

Hallows, D. A. "Budget Processes and Budgeting in the New Authorities." *Nursing Times* (4 Aug. 1982):1309-1311.

Hancock, C. "The Nursing Budget." *Nursing Mirror* (20 Oct. 1982):47-48.

Hicks, L. L., and Boles, K. E. "Why Health Economics?" *Nursing Economics* (May-June 1984):175-180.

Hutton, J., and Moss, D. "Budgetary Control—The Role of the Director of Nursing Services and Treasurers." *Nursing Times* (11 Aug. 1982):1364-1365.

Johnson, K. P. "Revenue Budgeting/Rate Setting." In *Handbook of Health Care Accounting and Finance*, ed. William O. Cleverly, 279-311. (Rockville, Md: Aspen, 1982.)

La Violette, S. "Classification Systems Remedy Billing Inequity." *Modern Healthcare* (Sept. 1979):32-33.

Lyne, M. "Grasping the Challenge." *Nursing Times* (23 Nov. 1983):11-12.

Marriner, A. "Budgetary Management." *The Journal of Continuing Education in Nursing* (Nov.-Dec. 1980):11-14.

McCarty, P. "Nursing Administrators Control Millions." *The American Nurse* (20 Sept. 1979):1, 8, 19.

Narayanasamy, A. "Evaluation of the Budgeting Process in Nurse Education." *Nurse Education Today* (Aug. 1990):245-252.

Orem, D. E. *Nursing Concepts of Practice.* 2d. ed. (New York: McGraw-Hill, 1980.)

Rowsell, G. "Economics of Health Care." *AARN Newsletter 37* No. 7 (July-Aug. 1981):6-8.

Ruskowski, U. "A Budget Orientation Tool for Nurse Managers." *Dimensions in Health Service* (Dec. 1980):30-31.

Seawell, V. L. *Chart of Accounts for Hospitals: An Accounting & Reporting Reference Guide.* (Burr Ridge, Ill: Probus, 1994.)

Sonberg, V., and Vestal, K. E. "Nursing as a Business," *Nursing Clinics of North America 18* No. 3 (Sept. 1983):491-98.

Suver, J. D. "Zero-Base Budgeting." In *Handbook of Health Care Accounting and Finance*, ed. William O. Cleverly (Rockville, Md: Aspen, 1982):353-376.

Swansburg, R. C., Swansburg, R. J., and Swansburg, P. W. *The Nurse Manager's Guide to Financial Management* (Rockville, Md: Aspen, 1988).

Thurgood, J. "Definitions and Explanations of the New Financial Vocabulary." *British Journal of Nursing* (Mar. 1993):295-296.

Trofino, J. "Managing the Budget Crunch." *Nursing Management* (Oct. 1984):42-47.

University of South Alabama Medical Center. *Hospital and Health Care Complex Cost Report Certification and Settlement Summary (Medicare Cost Report [MCR])* (Mobile, Ala: University of South Alabama Medical Center, annual).

Ward, D. L. "Operational Finance and Budgeting." In *The Managed Care Handbook* 2d. ed., ed. P. R. Kongstvedt (Gaithersberg, Md: Aspen, 1993):281-298.

Webster's New Twentieth Century Dictionary, Unabridged, 2d ed. (New York: Simon and Shuster, 1979):236.

2

Personnel Budgeting Including Staffing

Most budgets for nursing personnel are based on quantitative workload measurements such as a patient-acuity system. It is usually a computer software program that produces staffing requirements by shift and by day. It produces an acuity index for each patient and the formula indicates needed staff by level of qualifications (RN, LPN, nursing assistant) and by shift. It also compares actual staffing with that required and can be summarized by month and year. Each day at a given time a clerk enters each patient's acuity rating, as determined by a registered nurse, into a computer terminal. To promote objectivity of the ratings, RNs should be trained to use the same procedures when evaluating each patient. Quality-assurance tests compare the trainer's ratings with those done by registered nurses.

Exhibit 2.1 is a nursing personnel budget based on a patient-acuity rating system. The average daily census (ADC) is obtained from records produced in the admissions office. It is the result of dividing the total patient days for a unit for one year by 365 days. Census reports are computer-generated on a daily, monthly, and annual basis.

Acuity is the result of the sum of all acuities for one year divided by 365 days. This figure is also computer-generated daily, monthly, and annually. The nursing hours are generated from the acuity standard listed in item 1 of Exhibit 2.1. Application of a staffing formula for preparing the personnel budget for a specific unit is illustrated in Exhibit 2.2.

In planning the personnel budget, the nurse manager has quantitative information related to staffing and can accurately predict the number of full-time equivalents (FTEs) needed for patient care. Other considerations must be weighed at the same time. Will there be a pay increase next year? If so, it must be calculated and budgeted. Will fringe benefits increase or decrease? They must also be budgeted. If new programs are being implemented, do they require additional labor power? Will this labor power come from cutbacks in other programs or from added FTEs? See Exhibit 2.3 for adding new positions to the budget.

Careful planning ensures that the nurse administrator controls the nursing budget. It also ensures that the nurse administrator has a handle on the total

EXHIBIT 2.1   Nursing Personnel Budget

Nursing Budget

1. The attached personnel budget for all nursing units is based on a patient-acuity rating system purchased from Medicus Systems. The standard is:

Acuity	Nursing hours per patient needed during 24-hour period
.5	0–2 hours
1.0	2–4 hours
2.5	4–10 hours
5.0	10–24 hours

2. The staffing formula is

$$\frac{\text{Average census} \times \text{nursing hours} \times 1.4 \times 1.14}{7.5}$$

3. The total nursing personnel needed includes ward clerks and units not using a patient-acuity rating system:

Unit	ADC	Acuity	NSG/HRS	RN	LPN	NA	Other	Total
Maternal Child								
3rd	31.8	0.9	4	14	9	4	5	32
Peds	22.0	1.3	4.5	16	5	0	4	25
PICU	4.4	3.4	12	11	0	0	2	13
ICN	21.7	2.9	12	41	7	6	4	58
Inter.	11.9	2.3	4.5	6	4	1	1	12
NBN	19.7	1.0	4	9	6	1	3	19
Del. Rm.	—	—	—	20	3	1	4	28
Play Rm.	—	—	—	—	—	—	1	1
Totals				117	34	13	24	188
Medical								
5 No.	14.3	1.3	4.5	11	3	0	3	17
5 So.	22.1	1.3	4.5	12	5	4	3	24
CRU	3.6	—	4.5	6	—	1	1	8
8th	25.1	1.7	4.5	15	7	2	3	27
MICU	7.2	4.0	12	18	0	0	3.5	21.5
CCU	6.5	3.0	12	16	0	0	1	17
Telemetry	—	—	—	—	1	5	0	6
Totals				78	16	12	14.5	120.5
Surgical								
9th	16.2	1.2	4.5	11	2	2	3	18
6 Surg.	26.5	1.6	4.5	16	6	3	3	28
6 Ortho.	23.5	1.5	4.5	15	4	4	3	26
SICU	6.4	3.8	12	17	0	0	2	19
B.U.	3.7	2.8	12	8	2	0	1	11
Ortho Tech	—	—	—	—	—	—	1	1
Totals				67	14	9	13	103
Psychiatry								
7th	23.5	—	5.5	11	4	11	6	32
OR/RR/EAU/ED								
OR	—	—	—	21	13	4	2	40
RR/EAU	—	—	—	16	0	1	2	19
ED	—	—	—	25	0	7	8	40
Totals				62	13	12	12	99

EXHIBIT 2.1 Nursing Personnel Budget *(Continued)*

Unit	ADC	Acuity	NSG/HRS	RN	LPN	NA	Other	Total
			Administration					
N/S Adm.	—	—	—	13	0	0	3.5	16.5
Staff Dev.	—	—	—	8.5	0	0	1	9.5
Health Nurse	—	—	—	1	—	—	—	1
CVICU								
Pool	—	—	—	4.5	12	18	2	36.5
Totals				27	12	18	6.5	63.5
Totals				362	93	75	76	606

Note: The formulary budget is based on actual ADC for 12 months (July–June). All positions above formula calculations are placed in CVICU budgeted cost center and held vacant.

Source: Courtesy of the University of South Alabama Medical Center, Mobile, Alabama.

dollar amount that will be expended on personnel and that will be generated (income) by personnel.

In the budgeting process, personnel account for the largest portion of the nursing budget. When one is preparing budgets for clinics, emergency departments, recovery rooms, operating rooms, and delivery rooms, it is important to have quantitative data. These include number of visits, procedures, deliveries, and the like. Records of lengths of time required for each activity can be taken by using management engineering techniques in which visits, procedures, or other activities are charted over a period of time.

For these types of departments, data should be collected over a representative period to show the actual hours worked by shift and by day. These data indicate fluctuations in the workload by shift and by day of the week. A second

EXHIBIT 2.2 Calculating the Nursing Personnel Budget

The staffing formula is

$$\frac{\text{Average daily census} \times \text{nursing hours} \times 1.4 \times 1.14}{7.5}$$

Example: 3rd Floor
Average daily census = 31.8
Nursing hours = 4 (per 24 hours)
1.4 is a constant representing 7 days in a week with a full-time worker working 5 days in a week:
$7 \div 5 = 1.4$
1.14 is a constant representing an allowance of 0.14 FTE for vacation, illness, etc. for each 1.0 FTE
7.5 represents one workday

$$\frac{31.8 \times 4 \times 1.4 \times 1.14}{75} = 27 \text{ FTEs}$$

Note: According to Exhibit 2.1, there are 14 RNs, 9 LPNs, and 4 NAs (27 FTEs) budgeted for 3rd Floor. The Other column represents ward clerks or other non-nursing personnel not included in the formula. While quantitative measurements justify a full complement of nursing personnel, the budget committee can reduce this number. Note that ICN has been reduced from the formula calculation by 1.0 FTE.

Source: Courtesy of the University of South Alabama Medical Center, Mobile, Alabama.

EXHIBIT 2.3   New Position Questionnaire, Budget Year _____

1. Department _____ Department number _____
2. Position class, title _____ Position FTE _____
3. Minimum starting salary _____ Expected starting date _____
4. Permanent _____ Temporary _____ If temporary, ending date _____
5. Describe briefly the new position responsibilities:

_____

_____

_____

_____

Need for new position

6. New service _____ Increased volume _____
   If new service, complete question 7.
   If increased volume, complete question 8.
7. Describe the new service to be provided and estimate new revenues.

_____

_____

_____

_____

_____

8. Document increased volume and provide staffing analysis for your department.

_____

_____

_____

(Attach additional pages if necessary.) _____

_____

_____

Source: Courtesy of the University of South Alabama Medical Center, Mobile, Alabama.

data sheet records the number of patients in the department at any one time, including those patients in a holding status. Conversion of these data into graphs provides the following information to compare staffing with workload:

- the current nursing hours available per patient visit
- fluctuation in available hours by shift and day
- fluctuation in workload by time of day
- fluctuation in ratio of staffing levels to patient load[1]

In considering an emergency department, Piper indicates that the basic staffing should be calculated to handle a "critical mass," the staffing level required to handle an unexpected emergency. In addition to quantitative data, the nurse administrator should collect qualitative data from the staff to assist in containing stress, determining mix of staff, and improving support services. Data can be compared with those from other institutions. The result can then be translated into personnel dollars.[2]

In the process of budgeting the nurse manager knows how much each decision will cost, and whether it involves numbers and kinds of personnel or amounts and kinds of supplies and equipment. Few nurse managers have the luxury of a budget that provides all of the resources that can be used. Hard decisions have to be made. They are easier to substantiate when workloads are quantified. In the personnel area, if the patient-dependency or patient-acuity

system is reliable and valid, and has quality checks on the raters, it will pro-vide data that justifies the personnel budget. When the number of highest acuity-level adult patients increases from 24 to 32 per shift and day, the budget must be adjusted. Comparisons must be made to determine whether other levels have decreased. Estimates must be made as to whether the increases and de-creases are permanent or temporary. Then the budget decisions are made.

Nurse managers study fluctuation trends in patient census as data for mini-mum staffing to determine the percentage of time to staff one nurse less and the percentage of time to staff one nurse more per shift. The salary expense for the one time that one nurse less per shift is needed should be subtracted. The salary expense for the time one nurse more per shift is needed should be added. The result is an improved salary expense budget (see Exhibit 2.4).

Strategies to reduce budget overages include

- maintaining good retention of staff
- using nurse extenders to perform non-RN functions
- monitoring and controlling unscheduled absenteeism
- implementing an effective on-call system
- instituting a "flex-team" model in related clinical areas to avoid overtime and agency nurse expenses
- creating a large pool of part-time nurses
- budgeting according to trend
- negotiating for a reasonable budget that considers turnover and orientation[3]

Nonproductive FTEs

Nonproductive FTEs are hours for which an employee is paid but does not work. Nonproductive FTEs include vacation days, holidays, sick days, education and training time, jury duty, funerals, and military leave. These nonproductive hours must be determined and added to personnel expenditures as replacement FTEs. A full-time equivalent is based on 2080 hours per year. If the nonproductive FTE average is to be used for personnel budgeting, it will be provided by the human resource department payroll section. For example,

Average vacation FTE	12.5 days
Average holiday FTE	7.0 days
Average sick days FTE	3.5 days
Average training and education FTE	3.0 days
Average other leave FTE	1.5 days
Total	27.5 days or 220.0 hours

The total work time is 2080 hours, less 220 hours, so the actual work time is 1860 hours. The percentage of nonworked to total hours paid is 10.6 percent. The percentage of nonworked to worked hours is 11.8 percent.

A cost-center manager prepares the budget according to management rules. These should include a budget for replacement FTEs to cover nonproductive FTEs by assigning a fixed amount to each person's paid time off. An option is to determine percentage of nonproductive FTEs and add this total to the bud-get. This information is then used for staffing determination, taking into consid-eration seasonal fluctuations for vacations, census, and other pertinent factors.[4]

EXHIBIT 2.4   Budgeting for Fluctuating Census

Staffing	Census	%	Total Days	Required Hours/Day	Total Hours Required	Budgeted Labor Rate	Salary Expense Budget
Minimum staffing	9	100.00%	365	12	39,420	$17	$670,140
1 less nurse/shift	<6	4.98%	(18)	24	(432)	$17	($7,344)
1 more nurse/shift	>9	39.99%	146	24	3,504	$30	$105,120
Total					42,492		$767,916

Source: E. Tzirides, V. Waterstraat, and W. Chamberlin. "Managing the Budget with a Fluctuating Census." *Nursing Management* (March 1991): 80H. Reprinted with permission of Springhouse Corporation.

To provide for fluctuations in personnel costs, a personnel pool can be established. This can consist of permanent or temporary FTEs, part-time workers, persons who work flexible hours, a mixture of RNs, LPNs, nursing assistants, and clerks, and can provide for all shifts and days of the week. An effective as-needed (PRN) pool is well managed by one line manager or staffing director. Its personnel require staff development programs and concern for managing them as a unique workforce of human beings. The nurse manager or administrator determines the level of service and then expresses it in financial terms to produce a budget. Personnel pools can be decentralized to cost centers.

Staffing Philosophy

Staffing is certainly one of the major problems of any nursing organization, whether it be a hospital, nursing home, home health care agency, ambulatory care agency, or another type of facility. Aydelotte has stated that "nurse staffing methodology should be an orderly, systematic process, based on sound rationale, applied to determine the number and kind of nursing personnel required to provide nursing care of a predetermined standard to a group of patients in a particular setting. The end result is prediction of the kind and number of staff required to give care to patients."[5]

The staffing process is complex. Components of the staffing process as a control system include a staffing study, a master staffing plan, a scheduling plan, and a nursing management information system (NMIS). The NMIS includes these five elements:

1. quality of patient care to be delivered and its measurement
2. characteristics of the patients and their care requirements
3. prediction of the supply of nurse power required for items 1 and 2
4. logistics of the staffing program pattern and its control
5. evaluation of the quality of care desired, thereby measuring the success of the staffing itself[6]

West includes a position control plan and a budgeting plan as components of a staffing process (see Exhibit 2.5).[7]

Nurse staffing must meet certain regulations. Among these are legal requirements of Medicare. The Medicare Survey report is excerpted in Exhibit 2.6. This

EXHIBIT 2.5   Components of the Staffing Process

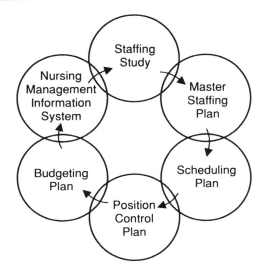

Source: M.E. West. "Implementing Effective Nurse Staffing Systems in Managed Hospitals." *Topics in Health Care Financing,* Vol. 6, 4 (Summer 1980): 15. Copyright © 1980 Aspen Publishers, Inc. Reprinted with permission.

legal standard is further supported by other standards such as those of the *Accreditation Manual for Hospitals,* which are reprinted in Exhibit 2.7.

Other standards include the ANA *Standards of Administrative Nursing Practice,* ANA *Standards of Clinical Nursing Practice,* and state licensing requirements. From all of these and from the expectations of the community, of nurses, and of physicians, the nurse administrator develops a staffing philosophy as a basis for a staffing methodology. Exhibit 2.8 shows staffing guidelines developed this way. Community expectations will be related to economic status, to local values and beliefs, and to local culture. Nurses' expectations usually relate to the same community standards and, in addition, to their perceptions of the practice of nursing and its components, to the results desired, and to the workload tolerated.

Nurse managers can discern from the nursing division's existing statements of purpose, philosophy, and objectives various values related to staffing. A staffing philosophy may encompass beliefs about using a patient-dependency system or patient-classification system to identify patients' needs. It may cover beliefs about use of skilled personnel as a core staff, with a float pool for supplemental staffing. It may also specify who will be responsible for hiring.[8]

Objectives of nurse staffing are excellent care and high productivity. Professional nurses can develop a statement of purpose that is comprehensive in stating the quality and quantity of performance it is intended to motivate. Purpose statements should be quantified.[9]

Current trends indicate extensive structural changes to come in the healthcare system. These changes include downsizing, mergers, closures, and increased ambulatory care services. Managers and clinical nurses will be faced

EXHIBIT 2.6   Medicare and Medicaid Regulations

482.23   Condition of participation: Nursing services.
The hospital must have an organized nursing service that provides 24-hour nursing services. The nursing services must be furnished or supervised by a registered nurse.

(a) *Standard: Organization.* The hospital must have a well-organized service with a plan of administrative authority and delineation of responsibilities for patient care. The director of nursing service must be a licensed registered nurse. He or she is responsible for the operation of the service, including determining the types and numbers of nursing personnel and staff necessary to provide nursing care for all areas of the hospital.

(b) *Standard: Staffing and delivery of care.* The nursing service must have adequate numbers of licensed registered nurses, licensed practical (vocational) nurses, and other personnel to provide nursing care to all patients as needed. There must be supervisory and staff personnel for each department or nursing unit to ensure, when needed, the immediate availability of a registered nurse for bedside care of any patient.

(1) The hospital must provide 24-hour nursing service furnished or supervised by a registered nurse, and have a licensed practical nurse or registered nurse on duty at all times, except for rural hospitals that have in effect a 24-hour nursing waiver granted under §405.1910(c) of this chapter.

(2) The nursing service must have a procedure to ensure that hospital nursing personnel for whom licensure is required have valid and current licensure.

(3) A registered nurse must supervise and evaluate the nursing care for each patient.

(4) The hospital must ensure that the nursing staff develops, and keeps current, a nursing care plan for each patient.

(5) A registered nurse must assign the nursing care of each patient to other nursing personnel in accordance with the patient's needs and the specialized qualifications and competence of the nursing staff available.

(6) Non-employee licensed nurses who are working in the hospital must adhere to the policies and procedures of the hospital. The director of nursing service must provide for adequate supervision and evaluation of the clinical activities of non-employee nursing personnel which occur within the responsibility of the nursing service.

(c) *Standard: Preparation and administration of drugs.* Drugs and biologicals must be prepared and administered in accordance with federal and state laws, the orders of the practitioner or practitioners responsible for the patient's care as specified under §482.12(c), and accepted standards of practice.

(1) All drugs and biologicals must be administered by, or under supervision of, nursing or other personnel in accordance with federal and state laws and regulations, including applicable licensing requirements and in accordance with the approved medical staff policies and procedures.

(2) All orders for drugs and biologicals must be in writing and signed by the practitioner or practitioners responsible for the care of the patient as specified under §482.12(c). When telephone or oral orders must be used, they must be

   (i) Accepted only by personnel who are authorized to do so by the medical staff policies and procedures, consistent with federal and state laws;

   (ii) Signed or initialed by the prescribing practitioner as soon as possible; and

   (iii) Used infrequently.

(3) Blood transfusions and intravenous medications must be administered in accordance with state law and approved medical staff policies and procedures. If blood transfusions and intravenous medications are administered by personnel other than doctors of medicine or osteopathy, the personnel must have special training for this duty.

(4) There must be a hospital procedure for reporting transfusion reactions, adverse drug reactions, and errors in administration of drugs.

Source: Reprinted with permission from *CCH Medicare and Medicaid Guide*, published and copyrighted © 1986 by CCH Incorporated, Riverwoods, Illinois.

with making staffing decisions to increase productivity. These decisions should be based on lessons learned during the past two decades about management of human resources or human capital.

Staffing Study

A staffing study should gather data about environmental factors within and outside the organization that affect staffing requirements.

EXHIBIT 2.7 JCAHO Standards

The following are JCAHO standards related to nurse staffing. Although the wording may change each year, the basic principles remain the same.

NC. 3.4.2 Nurse staffing plans for each unit define the number and mix of nursing personnel in accordance with current patient care needs.

NC. 3.4.2.1 In designing and assessing nurse staffing plans, the hospital gives appropriate consideration to the utilization of registered nurses, licensed practical/vocational nurses, nursing assistants, and other nursing personnel, and to potential contributions these personnel can make in the delivery of efficient and effective patient care.

NC. 3.4.2.2 The staffing schedules are reviewed and adjusted as necessary to meet defined patient needs and unusual occurrences.

NC. 3.4.2.3 Appropriate and sufficient support services are available to allow nursing staff members to meet the nursing care needs of patients and their significant other(s).

NC. 3.4.2.4 Staffing needs are adequate to support participation of nursing staff members, as assigned, in committees/meetings and in educational and quality assessment and improvement activities.

NC. 4.1 The plan for nurse staffing and the provision of nursing care is reviewed in detail on an annual basis and receives periodic attention as warranted by changing patient care needs and outcomes.

NC. 4.1.1 Registered nurses prescribe, delegate, and coordinate the nursing care provided throughout the hospital.

NC. 4.1.2 Consistent standards for the provision of nursing care within the hospital are used to monitor and evaluate the quality of nursing care provided throughout the hospital.

NC 5.1 Nursing services are directed by a nurse executive who is a registered nurse qualified by advanced education and management experience.

NC. 5.1.1 If the hospital utilizes a decentralized organizational structure, there is an identified nurse leader at the executive level to provide authority and accountability for, and coordination of, the nurse executive function.

Source: Copyright © 1995 *Comprehensive Accreditation Manual for Hospitals.* Joint Commission on Accreditation of Healthcare Organizations. (Oakbrook Terrace, IL.: 1994): 42, 51, 85. Reprinted with permission.

Aydelotte listed four techniques drawn from engineering to measure the work of nurses. All involve the concept of time required for performance.[10] These techniques are:

1. Time study and task frequency
   1.1 Tasks and task elements (procedures)
   1.2 Point and time started
   1.3 Point and time ended
   1.4 Sample size
   1.5 Average time
   1.6 Allowance for fatigue, personal variation, and unavoidable standby
   1.7 Standard time = step 1.5 + step 1.6
   1.8 Frequency of task × standard time = the measurement of nursing activity
   1.9 Total of all tasks × standard time = volume of nursing work
2. Work sampling (variation of task frequency and time). Procedure is as follows:
   2.1 Identify major and minor categories of nursing activities.
   2.2 Determine number of observations to be made.
   2.3 Observe random sample of nursing personnel performing activities.
   2.4 *Analyze observations.* Frequency occurring in a specific category = percentage of total time spent in that activity. Most work sampling studies sample direct care and indirect care to determine ratio.
3. Continuous sampling (variation of task frequency and time). Technique is the same as for work sampling except that:
   3.1 Observer follows one individual in the performance of a task.
   3.2 Observer may observe work performed for one or more patients if they can be observed concurrently.

EXHIBIT 2.8   University of South Alabama Medical Center Hospital Department of Nursing Staffing and Assignment Guidelines

SUBJECT: Staffing and Assignment

I.   Policy Statement

II.   Purposes

To provide a uniform system

1. for adequate staffing mix to meet acuity needs of patients.
2. to maintain equitable and consistent staffing for all professional and support groups within nursing.

III.   General Information

A. Appropriate resources are provided to meet patient needs. Indicators for patient outcomes are monitored on an ongoing basis through the Quality Assessment and Improvement Plan. These results are reviewed as part of the budget review process to determine if the same patient care needs are being met throughout the hospital. If outcomes are not acceptable and/or do not demonstrate improvement 5 and if insufficient information exists related to staffing, further investigation may be required.

B. Staffing requirements are projected by each Nurse Manager and weekly schedules are submitted to the Staffing Office. If there are vacancies, the Staffing Coordinators utilize in-house PRN personnel as well as other staff to provide coverage.

C. Daily staffing needs are determined by the skill level of employee, acuity measurement, census 5, and anticipated changes in activity. Adjustments are made each shift to meet the staffing requirement, as well as during the shift.

D. The staffing office is staffed by Staffing Coordinators on the 7–3 and 3–11 shifts, 7 days a week. Staffing for the 11–7 shift is provided by the 3–11 Shift Coordinator. Adjustments to increased acuity of patients or census variations are made by the Staffing Coordinator or Clinical Administrator providing house supervision.

E. Staffing is individualized and the acuity of patients is the primary concern when assignments are made. Consideration is given to the special needs of selected patients.

F. Support personnel, which includes ward clerks, telemetry technicians, wound care technicians, guest relation aides, and students are considered when staffing the unit.

G. The staffing is adjusted to meet patient needs as effectively as possible. At times it is necessary to reassign nursing personnel on a daily or temporary basis to meet these needs. Whenever possible nursing personnel will be reassigned to a unit within their nursing division, or to a like unit. PRN staff are expected to work where assigned. If scheduled for a Med/Surg Unit, they may be required to work any Med/Surg Unit.

H. Personnel will be clinically cross-oriented within each division to the individual nursing units.

I. If staff are reassigned to a unit outside of their division they are assigned as support working with regular unit staff. Licensed personnel reassigned out of their division are not assigned charge duties.

J. Nursing personnel will be floated based on their qualifications. Refusal to accept reassignment will be handled individually by the Director of Nursing or Assistant Administrator for Nursing. Negotiations between personnel is encouraged.

K. Regular scheduled staff members cannot be floated in lieu of overtime, PRN, or float staff. Regular staff may only be floated when no other (overtime, PRN, or float) staff is available.

L. When personnel are requested to work overtime, they can only be offered the option to work overtime within their division, i.e., Med/Surg or Critical Care. No agreement for overtime will be made that specifies one particular unit.

M. All scheduled overtime work will be approved by the Nurse Manager or Director of Nursing. Directors and Nurse Managers are ultimately responsible for monitoring overtime.

N. Mandatory meetings of nursing personnel are an extreme inconvenience to off-duty personnel. Personnel will be paid for hours worked when mandated to return for a meeting. Meetings must be approved by the Assistant Administrator prior to announcement.

Source: Courtesy of the University of South Alabama Medical Center, Mobile, Alabama.

4. Self-reporting (variation of task frequency and time).

4.1 The individual records the work sampling or continuous sampling on himself or herself.

4.2 Tasks are logged using time intervals or the time tasks start and end.

4.3 Logs are analyzed.

Many work sampling studies focus on procedures, ignore standards, and are lacking in objectivity, reliability, and accuracy. The techniques themselves are sound (see Exhibit 2.9).

According to West, "there are three cardinal rules for forecasting staffing requirements."[11] The first is to base staffing projections on staffing history; Exhibit 2.10 is a data sheet designed for this purpose. The data can be collected from the patient-classification system reports and census reports. Such data is readily available in most hospitals; some NMISs, such as Medicus, provide numbers of personnel required, including the mix of RNs, LPNs, and nursing assistants. Other data needed are sick time, overtime, holidays, and vacation time. The attrition rate is also important and will be discussed elsewhere. In some patient-classification systems, these considerations are built into the staffing formula.

The second cardinal rule for planning staffing needs is to review current staffing levels. Review of future plans for the institution is the third cardinal rule.[12] When clinical nurses are involved in staffing plans, they will have confidence in them. These staffing studies can be made with electronic spreadsheets.

Staffing requires much planning on the part of the nurse administrator. Data must be collected and analyzed. These data include facts about the product—patient care. They include diagnostic and therapeutic procedures performed by both physicians and nurses. They include the cognitive elements of professional nursing translated into the skills of professional nursing such as history-taking and assessment, nursing diagnosis and prescription, application of care, evaluation, recordkeeping, and all other actions related to primary health care of patients.

Basic to planning staffing of a division of nursing is the fact that qualified nursing personnel must be provided in sufficient numbers to ensure adequate, safe nursing care for all patients 24 hours a day, 7 days a week, 52 weeks a year. Each staffing plan must be tailored to the needs of the hospital and cannot be arrived at by a simple worker/patient ratio or formula.

Planning for staffing requires judgment, experience, and thorough knowledge of the requirements of the organization in which the individual nurse administrator is employed. It requires support of hospital administrators, physicians in charge of clinical services, and the nursing staff.

The basic requirement is unchanging, regardless of the type or size of the institution: plan for the kinds and numbers of nursing personnel that will give safe, adequate care to all patients and will ensure the work of nursing is productive and satisfying.

Changing and expanding knowledge and technology in the physical and social sciences, in the medical field, and in economics influence planning for staffing. Health-care institutions are treating more clients on an outpatient basis. New drugs, improved diagnostic and therapeutic procedures, and changes in reimbursement have decreased the length of hospital stays. Standards of the Joint Commission on Accreditation of Healthcare Organizations, the American Nurses' Association, and other professional and governmental organizations have required upgrading of health care.

Planning for staffing is influenced by changing concepts of nursing roles for clinical nursing practitioners and specialists. Decision making is being delegated to the lowest practical level. Ward clerks and unit managers have assumed duties formerly done by nursing personnel.

EXHIBIT 2.9 Work Sampling Study

Task or Procedure	Time Started	Time Ended	Minutes
		RN, LPN, NA (*circle one*)	
1. _____			
2. _____			
3. _____			
4. _____			
5. _____			
6. _____			
7. _____			
8. _____			
9. _____			
10. _____			

(A) Total number of tasks and procedures = _____
(B) Total minutes = _____

Average Time

Total minutes	÷	Total number of tasks and procedures	=	Average time per procedure or task
(B) _____	÷	(A) _____	=	(C) _____

Standard Time

Average time	+	Time allowed for fatigue, personal variation, and unavoidable standby	=	Standard time in minutes
(C) _____	+	(D) _____	=	(E) _____

Measurement of Nursing Activity

Standard time	×	Frequency of an individual task or procedure	=	Measurement of nursing activity
(E) _____	×	(F) _____	=	(G) _____

Volume of Nursing Work

Standard time	×	Total number of tasks and procedures	=	Volume of nursing work
(E) _____	×	(A) _____	=	(H) _____

Source: Adapted from: M. K. Aydelotte, *Nurse Staffing Methodology: A Review and Critique of Selected Literature.* (Washington, DC: U.S. Government Printing Office, January 1973).

Patient populations are changing as birth rates decline and longevity increases. Staffing plans are influenced by institutional missions and objectives related to research, training, and many specialties. They are influenced by personnel policies and practices related to vacations, time off, overtime, holidays, temporary workers, and other factors. They are influenced by policies and practices related to admission and discharge times of patients, assignment of patients to units, and intensive and progressive care practices.

The amount and kind of nursing staff required is also influenced by the degree to which other departments carry out their supporting services. This is particularly true during weekends, evenings, nights, and holidays. Staffing requirements should plan for nursing personnel to perform non-nursing duties such as dietary functions, clerical work, messenger and escort activities, and

EXHIBIT 2.10 Staffing History Data Sheet

Year _____ Month _____   Cost Center _____

Day	ADC	Patient Acuity	Personnel				
			Sick Hours	Overtime Hours	Holiday Hours	Vacation Hours	Other
1							
2							
· · ·	· · ·	· · ·	· · ·	· · ·	· · ·	· · ·	· · ·
31							
Average							

Source: Data adapted with permission from M. E. West, "Implementing Effective Nurse Staffing Systems in the Managed Hospitals," *Topics in Health Care Financing*, Summer 1980. Copyright © 1980 Aspen Publishers.

housekeeping. Whether these services should or should not be carried out by nursing personnel is not the point here; the point is that the degree to which the situation exists has to be considered in any planning. Nurse managers should avoid assuming responsibility for non-nursing services and encourage the appropriate departments to perform such services. When they do not, nurse managers should have a system of charging the provided services to the appropriate cost center, which then provides revenue to the nursing cost center.

Staffing plans are influenced by the number and composition of the medical staff and the medical services offered. Nursing requirements are affected by characteristics of patient populations determined by the size and capability of the medical staff. Special requirements of individual physicians; the time and length of their rounds; the required time, and the complexity, and number of tests, medications, and treatments ordered; and kind and amount of surgery all affect the quality and quantity of nursing personnel required and influence their placement.

Arrangement of the physical plant has a large impact on staffing requirements. Fewer personnel are needed for a modern, compact facility equipped with labor-saving devices and efficient working arrangements than for one that is spread out and has few or no labor-saving devices. Different staffing is required for a facility that is arranged functionally than for one that is not. If, for example, the surgical suite is not next to the birthing rooms, recovery room, and intensive care units, more staff is needed to meet acceptable standards of quality and safety. Many other architectural features must be considered, such as location of patient rooms in relation to the nursing stations; the location of specialized units, work rooms, and storage space; and the time required to transport patients to other sections of the hospital for diagnostic or therapeutic services such as radiography and nuclear medicine.

Staffing is further affected by the organization of the division of nursing. Plans should be reviewed and revised to organize the department for efficient and economic operation with written statements of mission, philosophy, and

objectives; sound organizational structure; clearly defined functions and responsibilities; written policies and procedures; effective staff development programs; and planned periodic system evaluation. Staffing plans for such a department are different from those for one that is loosely organized with overlapping functions and responsibilities, vague or conflicting policies, and poorly defined standards of nursing practice.

In addition, data to be analyzed will include numbers of admissions, discharges, transfers; the amount of supervision (in hours) of (assisting) personnel needed; patient teaching (in hours); emergency responses; mode of care delivery (team, primary, or other); and staff mix (ratios of RNs to LPNs to others).[13]

Staffing Activities

Price identified seventeen staffing activities and suggested that the nurse administrator identify by names the persons responsible for each of them. She further suggested that

1. each activity be specified as requiring nursing or non-nursing personnel, and
2. the category and position of the person who *should* be responsible for each activity be identified,
3. the one person ultimately responsible for each activity be identified,
4. this review (steps 1 through 3) be performed for the day shift, evening shift, night shift, and weekend and holiday shifts.

A modified Price format for gathering data and analyzing responsibility for staffing activities would cover the following: recruiting personnel; interviewing and screening; hiring RNs, LPNs, and nursing assistants; making assignments to clinical units; making assignments to shifts; preparing work schedules in advance; maintaining daily schedules; adjusting for staff absences and patients' needs; calculating turnover; calculating hours of care; checking time cards and payroll; developing policies; time spent in telephone communication; and monitoring compliance with contracts.[14]

Orientation Plan

A main purpose of orientation is to help the nursing worker adjust to a new work situation. Orientation should be a planned program carried out through a "buddy" system, a special in-service unit, or other method. Nursing tasks and skills for which each new nursing worker must be certified are usually included in orientation. Orientation increases productivity, because fewer personnel are needed when they are fully conversant with the work situation. Exhibit 2.11 is an example of an orientation plan.

Staffing Policies

Written staffing policies should be available to all personnel and should cover at least the following areas:

- vacations
- holidays

EXHIBIT 2.11 Nursing Orientation—Week 1

MONDAY	TUESDAY	WEDNESDAY	THURSDAY	FRIDAY
8:00–4:30	8:00–10:00 Introduction Philosophy Dress code Staffing Time/attendance Skills assessment	8:00–8:15 Computer Class Assignment	8:00–4:30 RN IV Therapy	8:00–8:45 Alabama Eye Center
Personnel Orientation				
Benefits		8:15–12:00 Code 1 CPR		8:45–9:30 Alabama Organ Center
Quality assurance				
Employee health	10:00–10:15 Break	12:00–1:00 Lunch		9:30–9:45 Break
Infection control				9:45–10:00 Nutrition Service
	10:15–12:15 Documentation	1:00–4:30 Clinical Skills RN/LPN BGM Emergency trach R. TPN dressing C.		
Fire & safety				10:00–11:00 Telephone System
	12:15–1:15 Lunch			11:00–12:00 Lunch
	1:15–4:30 MAR Medical Policies Medical Exam	NA BGM Vital signs Body mechanics Infection control Legal		12:00–4:30 Team Building

Source: Courtesy of the University of South Alabama Medical Center, Mobile, Alabama.

- sick leave
- weekends off
- consecutive days off
- rotation to different shifts
- overtime
- part-time personnel and temporary personnel
- use of "float" personnel
- exchangeability of staff
- use of special abilities of individual staff members
- exchanging hours
- personnel requests
- management requests
- the work week

Work Contracts

Each employee should have a work contract with the institution. The contract should state the date employment is to commence, the job classification, the hours of work, the rate of pay, whether the job is full time or part time, and all other specific points agreed on between the employee and the institutional representative. To be valid both parties must sign it. Work contracts may be superseded by union contracts.

Staffing Function

The staffing function should probably be centralized, because this removes a clerical burden from first-line nurse managers and provides more time for them to attend to direct patient care and nursing activities. All of the activities related to staffing should be developed into policies and procedures that reflect the thinking of nursing administration and can be performed by non-nurse employees. Obviously, nurse managers will remain involved in hiring, firing, and promotions, in consultation with their supervisors and human-resource specialists.

A sign of maladministration in nursing is too many levels of supervision. Often a professional nurse is employed at the departmental level to perform the function of scheduling, which is time consuming and can be done by non-nursing personnel. Price recommends that a non-nurse perform the staffing function, advised by professional nurses, as needed. The staffing employee should be a very competent person, that is, "a good business person, mature, effective in interpersonal relations, objective in dealing with personnel, fair and firm; one who can communicate effectively orally, by phone, and in writing, and finally, one who has above-average mathematical ability."[15]

Staffing the Units

Each patient-care unit should have a master staffing plan. This should include the basic staff needed on the unit for each shift. Basic staff is the minimum or lowest number of personnel needed to staff a unit. It includes fully oriented, and full- and part-time employees. The number may be based on examination of staffing records and expert opinions of nurse managers. It includes all categories: registered nurses, licensed practical nurses, and nursing technicians or assistants for each shift. Exhibit 2.12 shows a formula for determining a core staff per shift.

Next the number of *complementary* personnel are determined. They are scheduled as an addition to the basic group, but the total number in both groups is controlled by financial resources and the availability of personnel. Complementary personnel provide the flexibility to meet short-range and unexpected changes such as illnesses and census fluctuations. Complementary personnel are not ensured a permanent work-shift pattern and are usually scheduled for 4-week periods.

Float personnel are employees who are not permanently assigned to a station. They provide flexibility to meet increased patient loads, as well as unexpected personnel absences. The number and kinds of float personnel can be accurately determined from general monthly records that show absence rates, personnel turnover, and fluctuations in patient-care workloads. Float personnel may be assigned to a pool or by unit.

Some nurse administrators do not hire part-time nursing personnel, although they can be a cost-controlling factor in staffing because they do not receive the same benefits as full-time personnel. Part-time personnel are better motivated when they receive some benefits such as a number of holidays and vacation days proportionate to days worked and pay increases when they complete the aggregate days worked by full-time personnel. Their total hours worked can be controlled to fill actual shortfalls.

EXHIBIT 2.12 Formula for Estimating a Core Staff per Shift

The average daily census for a 25-bed medical-surgical unit over a 6-month period is 19 patients. The basic average daily hours of care to be provided are 5 hours per patient per 24 hours. How many total hours of care will be needed on the average day to meet these standards? 19 × 5 = 95 hours. If the work day is 8 hours, this means 95 ÷ 8 = 11.9 or 12 full-time-equivalent (FTE) staff are needed to staff the unit for 24 hours. An FTE is one person working full time (40 hours a week) or several persons who together work a total of 40 hours a week. A total of 12 FTEs × 7 days per week = 84 shifts per week, if the staffing is to be the same each day. If each employee works five 8-hour shifts per week, 84 ÷ 5 = 16.8 is the number of FTEs needed as basic staff for this unit.

The number of nursing personnel to cover sick leave, vacations, and holidays or other absences can also be determined and added to the basic staff. This information is determined from a study of personnel policies and use. It is frequently included in patient classification system formulas. Such additional staff may be provided from a float pool.

The next determination to be made is the ratio of RNs to other nursing personnel. If the ratio is determined as 1:1, how many of the basic staff of 16.8 should be RNs? One half of the total, which would be 8.4 RNs and 8.4 others (LPNs, nurse's aides, orderlies, or nursing assistants). A study of staffing patterns in 80 med-surg, pediatrics, and postpartum units in 12 Salt Lake City community hospitals recommends a mix of 58% RNs, 26% LPNs, and 16% aides.[16]

The final determination is how many personnel are needed for each shift. Warstler recommends proportions of: day—47%; evening—35%; and night—17%.[17] This means that for a total staff of 16.8 personnel, 8 would be assigned to days, 6 to evenings, and 2.8 to nights. This is obviously approximate; other patterns could also be chosen by the nurse administrator.

The number of complementary nursing personnel would be added to this basic staff. They could be a group of one RN, one LPN, and one other and assigned accordingly. They are entered into the following table as numbers in parentheses added to the figure for basic staff.

In today's reimbursement environment, complementary personnel may be budgeted as a pool. They may even exist only as a portion of basic personnel assigned to a pool.

Basic Staffing Plan for 25-Bed Medical-Surgical Unit

Category	Day	Evening	Night	Totals
RNs	4 + (1)	3	1.4	8.4 + (1)
LPNs	2	2 + (1)	1.4	5.4 + (1)
Others	2	1	0 + (1)	3 + (1)
Totals	8 + (1)	6 + (1)	2.8 + (1)	16.8 + (3)

Whatever the staffing policy, it should be arrived at through consultation with clinical nurses. The nursing department's personnel budget is also a master staffing plan. The process for developing a master staffing plan is depicted in Exhibits 2.12, 2.13, and 2.14. Once the basic staff for a unit is determined, as in Exhibit 2.12, it can be translated to a staffing board as in Exhibit 2.13. Exhibit 2.14 can be used for self-scheduling. Exhibits 2.13 and 2.14 represent staffing for 27 patients at 5 hours of care per patient per 24 hours.

Staffing Modules

Cyclic Scheduling

Cyclic scheduling is one of the best ways to meet the requirements of equitable distribution of hours of work and time off. A basic time pattern for a certain number of weeks is established and then repeated in cycles. Advantages of cyclic scheduling include the following:

- Once developed, it is a relatively permanent schedule, requiring only temporary adjustments from time to time.

EXHIBIT 2.13   Staffing Board

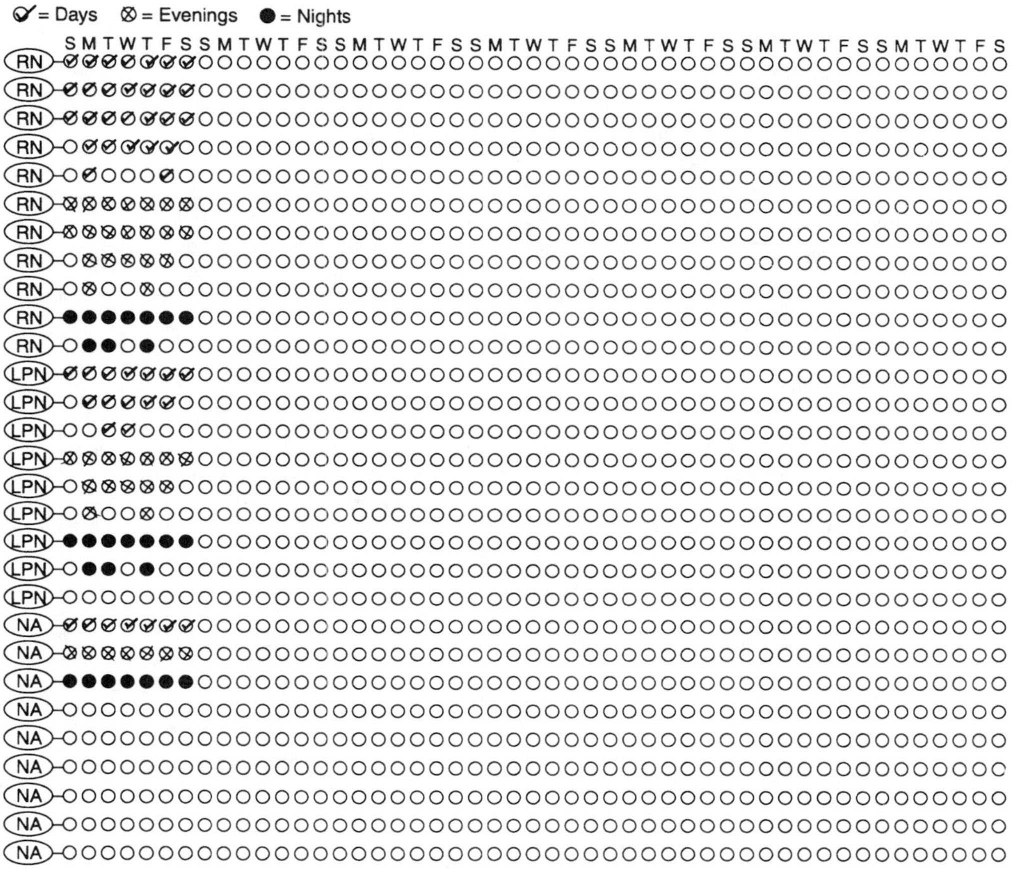

☑ = Days   ⊗ = Evenings   ● = Nights

	S M T W T F S	S M T W T F S	S M T W T F S	S M T W T F S	S M T W T F S	S M T W T F S	S M T W T F S

(Staffing board grid with peg holes for 29 persons across 7 weeks, rows labeled RN, LPN, NA)

Note: Left row of pegs are coded by category of personnel: RN, LPN, NA (Nursing Assistant). There are peg holes on the board for 29 persons for 7 weeks. Larger boards can be used. Pegs for scheduling would be color coded for shifts: day, evening, night, weekend, off, and so on.

- Nurses no longer have to live in anticipation of learning their new schedules to know their time off-duty, because it can be scheduled for as long as 6 months in advance.
- Personal plans can be made in advance with a reasonable degree of reliability.
- Requests for special time off are kept to a minimum.
- It can be used with rotating, permanent, or mixed shifts and can be modified to allow fixed days off and uneven work periods, based on personnel needs and preferences.
- It can be modified to fit known or anticipated periods of heavy workloads and can be temporarily adjusted to meet emergencies or unexpected shortages of personnel.

Because it is relatively inflexible, cyclic scheduling only works with a staff that rotates by policy and personal choice. It is not generally accepted by personnel who need flexible scheduling to meet their needs related to families, educational pursuits, and similar demands.

EXHIBIT 2.14 Self-Scheduling Format

	S	Initials	M	Initials	T	Initials	W	Initials	T	Initials	F	Initials	S	Initials
Week Jan 15 11a.m.	3 RNs 1 LPN 1 NA	JH	5 RNs 2 LPNs 1 NA		4 RNs 3 LPNs 1 NA		4 RNs 3 LPNs 1 NA		4 RNs 2 LPNs 1 NA		5 RNs 2 LPNs 1 NA		3 RNs 1 LPN 1 NA	
3p.m.	3 RNs 1 LPN 1 NA	JH	5 RNs 2 LPNs 1 NA		4 RNs 3 LPNs 1 NA		4 RNs 3 LPNs 1 NA		4 RNs 2 LPNs 1 NA		5 RNs 2 LPNs 1 NA		3 RNs 1 LPN 1 NA	
7p.m.	2 RNs 1 LPN 1 NA		4 RNs 3 LPNs 1 NA		3 RNs 2 LPNs 1 NA		3 RNs 2 LPNs 1 NA		4 RNs 3 LPNs 1 NA		3 RNs 2 LPNs 1 NA		2 RNs 1 LPN 1 NA	
11p.m.	2 RNs 1 LPN 1 NA		4 RNs 3 LPNs 1 NA		3 RNs 2 LPNs 1 NA		3 RNs 2 LPNs 1 NA		4 RNs 3 LPNs 1 NA		3 RNs 2 LPNs 1 NA		2 RNs 1 LPN 1 NA	
3a.m.	1 RNs 1 LPN 1 NA		2 RNs 2 LPNs 1 NA	JH	2 RNs 2 LPNs 1 NA	JH	1 RN 1 LPN 1 NA	JH	2 RNs 2 LPNs 1 NA	JH	1 RN 1 LPN 1 NA		1 RN 1 LPN 1 NA	
7a.m.	1 RN 1 LPN 1 NA		2 RNs 2 LPNs 1 NA	JH	2 RNs 2 LPNs 1 NA	JH	1 RN 1 LPN 1 NA	JH	2 RNs 2 LPNs 1 NA	JH	1 RN 1 LPN 1 NA		1 RN 1 LPN 1 NA	
Week 11a.m.														
3p.m.														
7p.m.														
11p.m.														
3a.m.														
7a.m.														

Each block represents 4 hours of staffing.
Names and Initials:
RN Jane Hatfield JH _____   _____   _____   _____
_____   _____   _____   _____
_____   _____   _____   _____

An infinite number of basic cyclic patterns can be developed, tailored to suit each unit. Exhibit 2.15 shows two variations. Patterns should reflect policy, workload factors, and staff preferences. Nursing personnel may use a staffing board (Exhibit 2.13) to develop a pattern and cycle satisfactory to them. The staffing board shows the numbers of nursing personnel required for each day of the week for seven weeks. According to the basic staffing plan, four RNs are needed on Tuesdays, Wednesdays, and Thursdays, but only three RNs are needed on Saturdays and Sundays, so the fourth RN (FTE) could be used on Mondays and Fridays because the standard indicated that these were high-volume work days. Also, only two RNs are needed on Saturday and Sunday evenings, and four are needed on Monday and Thursday evenings. One RN is needed on Sunday, Wednesday, Friday, and Saturday nights, but two are needed on Monday, Tuesday, and Thursday nights. Similarly, basic staffing for LPNs and others are shown on the staffing board. These numbers are then transferred to the self-scheduling format shown in Exhibit 2.14.

EXHIBIT 2.15   Cyclic Schedules

Minimum Basic Schedule

week	|1|							|2|							|3|							|4|						
	S	M	T	W	T	F	S	S	M	T	W	T	F	S	S	M	T	W	T	F	S	S	M	T	W	T	F	S
1	N	N	N	N	N	–	–	–	–	E	E	E	E	E	E	E	–	–	D	D	D	D	D	D	–	–	N	N
2	D	D	D	–	–	N	N	N	N	N	N	N	–	–	–	–	E	E	E	E	E	E	E	–	–	D	D	D
3	E	E	–	–	D	D	D	D	D	D	–	–	N	N	N	N	N	N	N	–	–	–	–	E	E	E	E	E
4	–	–	E	E	E	E	E	E	E	–	–	D	D	D	D	D	D	–	–	N	N	N	N	N	N	N	–	–
charge	–	D	D	D	D	D	–	–	D	D	D	D	D	–	–	D	D	D	D	D	–	–	D	D	D	D	D	–
N	1	1	1	1	1	1	1	1	1	1	1	1	1	1	1	1	1	1	1	1	1	1	1	1	1	1	1	1
D	1	2	2	1	2	2	1	1	2	2	1	2	2	1	1	2	2	1	2	2	1	1	2	2	1	2	2	1
E	1	1	1	1	1	1	1	1	1	1	1	1	1	1	1	1	1	1	1	1	1	1	1	1	1	1	1	1

Eight-Week Cycle—Mixed Shifts

week		|1|							|2|							|3|							|4|						
		S	M	T	W	T	F	S	S	M	T	W	T	F	S	S	M	T	W	T	F	S	S	M	T	W	T	F	S
Permanent shifts	1	N	N	N	–	–	N	N	N	N	–	–	N	N	N	N	N	N	–	–	N	N	N	N	–	–	N	N	N
	2	N	N	N	N	N	–	–	–	–	N	N	N	N	N	N	N	N	N	N	–	–	–	–	N	N	N	N	N
	3	E	E	E	E	E	–	–	E	E	E	E	E	–	–	E	E	E	E	E	–	–	E	E	E	E	E	–	–
	4	–	–	E	E	E	E	E	–	–	E	E	E	E	E	–	–	E	E	E	E	E	–	–	E	E	E	E	E
	5	E	E	–	–	D	E	E	E	E	–	–	D	E	E	E	E	–	–	D	E	E	E	E	–	–	D	E	E
Rotate	6	D	–	–	N	N	N	N	N	N	N	N	–	–	D	D	D	D	D	D	–	–	–	D	D	D	–	D	D
	7	–	D	D	D	D	D	–	–	D	D	D	–	D	D	D	–	–	N	N	N	N	N	N	N	N	–	–	D
	8	–	D	D	D	–	D	D	D	D	D	D	D	–	–	–	D	D	D	D	D	–	–	D	D	D	–	D	D
Leave relief	9	D	D	D	D	D	–	–	–	D	D	D	D	D	–	–	D	D	D	–	D	D	D	D	D	D	D	–	–
	10	–	–	D	D	D	D	D	D	D	–	D	D	D	–	–	–	D	D	D	D	D	D	D	–	D	D	D	–
Assistant	11																												
Charge	12																												

		|5|							|6|							|7|							|8|						
		S	M	T	W	T	F	S	S	M	T	W	T	F	S	S	M	T	W	T	F	S	S	M	T	W	T	F	S
	1	N	N	N	–	–	N	N	N	N	–	–	N	N	N	N	N	N	–	–	N	N	N	N	–	–	N	N	N
	2	N	N	N	N	N	–	–	–	–	N	N	N	N	N	N	N	N	N	N	–	–	–	–	N	N	N	N	N
	3	E	E	E	E	E	–	–	E	E	E	E	E	–	–	E	E	E	E	E	–	–	E	E	E	E	E	–	–
	4	–	–	E	E	E	E	E	–	–	E	E	E	E	E	–	–	E	E	E	E	E	–	–	E	E	E	E	E
	5	E	E	–	–	D	E	E	E	E	–	–	D	E	E	E	E	–	–	D	E	E	E	E	–	–	D	E	E
	6	–	D	D	D	–	D	D	D	D	D	D	D	–	–	–	D	D	D	D	D	–	–	D	D	D	–	D	D
	7	D	D	D	D	D	–	–	–	D	D	D	D	D	–	–	D	D	D	–	D	D	D	D	D	D	D	–	–
	8	D	–	–	N	N	N	N	N	N	N	N	–	–	D	D	D	D	D	D	–	–	–	D	D	D	D	D	–
	9	–	D	D	D	–	D	D	D	D	D	D	D	–	–	–	D	D	D	–	D	D	D	D	D	D	D	–	–
	10	–	–	D	D	D	D	D	D	D	–	D	D	D	–	–	–	D	D	D	D	D	D	D	–	D	D	D	–
	11																												
	12																												

Note: N = nights, D = days, E = evenings; numbers are FTEs.

Source: Dept. of the Air Force, *USAF Hospital Nursing Service Manual* (Washington, DC: USGPO, 1971): 4-4–4-14.

The numbers of staff are noted by the nurse manager for each four hours of staffing. Nursing personnel insert their initials in each block according to the "givens" of staffing policies. Additional pages can be used to self-schedule four, six, or any number of weeks. Exhibit 2.14 illustrates a single week of scheduling. It can be expanded to cover any number of weeks.

Patterns should be reviewed periodically to see that they meet the purpose, philosophy, and objectives of the organization and the division of nursing, that they are practical with regard to the numbers and qualifications of personnel, that they are satisfactory to nursing personnel, that they meet patient needs, and that they use people effectively.

Scheduling records should be retained for a period of time, probably one year, because they provide valuable statistical planning information for staffing as well as historical information for questions related to personnel on duty when specific events occurred.

It has been stated that staffing policies should be established in specific areas. The following policies may be considered:

- Personnel are scheduled to work their preferred shifts as much as possible.
- Personnel choices are balanced to meet the needs of the unit and of other employees.
- An employee is allowed to make her or his own arrangements for special time off or exchange within specific personnel policies.
- Policies have been established for making schedule changes.
- Each employee has a copy of his or her work schedule.
- Consideration has been given to staffing during hours of clinical experience for students.
- There is a weekend and holiday schedule policy. It is a common practice in many organizations throughout the United States to plan alternate weekends off for nursing personnel. Weekend coverage can be by "weekends-only" employees; staffing levels can be influenced by hospital policies on admissions and discharges and weekend staffing policy.

Self-Scheduling

Self-scheduling is an activity that may make a staff happier, more cohesive, and more committed. It should be planned carefully on a unit (cost-center) basis. Planning may use either a self-directed work team or a quality circle approach. Self-scheduling matches staff to individual preferences. It has been found to shorten scheduling time and reduce conflicts, increase retention and job satisfaction, and reduce illness time, voluntary absenteeism, and turnover.

In one case, a nurse manager asked a nurse administrator how to reduce high absenteeism. The nurse manager had 12 RNs with absentee problems. There followed a discussion about self-scheduling and the procedures to use. Several months later the nurse manager called the nurse administrator to say that after self-scheduling had been implemented, only one of the 12 employees was an absentee problem. The problem with the other 11 had disappeared with self-scheduling. The nurse manager then successfully proceeded to self-scheduling with all other employees who requested it.

Self-scheduling leads to more responsible employees. It meets their personal goals—family, social life, education, child care, commuting, and others. It is an

example of participatory management with decentralized decision making. The planning must include the givens or rules, which should be minimal to meet legal and professional standards.[18]

Patient Classification Systems

A patient classification system (PCS) is essential to staffing nursing units of hospitals. It quantifies the quality of nursing care. In selecting or implementing a PCS, a representative committee of nurse managers and clinical nurses should be used. The committee can include a hospital administrator, which will decrease skepticism about the PCS.

Purposes

The committee will identify the purposes of the PCS to be purchased or developed. Among them are the following:

1. *Staffing.* The system will establish a unit of measure for nursing: *time.* This unit of measure will be used to determine both the numbers and kinds of staff needed. Perceived patient needs can be matched with available nursing resources.

2. *Tracking program costs and formulating the nursing budget.* A prescribed unit of time will be used to determine the actual cost of nursing services. Profits and losses of nursing can then be determined.

3. *Tracking changes in patient care.* A PCS gives nurse managers the ability to moderate and control delivery of care, adjusting intensity and cost according to patients' needs.

4. *Determining values for the productivity equation,* which is output divided by input. Reducing input cost reduces costs of each output (time unit). In the prospective payment system (PPS), this output measure has been the discharged patient. Outputs become the criteria for measuring nursing productivity, regardless of quality. A PCS provides workload indices as productivity measurements.

5. *Determining quality.* Once a standard time element is established, staffing is adjusted to meet the aggregate times. A nurse manager can elect to staff below the standard time to reduce costs. Thus the nurse manager makes a decision to reduce quality by reducing time and cost. It is best to do this in collaboration with clinical nurses. They are the personnel who are continually present and can assist with developing and applying more efficient procedures and protocols, such as rearranging the physical setting, and the assembling of equipment and supplies. Their involvement increases their trust and respect, improves their attendance and work habits, improves workforce stability, and reduces errors. Their input into decision making can be through product evaluation and selection, identification of non-nursing tasks to be done by lower priced workers, increased mechanization, and job evaluation.[19]

Nursing Management Information Systems for a PCS

Nursing Management Information Systems (NMISs) are described in more detail in chapter 5. A good NMIS is basic to a sound PCS. It provides shift reports of personnel needed and assigned, by type. It provides staffing and productivity data by unit and area. It provides average data on the intensity of care needed by class of patient. It provides the cost per time unit of patient care by class of patient.[20]

Desirable Characteristics of a PCS

The following characteristics are desirable for a PCS. Such systems should

- Differentiate intensity of care among definitive classes.
- Measure and quantify care to develop a management engineering standard.
- Match nursing resources to patient-care requirements.
- Relate item above to time and effort spent on the associated activity.
- Be economical and convenient to report and use.
- Be mutually exclusive, counting no item under more than one work unit.
- Be open to audit.
- Be understood by those who plan, schedule, and control the work.
- Be individually tailored as to the procedures needed for accomplishment.
- Separate requirements for registered nurses and other staff.[21]

Components of a PCS

The first component of a PCS is a method for grouping patients, or setting up classifications. Johnson indicates two methods of categorizing patients. Using *factor evaluation* each patient is rated on independent elements of care; each element is scored (weighted); scores are summarized; and the patient is placed in a category based on the total numerical value obtained. Using *prototype evaluation*, each patient is categorized according to a broad description of care requirements.[22]

Johnson describes a prototype evaluation with four basic categories and one category for a typical patient requiring one-to-one care. Each category addresses activities of daily living (ADL), general health, teaching, emotional support, treatments, and medications. Data are collected on average time spent on direct and indirect care (see Exhibit 2.16).

A second component of a PCS is a set of guidelines describing the way in which patients will be classified, the frequency of classification, and the method of reporting the data (see Exhibit 2.17). The third component of a PCS is the average amount of time required for care of a patient in each category (see Exhibit 2.18).

A method for calculating required staffing and required nursing-care hours is the fourth and final component of a PCS.

The formula is "the sum of the standard times for each category, multiplied by the number of patients in that category, plus the indirect care time, equals required hours of patient care. Dividing this value by 7.0 (number of hours staff actually work each shift) results in the number of staff required to work each shift."[23]

EXHIBIT 2.16   Classification Categories—Medical-Surgical Units

Category I—Self Care
1. Activities of daily living
   a. Eating—feeds self or needs little assistance.
   b. Grooming—almost entirely self-sufficient.
   c. Excretion—goes to bathroom alone or almost alone; not incontinent.
   d. Comfort—self-sufficient.
2. General health—good; admitted for a diagnostic procedure, simple procedure, or surgery that is simple or minor.
3. Teaching and emotional support—routine teaching for simple procedures, follow-up teaching or discharge teaching. No unusual or adverse emotional reactions. Patient may require orientation to time, place, and person once per shift.
4. Treatments and medications—none or simple medications or treatment.

Category II—Minimal Care
1. Activities of daily living
   a. Eating—needs help in preparing food, positioning, or encouragement to eat; can feed self.
   b. Grooming—can do majority of care unassisted or with minimal assistance.
   c. Excretion—needs help getting to bathroom or using urinal; not incontinent or experiences occasional stress incontinence or dribbling.
   d. Comfort—turns self or with minimal encouragement and assistance.
2. General health—mild symptoms including more than one mild illness; requires monitoring of vital signs, diabetic urines, uncomplicated drainage, or infusion.
3. Teaching and emotional support—needs 5–10 minutes per shift for teaching or emotional support. Patient may be mildly confused, belligerent, or agitated, but is well controlled by medications, frequent orientation, or restraints.
4. Treatments and medications—requires 20–30 minutes per shift. Needs evaluation of effectiveness of medication or treatment frequently; may require observation q 2 h for mental status.

Category III—Moderate Care
1. Activities of daily living
   a. Eating—needs to be fed but can chew and swallow.
   b. Grooming—unable to do much for self.
   c. Excretion—needs bedpan or urinal placed or removed; can only partially turn or lift self; incontinent two times each shift.
   d. Comfort—completely dependent and needs turning but can be turned by one person.
2. General health—acute symptoms may be impending or subsiding; requires monitoring and evaluation of physiological or emotional state q 2–4 h. Has continuous drainage or infusion which requires monitoring q 1 h.
3. Teaching and emotional support—requires 10–30 minutes per shift; very apprehensive or mildly resistive to teaching. Patient may be confused, agitated, or belligerent, but is fairly well controlled by medications, frequent orientation, or restraints.
4. Treatments and medications—requires 30–60 minutes per shift; requires frequent observation for side effects or allergic reaction; may require observation q 1 h for mental status.

Category IV—Extensive Care
1. Activities of daily living
   a. Eating—cannot feed self; difficulty chewing and swallowing; may require tube feeding.
   b. Grooming—complete bath, hair care, oral care; patient cannot assist at all.
   c. Excretion—incontinent more than two times a shift.
   d. Comfort—cannot turn self or assist with turning; may require two people to turn.
2. General health—seriously ill; exhibits acute symptoms such as bleeding and/or fluid loss, acute respiratory episodes, or other episodes requiring frequent monitoring and evaluation.
3. Teaching and emotional support—requires more than 30 minutes per shift for teaching of very resistive patients or care and support of patients with severe emotional reactions. Patient may be confused, belligerent, or agitated, and is not controlled by medications, frequent orientation, or restraints.
4. Treatment and medication—requires more than 60 minutes per shift; elaborate treatments done more than once per shift or requiring two persons; may require observation more frequently than q 1 h for mental status.

Category V—Intensive Care
Requires one-to-one observation or continuous monitoring each shift.

Source: K. Johnson. "A Practical Approach to Patient Classification." *Nursing Management* (June 1984): 40. Reprinted with permission of Springhouse Corporation.

The Commission for Administration Services in Hospitals (CASH) system of patient classification appears to be a prototype. CASH is a patient-classification design that rates patents by intensity of care and establishes a category relating to nursing hours required based on patients' ability to feed and bathe themselves with supervision, mobility status, special procedures and treatments, and observational, institutional, and emotional needs. This

EXHIBIT 2.17 Directions for Classifying Patients

1. Patient classification will be reviewed one time each shift by the charge nurse or her designee on the 7–3 and 3–11 shifts.
2. Classification is made by comparing the individual patient with each category. If a charge nurse is unsure as to what category a patient belongs she should refer to the ADL indicator only and classify by those guidelines.
3. The cue sheet is only a guideline. It is not expected that every patient will be classified in the same category by disease entity alone.
4. After the category is selected, the charge nurse will place a number on the Kardex to denote that patient's classification
   Self-care — I
   Minimal care — II
   Moderate care — III
   Extensive care — IV
   Intensive care — V
5. The charge nurse (or designee, i.e., secretary) will tally the number of patients in each category. The nursing office will call for the tallies at about 1 P.M. and 9 P.M.
6. Patients who have private-duty nurses and sitters are classified according to the level of care the staff on the unit must provide to the patients.

Source: K. Johnson. "A Practical Approach to Patient Classification." *Nursing Management* (June 1984). Reprinted with permission of Springhouse Corporation.

EXHIBIT 2.18 Data Collection—Standard Care Hours per Patient Category

Directions: Consider a patient for whom you have cared today in each of the following categories. Indicate, to the best of your ability, the amount of time that was required to care for the patient. If you did not care for a patient in one of the categories this shift, please leave that category blank. Your cooperation in completing these forms is appreciated.

Category I	—Self-care	_____ minutes
Category II	—Minimal care	_____ minutes
Category III	—Moderate care	_____ minutes
Category IV	—Extensive care	_____ minutes

Check one: **Fill in blank:**

RN	_____	_____ Shift
LPN	_____	_____ Unit
Aide/Attendant	_____	_____ Date

Please leave this form in the area designated for that purpose on the nursing unit.

Source: K. Johnson. "A Practical Approach to Patient Classification." *Nursing Management* (June 1984). Reprinted with permission of Springhouse Corporation.

design is quantified by determining the nursing-care time associated with the critical indicators. The GRASP® system of patient classification uses a workload measurement design to evaluate the categories of tasks that nurses perform in providing patient care and identifies how much nursing time is required for each task. The time is then totalled.[24] GRASP® is a factor evaluation design, as is Medicus.

There is only general agreement that three to five categories of patient acuity are sufficient for a PCS. Alward argues that four categories best reduce variance and statistical probability of error. She also states that the factor-evaluation instrument is better than the prototype system because it prevents ambiguity or overlap among the categories.[25]

Examples

Nursing Models

A PCS based on a model of nursing is rare. Auger and Dee describe one based on the Johnson Behavior System Model, which has eight behavioral subsystems: ingestive, eliminative, affiliative, dependency, sexual, aggressive-protective, achievement, and restorative (see Exhibit 2.19).

Patients' behaviors and nursing interventions were rank ordered for four categories of patient acuity (see Exhibit 2.20).

EXHIBIT 2.19   Definitions and Behavioral Characteristics of Behavioral Subsystems

Subsystem	Definition	Critical Behavioral Characteristics
Ingestive	Behaviors associated with the intake of needed resources from the external environment including food, information, and objects, for the purpose of establishing an effective relationship with the environment	Food/fluid intake; sensory perception; mental status
Eliminative	Behaviors associated with the release of physical waste products	Bowel/bladder patterns; hygiene
Affiliative	Behaviors associated with the development and maintenance of interpersonal relationships with parents, peers, authority figures; establishes a sense of relatedness and belonging with others	Attachment behaviors; interpersonal relationships; communication skills
Dependency	Behaviors associated with obtaining assistance from others in the environment for completing tasks and/or emotional support; includes seeking of attention, approval, recognition	Basic self-care skills; emotional security
Sexual	Behaviors associated with a specific sexual identity for the purpose of pleasure and procreation	Knowledge and behavior congruent with biological sex
Aggressive-Protective	Behaviors associated with real or potential threat in the environment for the purpose of ensuring survival	Protection of self through direct or indirect acts; identification of potential danger
Achievement	Behaviors associated with mastery of oneself and one's environment for the purpose of producing a desired effect	Problem-solving activities; knowledge of personal strengths and weaknesses
Restorative	Behaviors associated with maintaining or restoring energy equilibrium; relief from fatigue, recovery from illness, and so on	Sleep behavior; leisure/recreational activities; sick-role behavior

Source: J. A. Auger and V. Dee. "A Patient Classification System Based on the Behavioral System Model of Nursing: Part 1." *Journal of Nursing Administration* (April, 1983): 40. Reprinted with permission of Lippincott-Raven Publishers.

Patient behaviors and nursing intervention criteria, by category for eliminative and affiliative subsystems are given in Exhibit 2.21.

Fourteen pairs of observers were used to rate each subsystem of behavior for all patients present on the unit during the shift. Observers agreed on independent ratings of patient behavior for the eight subsystems. Employees were trained to do patient ratings. New employees rate patients differently, indicating a need to develop a common frame of reference for all observer-raters. This system applies to psychiatric patients, but indicates the necessity for rating psychosocial factors of all patients.[26]

Auger and Dee list four advantages to relating nursing models to PCSs:

1. Providing a frame of reference for the systematic assessment of patient behaviors and the development of nursing intervention
2. Providing a frame of reference for all practitioners in the clinical setting
3. Providing a theoretical framework of knowledge and behavior
4. Providing for consistency and continuity of care

EXHIBIT 2.20   General Framework for Categorization of Nursing Care Requirements

Patient Behaviors	Nursing Interventions

Behaviors that are
  a. healthy
  b. appropriate to developmental stage
  c. adaptive to environment
Behavioral subsystems that are currently inactive
Physical health status: normal
	I Maintain and support healthy, developmentally appropriate behaviors.
	Reinforce independent behaviors in adaptive areas.
	Provide general supervision.

Behaviors that are
  a. inconsistent
  b. in process of being learned
  c. may or may not be appropriate to developmental stage
  d. maladaptive to the environment
Physical health status: chronic or acute health problem of minor significance, such as a cold
	II Provide moderate/periodic supervision.
	Maintain behavioral programs designed to modify maladaptive behaviors and maintain new adaptive behaviors.
	Structure environment as needed to provide limits on behaviors.
	Provide care in the context of group setting.
	Provide nursing care appropriate to illness and handicaps.
	Implement medical regime.

Behaviors that are
  a. severely maladaptive to the environment
  b. not appropriate to developmental stage
Physical health status: chronic or acute health problem of major significance, such as seizures
	III Provide direct supervision.
	Implement behavioral programs designed to modify maladaptive behaviors.
	Initiate teaching of new behaviors.
	Reinforce healthy adaptive behaviors.
	Structure environment to provide limits on behaviors.
	Provide intensive nursing care appropriate to illness and handicaps.
	Critical activities: new admissions, seclusion and restraint, electroconvulsive therapy

Category III and IV behavior in one or more subsystems of acute intensity and/or frequency: includes self-destructive acts and aggression toward others	IV Provide care on a one-to-one basis for 8 hours per shift—that is, suicide observation.

Source: J. A. Auger and V. Dee. "A Patient Classification System Based on the Behavioral System Model of Nursing: Part I." *The Journal of Nursing Administration* (April, 1983): 41. Reprinted with permission of Lippincott-Raven Publishers.

Dee and Auger emphasize orientation and teaching of all new personnel so the system will be effective. This is true of all PCSs, including their use to make decisions about admissions.[27]

Research

A research study was conducted at a 1000-bed acute-care, urban, university-affiliated hospital in Canada. The purpose of the research was to examine whether three methods of patient classification estimate the same hours of care when applied to the same patient population. The three PCSs used were GRASP®, PRN (Project Research in Nursing), and Medicus, all factor-type evaluation designs.

The PRN, which was developed in Canada, includes 154 care activities, organized within a needs approach model adapted from the Henderson model.

GRASP® assumes that 15 percent of activities in which nurses are involved take up 85 percent of their time. Classification instruments are developed around these activities and are hospital specific.

EXHIBIT 2.21   Samples of Level III Categorization Criteria for Two Behavioral Subsystems

Eliminative Subsystems

Patient Behaviors	Nursing Interventions
1. Absence of bowel control	1. Implement behavioral program for toilet training, bed-wetting, and encopresis.
2. Absence of bladder control	2. Total care of eliminative needs: diapers, colostomy care, drains, and so on
3. Absence of established pattern of elimination or disruption of established pattern resulting in dehydration	3. Teach self-care, independent skills related to hygiene/eliminative tasks.
4. Failure to dispose of body wastes in sanitary manner: for example, fecal smearing	4. Direct supervision of hygiene care.
5. Excessive diaphoresis	5. Attend closely to changes in elimination pattern for signs and symptoms of physical problems.
	6. Provide medications, as ordered by physician.

Affiliative Subsystem

Patient Behaviors	Nursing Interventions
1. Absence of emotional attachment to others or excessive intense attachments	1. Provide regular, intensive one-to-one interactions to establish relationship.
2. Failure to establish or maintain relationships on an individual basis	2. Implement behavioral program to increase frequency of interactions with staff/family/peers.
3. Failure to establish or maintain relationships in group interactions	3. Implement behavioral program to increase participation in group activities.
4. Failure to initiate/maintain effective communication: verbal, nonverbal, and written	4. Promote adaptation to change by planning and limiting number of changes.
5. Indiscriminate attachment to others	5. Limit contact with family when indicated; provide information regarding denial of rights.
6. Resistant to change in milieu or daily routine	6. Implement behavioral program to develop basic communication skills and role model interactional techniques.
7. Unable to express positive/negative feelings in direct way; denial of feelings.	7. Assist in identification and expression of positive/negative feelings.
8. Lack of awareness of personal space	

Source: J. A. Auger and V. Dee. "A Patient Classification System Based on the Behavioral System Model of Nursing: Part I." *The Journal of Nursing Administration* (April, 1983): 41. Reprinted with permission of Lippincott-Raven Publishers.

The Medicus model has its origins in operations research, with approximately 37 condition indicators rated daily. PRN and Medicus require modification to account for layout and other physical differences among workplaces.

The mean hours of care estimated by each classification system is presented in Exhibit 2.22. It can be seen that for the average patient on the average day, PRN predicted more care (9.06 hrs) than Medicus or GRASP® (6.63 and 6.57, respectively). There was no significant difference between GRASP® and Medicus systems in mean estimates of total care ($t = 1.05$, $p = 0.30$).

From Exhibit 2.23 it can be noted that PRN predicted on average, more direct-care time (4.51 hours per patient) than did GRASP® or Medicus (3.35 and 3.22, respectively). GRASP® estimated an average of 0.13 more hours of direct care than did Medicus. All three systems demonstrated significant differences in direct-care time estimates ($P < 0.0001$). PRN fairly consistently estimated more hours of direct care than the other two systems. Medicus tended to estimate more hours than GRASP® in ICU settings but fewer in non-ICU settings.

EXHIBIT 2.22   Means of Total Nursing-Care Hours by Different Classification Systems*†

	$\overline{X}$	SD	Min	Max	SEM	CV
Medicus	6.63	6.18	1.75	31.9	0.14	0.93
PRN	9.06	7.04	0	36.0	0.15	0.77
GRASP®	6.57	5.21	1.4	22.5	0.12	0.79

* Result of Paired *t*-tests:

PRN–Medicus	$t = 35.50$	$p = 0.0001$
Medicus-GRASP®	$t = 1.05$	$p = 0.30$
PRN–GRASP®	$t = 32.40$	$p = 0.0001$

† $N = 2002$

Source: L. O'Brien-Pallas, P. Leatt, R. Deber, and J. Till. "A Comparison of Workload Estimates Using Three Methods of Patient Classification." *Canadian Journal of Nursing Administration* (September-October 1989): 20. Reprinted with permission.

Summarizing the results of the study, it is clear that:

- Different PCSs generate different estimates of hours of care and related nursing workload.
- PRN predicts more hours of care than Medicus or GRASP®.
- The GRASP® PCS will estimate fewer hours of care than Medicus or PRN; therefore, it is the least costly of the three.
- The Medicus PCS will estimate fewer hours of care than the PRN, so is less costly than PRN. However, it is more costly than GRASP®.
- PRN has construct validity.[28]

In-House versus Purchased PCSs

Purchased PCSs are very expensive and must be modified for specific hospitals. An in-house PCS can be developed using work-analysis techniques. Methods for developing such systems are described in several references; most use observation or self-reporting techniques. In the latter personnel are trained to list activities they perform at timed intervals. Observation on a continuous or internal basis can be costly in time and money. Self-reporting is cheaper but employees must be trained.[29]

Alward states that it is more realistic to use the budget to determine staffing. She suggests selecting a prototype or factor-evaluation classification instrument and revising it to conform to the division's nursing practice.[30]

Nyberg and Wolff describe a PCS that calculates the total time, direct and indirect, needed to care for each patient by unit, shift, and job classification. The required time is compared with actual and budgeted nursing time per patient. This system has been used for several years and has been found to identify patient-care trends, improve efficiency of staffing, and justify budgeting changes. It is used for utilization review: it considers admitting and working diagnoses, surgical procedures, physician-consultants, patient classifications, and a list of all daily nursing activities. If hospitalization is not justified, a chart review is done. This computerized system determines nursing costs per patient by unit, Medicare patients and non-Medicare patients by diagnosis, and average and total costs of Medicare and non-Medicare patients. In one two-week period, Medicare patients required 10 percent more nursing

EXHIBIT 2.23   Means of Direct Nursing-Care Hours by Different Classification Systems*†

	X̄	SD	Min	Max	SEM	CV
Medicus	3.22	3.36	0.79	17.9	0.08	1.04
PRN	4.51	3.77	0	18.29	0.08	0.84
GRASP®	3.35	2.66	0	13.81	0.06	0.79

* Result of Paired *t*-tests:

PRN–Medicus	$t = 38.16$	$p < 0.0001$
Medicus-GRASP®	$t = -4.08$	$p < 0.0001$
PRN–GRASP®	$t = 32.14$	$p < 0.0001$

† $N = 2002$

Source: L. O'Brien-Pallas, P. Leatt, R. Deber, and J. Till. "A Comparison of Workload Estimates Using Three Methods of Patient Classification." *Canadian Journal of Nursing Administration* (September-October 1989): 21. Reprinted with permission.

resources per day and 40 percent more nursing time for their entire hospital-ization. If this finding holds true in other hospitals, nurse managers can use the data to petition for increased Medicare reimbursement.[31]

Microcomputer Models

Microcomputer models of PCSs exist. One of them, described by Grazman, has modules for planning nursing care and dealing with the budget. This system projects the number of hours of care, for each of four patient levels, that will meet budgetary and program delivery constraints of the staffing parameters. It is a staffing system that addresses the "demand" function based on planning, and the "management" function based on a blend of planning and actual situations. Thus, the input variables can be changed and the budget renegotiated. This model plans nursing time and resource allocation daily, based on patient case mix and census. It gives the head nurse control over resources.[32]

Adams and Duchene describe a PCS that includes nursing diagnosis with related etiology, nursing care goals, and potential patient outcomes. It is an in-house system, the advantages of which include

- knowledge of the data tool,
- capability of altering the system to accommodate changes in procedural time standards,
- ability to make changes in staffing levels, and
- ability to make percentage alterations of time given to indirect activities.

It produces a plan of care, with acuity as the basis of determining nurse staffing needs.[33]

Problems with PCSs

One of the major challenges of PCSs is to maintain reliability and validity. This can be done through continuing education and quality assurance (QA) checks. A calendar can be established to have external personnel (from staff development or another nursing department or unit) repeat the classification done by unit personnel (rater reliability). This can be done monthly or more often, depending on the results. Patients can be monitored on different days

and different shifts, with a stratified random sample of about 15 or 20 percent of the patient census. Simple percentage agreement of 90 percent or higher indicates satisfactory reliability. If agreement is below 80 percent, the system should be reviewed and adjusted.

A calendar can also be established to take a unit rotation work sample to determine whether procedures or tasks change with time and technology. This can be an annual spot check. Validating of PCSs varies. A questionnaire can be used to evaluate nursing staff's satisfaction with hours of care. Validity can also be tested using an expert panel of nurses. Patient-category descriptions or critical indicators of nursing intervention and patient requirement lists should be reviewed annually against standards. The PCSs must be altered if results of QA checks or work samples so indicate.

Orientation and continuing education are the best methods of assuring reliability and validity. The nursing staff must find the PCS credible. If they believe that the classifications are accurate and useful, they will try to rate patients accurately. They need periodic classes to update them and keep them well informed. Managers must support the use of a valid and reliable PCS; it indicates the institution's commitment to quality patient care.

Nursing should orient other department heads and physicians to the use of PCSs. Admissions and placements of patients are related to PCS outcomes.[34]

Practicing nurses want the PCS to prove the need for more staff. Managing nurses want it to validate staffing and scheduling, and to promote variable staffing. These objectives must be kept in harmony.

Modified Approaches to Nurse Staffing and Scheduling

Many approaches to nurse staffing and scheduling are being tried in an effort to satisfy the needs of employees and meet workload demands for patient care. These include game theory, modified workweeks (10- or 12-hour shifts), team rotation, "premium day" weekend nurse staffing, and "premium vacation" night staffing. Such approaches should support the underlying purpose, mission, philosophy, and objectives of the organization and the division of nursing, and should be well defined by staffing philosophy and policies. Nurses are like other workers in one respect: they would like to live as normal a home life as possible. But shifts have to be staffed and patient-care needs met. The successful nurse executive will try to accommodate both by using the best administrative staffing methodology available, considered from the economic or cost/benefit viewpoint.

Dissatisfaction with staffing and scheduling are reasons for turnover and poor retention. Understaffing has a negative effect on staff morale, delivery of quality care, and the nursing practice modality. It can close beds. It causes absenteeism as a result of staff fatigue, burnout, and professional dissatisfaction. On the other hand, nurse managers want to receive value for their money. There are economic constraints, which are further stretched by the costs of recruiting, hiring, and orienting new nurses and for overtime and temporary hires, when the environment creates turnovers and absenteeism. Overstaffing is expensive and also has a negative effect on staff morale and productivity. Staffing and

scheduling must balance the personal needs of nurses with the economic and productivity needs of the organization.[35]

Modified Workweeks

Modified workweek schedules using 10- and 12-hour shifts and other methods are commonplace, but a nurse administrator should be sure they fulfill the staffing philosophy and policies, particularly with regard to efficiency. Also, they should not be imposed upon the nursing staff, but should show a mutual benefit to employer, employee, and ultimately the clients served.

The 10-Hour Day

One modification of the workweek is four 10-hour shifts per week in organized time increments. A problem of this model is time overlaps of 6 hours per 24-hour day. The overlaps can be used for patient-centered conferences, nursing-care assessment and planning, and staff development. Also, the overlap can be scheduled to cover peak workload demands, which can be identified by observation, consensus, or self-recording by professional nurses. It can be done by hour or by a block of 3 to 4 hours. Starting and ending times for the 10-hour shifts can be modified to provide minimal overlaps, the 4-hour gap being staffed by part-time or temporary workers. The staffing board in Exhibit 2.13 can be used to solve these problems.

Longer workdays can decrease overtime because of overlapping shifts, and absenteeism and turnover are decreased because nurses have more days off. All of these factors decrease costs. However, such a system can increase staffing needs if mechanisms are not used to maintain productivity. Some organizations use a 7-days-on, 7-days-off schedule, but pay for the actual 70 hours worked during the 2-week period.[36]

The 4-day, 10-hour work schedule for night nurses was studied in a hospital that had difficulty recruiting qualified nurses to the night shift. It had been perceived that 10-hour shifts had stabilized staffing in the intensive care unit, with increased productivity and decreased turnover. Turnover on the night shift had been 70 percent for an 8-month period. Positions stayed vacant longer than for other shifts and sick time was higher, which increased recruitment and orientation time. Nurses were involved in planning the 4-day, 10- hour night-shift schedule. Night nurses agreed to use overlap hours to assist with day-shift care. The day shift agreed to reduce staff by one FTE. Plans were discussed with and accepted by the union. Making assignments of personnel and meeting schedules were addressed and resolved through participatory management.

The results included reduced sick time on the 10-hour shift, reduced turnover, increased incentive, increased requests for night shift, and decreased labor hours[37] (see Exhibit 2.24).

The 12-Hour Shift

A second scheduling modification is the 12-hour shift, according to which nurses work 7 shifts in a 2-week period: 3 on, 4 off; 4 on, 3 off. They work a total of 84 hours and are paid for 4 hours of overtime. Twelve-hour shifts and

EXHIBIT 2.24 A Graph Comparing Casual Absenteeism on One Unit with Different Schedules

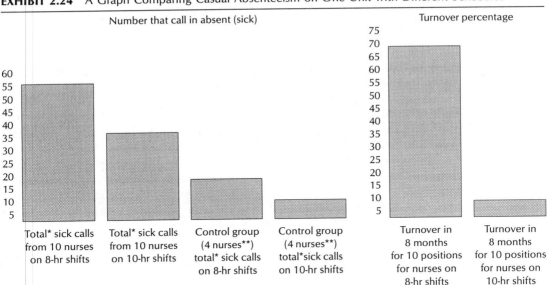

* 8-month period
** Same nurses

Source: J. A. Ricci. "10-Hour Night Shift: Cost vs Savings." *Nursing Management* (January 1984): 38. Reprinted with permission.

flexible staffing have been reported to have improved care and saved money because nurses can manage their personal lives better.[38]

Vik and MacKay report a study of the quality of care by nurses who worked 12-hour versus 8-hour shifts. It was a matched study of three units each. The Quality Patient-Care Scale was the measuring instrument. The "quality of care received by patients on the 8-hour shift units was significantly higher than that received by patients on the 12-hour shift units."[39] Shift patterns worked by nurses do affect the care received by patients. However, recruitment and retention of nurses can balance reduced quality of care when vacancies are high. This was a limited study and needs replication.

A research study was done to measure the effect on critical thinking of fatigue from 12-hour shifts. Researchers used the Industrial Fatigue Research Committee of the Japanese Association of Industrial Health checklist to test fatigue. They used the Three Minute Reasoning Test Based on Grammatical Transformation described by Baddeley to measure critical thinking. The sample included 94 Registered Nurses and 23 Licensed Practical Nurses (68 worked 8-hour shifts and 49 worked 12-hour shifts) in one hospital. The findings showed "no significant differences between levels of fatigue and critical thinking ability in nurses working 8- and 12-hour shifts."[40]

There is a break-even point for costs. It is the point at which decreased costs of recruiting, absenteeism, retention, and overtime equal the shift losses (4 hours/2 weeks) from 12-hour scheduling since no combination of 12-hour shifts adds up to 40 hours a week or 80 hours during 2 weeks.[41]

The Weekend Alternative

Another variation of flexible scheduling is the weekend alternative. Nurses work two 12-hour shifts (24 hours) and are paid for 40 hours plus benefits. They can use the weekdays for personal needs and pursuits such as going to school. There are several variations of the weekend schedule. Monday-through-Friday nurses have all weekends off.

Metcalf reports a test of the 12-hour weekend plan of two shifts on Saturday and Sunday, 7:00 A.M. to 7:00 P.M. and 7:00 P.M. to 7:00 A.M. The day shift was paid at the rate of 36 hours of pay for 24 hours worked. The night shift was paid at the rate of 40 hours of pay for 24 hours worked.

The sample included RNs, LPNs, and nurses' aides. Employed staff could volunteer for the shift and new staff were required to work it; this was not a weekends-only schedule. Full-time staff participating in it had two out of three weekends off. Results showed that only 3 percent of the total sample wanted the schedule discontinued, while 75 percent perceived weekend staffing as better.

Although illness and other absences increased by 19 percent, this negative finding was outweighed by positive ones. Recruiting improved, with vacancy rates dropping from 13 to 7 percent of budgeted positions. Use of agency personnel was cut in half and salary costs did not increase. Staffing and morale both improved. Problems were addressed to improve the plan.[42]

Other Modified Approaches

Team rotation is a method of cyclic staffing in which a nursing team is scheduled as a unit. It is used when the nursing modality is team practice.[43]

Premium-day weekend staffing is a scheduling pattern that gives a nurse an extra day off duty, called a *premium day*, if he or she volunteers to work one additional weekend within a 4-week scheduling block. This staffing technique could be modified to give the nurse a premium day off for every additional weekend worked beyond those required by nurse staffing policy. This technique does not add directly to hospital costs.[44]

Premium-vacation night staffing follows the same principle as premium-day weekend staffing. An example would be the policy of giving an extra 5 working days of vacation to every nurse who works a permanent night shift for a specific period of time—3 months, 4 months, or 6 months.

A study by Imig, Powell, and Thorman indicated that while flexible staffing filled vacant positions, it did not increase payroll costs, hours per patient day, or overtime, and it decreased absenteeism by 60 percent. The hospital in this study returned to 8-hour shifts because primary nursing was threatened. In this particular study there was *no change* in medication errors, patient and staff injuries, quality of care, complaints, recruitment, and staff attitudes from before to 6 months after flexible staffing. Also, use of agency nurses was not reduced.[45]

A Flexible Role: Resource Acuity Nurse

At West Virginia University Hospital, nurse executives established a resource acuity nurse position to provide greater flexibility and assure adequate staffing

during peak workload periods. The executives envisioned having nurses available to provide immediate relief to units whenever the greatest care needs arose. The resource acuity nurse would stay there for as long as needed.

The nurse managers developed guidelines for undertaking the resource acuity nurse responsibilities:

- assisting with such special procedures as central line placement and extensive dressing changes
- supporting nursing staff when many patients were returning from the operating room
- assisting in cardiac arrests or other emergency situations
- transferring unstable patients to the intensive care units

This program has enabled the hospital to better meet the staffing needs of units whenever workload increases. Since the position was established, nurses' morale has improved because short-term help is more readily available and is more equitably distributed among units.[46]

Flexible Hours

Other programs of flexible hours are used at

- *Metropolitan Life*, where 90 percent of 28,000 administrative employees can begin work between 7:30 A.M. and 10:00 A.M.;
- American Express's travel group, which has instituted job sharing, shorter workweeks, compressed workweeks, and telecommuting; and
- Federal Express's treasury and credit departments, where one-third of the employees work at home.

Clerical personnel tend to opt for working at home whereas professionals fear it will make their jobs less critical.[47]

Positive Aspects

Nurses of the 1990s want flexible scheduling to better accommodate their personal lives. Flexible time (frequently called *flextime*) schedules have become an increasingly important aspect of employment practices since 1980 when 11.9 percent of all nonfarm wage earners and salaried workers were reported to be on such schedules. They have resulted in improved attitudes and increased productivity as employees have gained more control over their work environments. Employees have been able to adjust to their own "bioclocks." Transportation has become more efficient and flexible. Employees have better control of work activities.[48]

A study that compared staggered work hours to fixed work hours done by the New York state government to control weaknesses of previous studies, showed that:

1. The greatest level of satisfaction and the least dissatisfaction with the workday was expressed by employees in agencies with the greatest flexibility in scheduling.
2. Employees in agencies with fixed schedules expressed the strongest dissatisfaction and lowest level of satisfaction.
3. Decreased commuting time may improve satisfaction with flextime.[49]

Flexible scheduling improves recruiting, reduces absenteeism, and increases retention. There are many flexible scheduling variations available. Before using them, nurse managers should establish philosophy and set objectives.

Negative Aspects

Among the disadvantages of 10- and 12-hour days are

- minimum weekend staffing (or excess staff on weekends)
- unsafe travel times
- shift overlaps that decrease total number of personnel on duty
- costs for overtime
- fatigue
- strain on family life
- increased staffing due to elimination of shifts, if the schedule is not carefully planned
- if required by state law overtime pay for hours worked in excess of 8 in a day and 40 in a week
- less continuity of care
- less communication among staff
- developing, maintaining, and explaining the master schedule
- modification of primary assessing[50]

Working night shifts, split shifts, or extended shifts may create problems, including sleeping on the job, conflicts with family members on other shifts, muddy thinking, and poor memory. Experts suggest the following ways to handle late or rotating shifts:

- If possible, consistently work one shift all the time.
- If the latter is not possible, rotate shifts clockwise, one shift for a week, with 48 hours between changing shifts.
- Avoid caffeine, alcohol, nicotine, or other sleep-disturbing chemicals for several hours before bedtime. Follow the workday routine on days off, insofar as possible.
- Prepare for a new shift by splitting time between sleep and wakefulness.[51]

Cross-Training

Cross-training of nursing personnel can improve flexible scheduling. Nurses need to be prepared to function effectively in more than one area of expertise. They can be kept in similar clinical specialties or families of clinical specialties. Cross-training requires complete orientation and ongoing staff development to prevent errors and increase job satisfaction, and should be done both for unit-assigned nurses and pool nurses. There should be policies, job descriptions, and performance evaluations. Pools can be in-house, or in supplemental staffing agencies that provide full-time and part-time nurses. Benefits can be prorated or employees can choose increased pay instead of benefits.

Temporary Workers

Nurses have been doing temporary work for two decades or more. They went to staffing agencies because they wanted control over their lives, personal and professional. It was the only way they could get such control until nurse managers

and hospital administrators realized the need to apply the science of behavioral technology, including human resource management, to nursing.

Many organizations are downsizing to make themselves more productive by decreasing overhead costs. One result of downsizing is the use of contract or external workers. Kanter reports the following about temporary workers:

1. The number of people employed by temporary agencies in the United States as a whole rose from 400,000 to 804,000 between 1982 and 1986. Although not all of them worked for temporary agencies, 4,625,000 persons worked part time in 1994 for economic reasons. Another 26,226,000 worked part time for noneconomic reasons.

2. According to Bureau of Labor Statistics data, "the number of American workers whose primary income was earned in temporary jobs rose from 471,800 to 835,000 from 1983 to 1986."

3. More than 50 percent of new jobs created between 1980 and 1989 went to contingent workers.

4. "By the year 2000, the Bureau of Labor Statistics indicates, about 80 percent of jobs will be in the service sector that uses 75 percent of temporary employees."

5. Temporary agencies have become big corporations. Norrell Corporation had 310 offices with $308.5 million in sales in 1987—and 130,000 "employees."

6. Demand for professional knowledge and services is being handled by temporary services.

7. The corporate ladder is collapsing from the weight of middle management, hence middle management is being eliminated.

8. Success in a career comes with a reputation of completing projects successfully. The professional must have value in the job marketplace.

9. Downsizing, combined with a trend toward a contract labor force, have been responsible for 6 million Americans experiencing downward mobility between 1981 and 1986.[52]

The lesson for nursing personnel is to gain a reputation for competence in more than one clinical area or in more than one of the areas of clinical practice, teaching, research, and management.

Some analysts predict that by the year 2000, one-half of working Americans, some 60 million people, will have joined the ranks of freelance providers of skills and services. By 1994, 21 million Americans worked part time; 6.4 million of them would rather have had full-time jobs.

Part-timers fill slots at every level of the organization. Twenty percent of 18 million jobs created since 1983 are part-time. A disposable work force that is not empowered may not be motivated, creative, or independent.[53]

Workforces in today's organizations are leaner and meaner. Temporary employees include engineers, chemists, and systems analysts. Of 75,000 temporaries working for Uniforce Temporary Services, one-third have elected to

make a career of it. They like to try out new companies and new locations. Many temporaries do so because of conflicts between work and personal life. This has been true of nurses for many years.

Trial work periods are more effective for hiring the right person than are job interviews. A trial work period allows both employer and employee to decide whether to make it permanent. Temporary employees prevent hiring mistakes by employers and employees. A negative aspect is that few fringe benefits are provided.

Potential temporaries should become informed about the temporary agency by asking others who have used it, screening the agency by telephone for customer treatment, visiting the agency on a busy Monday morning, and then interviewing with an agency's hiring official.[54]

Strategic Staffing

Accounting firms have developed a concept of strategic staffing as an approach to downsizing. Strategic staffing analyzes a unit's staffing needs, based on long-term objectives for the unit and the organization, to find a combination of permanent and temporary employees with the best skills to meet these needs. Temporary staffing may protect the jobs of permanent or core employees when the temporary employee covers a vacancy while the position or job is analyzed.

Temporary employees may want to sample the work. A variety of professional occupations are represented in the temporary workforce. Temporary workers provide relief for overworked permanent employees; many do one-time projects, including internal audits and forensic accounting. They work as trainers of permanent employees. Using temporary employees controls personnel expenses such as benefits, rehiring, and training.

To make strategic staffing work, managers should study staffing annually, looking at workload peaks and values, the financial blueprint, and communicating with providers and the staff.

The warning signs that strategic staffing is required include excessive overtime, high turnover, excessive absenteeism, and employees whose skills do not match job requirements, absence of regular staffing planning, missed deadlines, last-minute staffing with temporary employees, absence of a budget line for temporary employees, absence of communication with the human resource department, and low employee morale. To get the best temporary workers may require consultation with specialized temporary firms.[55]

Temporary workers are cost effective for small businesses because they eliminate the expense of a human relations department. For large businesses they are cost effective for the flexibility attendant with seasonal and short-term work. Also, it enables employers to evaluate employees for permanent jobs.[56]

Transfer Fair

One hospital held a "transfer fair" to place staff quickly and fairly when downsizing. The key participants were

- managers with vacancies,
- recruitment staff with a list of vacancies,

- employee relations staff to answer personnel policy questions, and
- staff affected by downsizing.

Each affected staff member made three choices. Seniority then determined placement, with decisions being made in 48 to 72 hours.

The atmosphere and tone of a transfer fair is gracious, welcoming, professional, relaxed, and supportive. Planners prepare well and make the fair convenient for all shifts. Refreshments are served and top nursing administrators attend.[57]

Scheduling with Nursing Management Information Systems

The duty schedule does not always match personnel with preferences. This is one major dissatisfaction among clinical nurses. Their satisfaction can be improved by posting the number of nurses needed by time slots and allowing them to select their own time slots. The staffing board shown in Exhibit 2.13 can be used.

Staffing is a major reason for having an NMIS. A microcomputer can be used for a cyclical schedule as well as single rotation to show: number of nurses required, by time slots; restrictions; off-duty policy; and paired days-off.[58]

Hanson defines a management information system (MIS) as "an array of components designed to transform a collective set of data into knowledge that is directly useful and applicable in the process of directing and controlling resources and their application to the achievement of specific objectives."[59]

Information stimulates action through management decision making. Data do not; they must be processed to be useful. Information must be timely to be useful. The process for establishing an MIS is:

1. State the management objective clearly.
2. Identify the actions required to meet the objective.
3. Identify the responsible position in the organization.
4. Identify the information required to meet the objective.
5. Determine the data required to produce the needed information.
6. Determine the system's requirement for processing the data.
7. Develop a flowchart.[60]

Refer to chapter 4, Computers, Information Systems, and Nursing Management, for a more detailed discussion.

Productivity

Productivity is commonly defined as outputs divided by inputs. Hanson translates this definition into:

$$\frac{\text{Required staff hours}}{\text{Provided staff hours}} \times 100 = \text{productivity}$$

To illustrate,

$$\frac{380.50 \text{ required staff hours}}{402.00 \text{ provided staff hours}} \times 100 = 94.7 \text{ percent productivity}$$

Productivity can be increased by decreasing the provided staff hours while holding the required staff hours constant or by increasing required staff hours. This data becomes information when related to an objective that allows for some variances.[61] Because resources for health care are limited, the nurse manager is faced with the task of motivating clinical nurses to increase productivity.

Productivity in nursing is related both to how efficiently clinical nurses deliver nursing care and to how effective that care is relative to its quality and appropriateness. Brown indicates that productivity in the United States has declined. He cites, as evidence of this claim, increased labor costs without corresponding increases in performance. This is due to such factors as inexperienced workers, technological slowdown due to outdated equipment and reduced amounts of research and development, government regulations, a diminished work ethic, increased size and bureaucracy in business and industry, and erosion of the managerial ethic.[62]

Measuring Productivity

In developing a model for an MIS, Hanson indicates several formulas for translating data into information. In addition to the productivity formula, he indicates that hours per patient day (HPPD) is another data element that is meaningful when information is available for an extended period of time. HPPD is determined by the formula

$$\frac{\text{Staff hours}}{\text{Patient days}} = \text{HPPD}$$

For example,

$$\frac{52,000 \text{ staff hours}}{2883.5 \text{ patient days}} = 18.03 \text{ HPPD}$$

Staff hours are calculated as

52,000 staff hours = 25 FTEs × 2080 work hours per year

Patient days are based on the following:

2883.5 patient days = 7.9 average daily census (ADC) × 365

No allowance is made for personal time such as coffee breaks, meals, vacations, holidays, sick time, or decreased census time. The figure of 18.03 HPPD may be a high value even for intensive care.

Another useful formula is

$$\frac{\text{Provided HPPD}}{\text{Budgeted HPPD}} \times 100 = \text{budget utilization}$$

or,

$$\frac{18.03 \text{ provided HPPD}}{16.0 \text{ budgeted HPPD}} \times 100 = 112.7 \text{ percent budget utilization}$$

This would be over budget if the provided hours had been net of personal time. Since they were not, the HPPD provided may be highly productive. The adequacy of the budget is determined by the following formula:

$$\frac{\text{Budgeted HPPD}}{\text{Required HPPD}} \times 100 = \text{budget adequacy}$$

or,

$$\frac{16.0 \text{ budgeted HPPD}}{18.03 \text{ required HPPD}} \times 100 = 88.74 \text{ percent budget adequacy}$$

Obviously, if the required HPPD is equal to the provided HPPD and exceeds the budgeted HPPD, productivity is artificially high because of the inadequate budget.[63] Staffing should be defined in terms of the HPPD goals, which should be related to productivity, budget utilization, and budget adequacy. Whether it is effective depends on measurement of quality of outcomes.

Artinian, O'Connor, and Brock measured nursing productivity by using the number of physicians' orders written during a specific period as an estimate of nursing services provided for a particular patient. They counted the number of patient contacts generated by each physician order and separated them for licensed and unlicensed nursing personnel. Nurses were asked to summarize and enumerate changes in nursing care during the preceding 5 years, and the changes related to physicians' orders were selected. They did not measure independent nursing functions or indirect care, assuming the latter to be similar to direct care. A pilot study to show whether the sickest patients generated the most nursing contacts indicated these results:

1. Three *not* acutely ill patients had 59.5 licensed nurse contacts and 47.5 non-licensed nurse contacts in 5 days.
2. Three acutely ill patients had 302.7 licensed nurse contacts and 58.3 non-licensed nurse contacts in 5 days.
3. There was a 103 percent increase in licensed nurse-patient contact from 1975-1976 to 1981-1982. This was statistically significant. It converted to a 27 percent increase in the nursing productivity index.[64]

One could conclude that the more acutely ill patients are, the more licensed nurse contacts they require.

Davis indicates that productivity in nursing is the volume and quality of products divided by the cost of producing and delivering them. It is directly related to what nurses do and how they do it. Systems have been developed to determine nursing cost per patient per shift. For example, at University Hospitals of Cleveland, the following formula is used:

Nurse competence rank × hourly salary × required nursing hours × care acuity = the nursing cost per patient

For example,

Clinician III × $17.50 × 3 hours × 5 = $787.50 per shift.[65]

Smith, Mackey, and Markham developed a productivity monitoring system for the recovery room. The performance ratio was the required FTEs divided by

worked FTEs. The data were used to decide whether to fill vacant positions and to develop a budget.[66]

Mailhot reported an analysis of problems in an operating room: poor physical environment, inadequate financial support, poor systems, and low morale. The department was overstaffed by 10 FTEs. Task forces brainstormed and held open forums to solve the problems. They used Lewin's force field analysis, putting complex alternatives through an outcome matrix, developing evaluation tools, and using pilot projects to test all changes. They made 87 changes in 1 year (see Exhibit 2.25).

In addition they marketed services to patients and surgeons, provided management training for operating room managers, analyzed operating room procedures, and once every 6 weeks held an "open day" during which each staff person could see the director. They reduced the staffing by 38 FTE positions and the budget by $1.5 million in 3 years. Job satisfaction surveys indicated improvement.[67]

Because high input for low output produces low productivity and high output for low input produces high productivity, the objective of a nursing model of productivity is low input for high output.

The first step in improving productivity is to study or measure it as it exists. At one hospital the personnel of the education department decided to improve their productivity. They considered a time-based method versus a value-based method to develop a productivity system.

A time-based method of productivity considers the length of time it takes to do each task. The steps of a time-based method are to review the literature, do a time study, and then compare the results with the literature. This is done for activities unique to the unit. Units are then assigned to each activity according to the estimated time for completing it. The time-based method does not give priority to activities.

A value-based system considers the value of activities to the institution. Steps for developing a value-based system of productivity include listing activities, grouping them by their value to the institution, and assigning units of productivity. The human resources department should be involved in developing a productivity system.

Exhibits 2.26 and 2.27 demonstrate tools for collecting data for a value-based productivity system used by the McKay-Dee education department at McKay-Dee Hospital Center, Ogden, Utah.[68]

Differences among Productivity Models

Producers of services do not fit the same productivity models as do producers of material goods. There is marked discretion in determining both expected and actual roles of nurses who do not produce physical outputs. This is one reason that such nursing prescriptions as "emotional support" are difficult to measure. Patient outputs or outcomes can be measured by client satisfaction as well as by client condition on discharge. There has been greater emphasis on nursing process than on nursing outcome. Haas defines *efficiency* as "the proportion between personnel assigned and time spent to materials expended, as well as to capital and management employed, for the greatest economy in use." Productive nurses must balance their personal energies and their institution's resources with their effectiveness.[69]

EXHIBIT 2.25 Examples of Major Operating Room Department Changes

Renovation	Restructuring of Department	Communication	Systems	Strategic Plan
Instrument room	Reorganized man- agement team	Nurse-physician committee	Materials manage- ment (established 5–7 day inventory)	Attained voting privileges on OR medical committee
Lounge locker room	Implemented RN specialization	OR delay reporting form	Equipment preven- tive maintenance program	Reallocated block time
Office space	Developed clinical ladder for RNs	Housewide staff exchange program	Established consign- ment program	Developed satellite ORs for same-day surgery
Fail-safe electrical project	Reclassified eight positions	Provide internal/ external consulta- tion	Held vendor fairs	Developed 5-year goals
Storage area	Revised job descrip- tions for all staff	Publish in OR and general nursing journals	Resolved phantom scheduling	Developed PERT chart for 1½-year master plan
Hospital modern- ization plan	Redesigned staff nurse orientation	Staff development programs	OR computer scheduling	Marketed new procedures/ equipment
	Developed and implemented management education series	Sought and attained medical director	Computerized utili- zation statistics program	Attained treatment room
	Assessed and modified all policies and procedures	Brought perfusion- ists under OR management	Computerized room- delay program	Established health fairs
	Hired staff specialists	Developed patient teaching tools	Restructured pricing	Initiated annual department/get- together
	Evaluated and purchased new scrubs	Developed staff teaching tools	Modified billing process	
	Initiated "open door" policy	Developed audio- visual modules for basic programs	Color-coded scrub clothes	
	Implemented director's "open days" with staff every 6 weeks	Initiated monthly meetings with staff and assistant head nurses	Established cost- containment committee	
	Supported 11 managers in their return to school		Established quality assurance committee	
	Initiated written commendations		Developed FTE con- trol mechanism	
			Restructured for DRGs	
			Developed equip- ment education plan	
			Began instrument repair/replace- ment program	
			Initiated environ- ment rounds	

Source: C. B. Mailhot. "Setting OR's Course Toward Greater Productivity." *Nursing Management,* October 1985. Reprinted with permission of Springhouse Corporation.

Curtin indicates that productivity in nursing is related to the application of knowledge. Professional productivity must be measured by means of efficacy, effectiveness, and efficiency in applying knowledge. She indicates objective measurements of these processes:

1. *Objective measures of efficacy*: years of formal education, levels of academic achievement, evidence of continuing education and skill development, and years of experience

EXHIBIT 2.26   Value-Based Productivity Form

NAME										DATE										
	SUNDAY			MONDAY			TUESDAY			WEDNESDAY			THURSDAY			FRIDAY			SATURDAY		
REQUIRED CLASSES	HRS	UNITS	#PRT	HRS	UNITS	#PRT	HRS	UNITS	#PRT	HRS	UNITS	#PRT	HRS	UNITS	#PRT	HRS	UNITS	#PRT	HRS	UNITS	#PRT
4 units x Hrs	♦♦♦	♦♦♦♦♦	♦♦♦♦	♦♦♦	♦♦♦♦♦	♦♦♦♦	♦♦♦	♦♦♦♦♦	♦♦♦♦	♦♦♦	♦♦♦♦♦	♦♦♦♦	♦♦♦	♦♦♦♦♦	♦♦♦♦	♦♦♦	♦♦♦♦♦	♦♦♦♦	♦♦♦	♦♦♦♦♦	♦♦♦♦
3 units x Hrs <5 part	♦♦♦	♦♦♦♦♦	♦♦♦♦	♦♦♦	♦♦♦♦♦	♦♦♦♦	♦♦♦	♦♦♦♦♦	♦♦♦♦	♦♦♦	♦♦♦♦♦	♦♦♦♦	♦♦♦	♦♦♦♦♦	♦♦♦♦	♦♦♦	♦♦♦♦♦	♦♦♦♦	♦♦♦	♦♦♦♦♦	♦♦♦♦
Orientation																					
Fire, Safety, Disaster																					
Hazardous Material																					
Infection Control																					
AIDS																					
NECESSARY TO FUNCTION	♦♦♦	♦♦♦♦♦	♦♦♦♦	♦♦♦	♦♦♦♦♦	♦♦♦♦	♦♦♦	♦♦♦♦♦	♦♦♦♦	♦♦♦	♦♦♦♦♦	♦♦♦♦	♦♦♦	♦♦♦♦♦	♦♦♦♦	♦♦♦	♦♦♦♦♦	♦♦♦♦	♦♦♦	♦♦♦♦♦	♦♦♦♦
4 units x Hrs	♦♦♦	♦♦♦♦♦	♦♦♦♦	♦♦♦	♦♦♦♦♦	♦♦♦♦	♦♦♦	♦♦♦♦♦	♦♦♦♦	♦♦♦	♦♦♦♦♦	♦♦♦♦	♦♦♦	♦♦♦♦♦	♦♦♦♦	♦♦♦	♦♦♦♦♦	♦♦♦♦	♦♦♦	♦♦♦♦♦	♦♦♦♦
3 units x Hrs <5 Part	♦♦♦	♦♦♦♦♦	♦♦♦♦	♦♦♦	♦♦♦♦♦	♦♦♦♦	♦♦♦	♦♦♦♦♦	♦♦♦♦	♦♦♦	♦♦♦♦♦	♦♦♦♦	♦♦♦	♦♦♦♦♦	♦♦♦♦	♦♦♦	♦♦♦♦♦	♦♦♦♦	♦♦♦	♦♦♦♦♦	♦♦♦♦
+2 units per Station	♦♦♦	♦♦♦♦♦	♦♦♦♦	♦♦♦	♦♦♦♦♦	♦♦♦♦	♦♦♦	♦♦♦♦♦	♦♦♦♦	♦♦♦	♦♦♦♦♦	♦♦♦♦	♦♦♦	♦♦♦♦♦	♦♦♦♦	♦♦♦	♦♦♦♦♦	♦♦♦♦	♦♦♦	♦♦♦♦♦	♦♦♦♦
ACLS																					
EKG																					
Critical Care																					
CPR Lecture																					
Computer																					
Management																					
Glucoscan																					
CEU .5 extra unit x Hrs																					
CPR CHECK OFF 2 units x Hrs																					
UPDATE CLASSES 3 units x Hrs 2 units x Hrs <5 Part																					
Departments																					
Clinical Instruction (one-to-one) 2 units X Hrs																					
Skill Lab 3 units x Hrs plus 2 units per station	♦♦♦	♦♦♦♦♦	♦♦♦♦	♦♦♦	♦♦♦♦♦	♦♦♦♦	♦♦♦	♦♦♦♦♦	♦♦♦♦	♦♦♦	♦♦♦♦♦	♦♦♦♦	♦♦♦	♦♦♦♦♦	♦♦♦♦	♦♦♦	♦♦♦♦♦	♦♦♦♦	♦♦♦	♦♦♦♦♦	♦♦♦♦
PROJECTS High value 2 units x Hrs		♦♦♦♦			♦♦♦♦			♦♦♦♦			♦♦♦♦			♦♦♦♦			♦♦♦♦			♦♦♦♦	
Lower value 1 unit x Hrs		♦♦♦♦			♦♦♦♦			♦♦♦♦			♦♦♦♦			♦♦♦♦			♦♦♦♦			♦♦♦♦	
COMMITTEES Meeting (1 unit x Hrs)		♦♦♦♦			♦♦♦♦			♦♦♦♦			♦♦♦♦			♦♦♦♦			♦♦♦♦			♦♦♦♦	
Work (2 units x Hrs)		♦♦♦♦			♦♦♦♦			♦♦♦♦			♦♦♦♦			♦♦♦♦			♦♦♦♦			♦♦♦♦	
ROUNDS (1 unit x Hrs)		♦♦♦♦			♦♦♦♦			♦♦♦♦			♦♦♦♦			♦♦♦♦			♦♦♦♦			♦♦♦♦	
PT/COMMUNITY EDUC. 4 units x Hrs 3 units x Hrs <5 Part																					
Units	♦♦♦		♦♦♦♦	♦♦♦		♦♦♦♦	♦♦♦		♦♦♦♦	♦♦♦		♦♦♦♦	♦♦♦		♦♦♦♦	♦♦♦		♦♦♦♦	♦♦♦		♦♦♦♦
PARTICIPANTS	♦♦♦	♦♦♦♦		♦♦♦	♦♦♦♦		♦♦♦	♦♦♦♦		♦♦♦	♦♦♦♦		♦♦♦	♦♦♦♦		♦♦♦	♦♦♦♦		♦♦♦	♦♦♦♦	
PARTICIPANT HOURS	♦♦♦	♦♦♦♦		♦♦♦	♦♦♦♦		♦♦♦	♦♦♦♦		♦♦♦	♦♦♦♦		♦♦♦	♦♦♦♦		♦♦♦	♦♦♦♦		♦♦♦	♦♦♦♦	

COMMENTS

GRAND TOTAL

UNITS _____

NO. OF PARTS _____

PART. HRS _____

*PRODUCTIVITY % _____

HOURS   APL   VAC   HOLIDAY   *Average is based on a 40-hr week; divide hours worked into value productivity to determine percent

Source: C. R. Waterstadt and T. L. Phillips. "A Productivity System for a Hospital Education Department." *Journal of Nursing Staff Development* (May/June 1990): 142. Reprinted with permission.

2. *Objective measures of effectiveness*: demonstrated ability to execute job-related procedures, correctly prioritized activities, performance according to professional and legal standards, appropriate information clearly and concisely recorded, and cooperative working with others

3. *Objective measures of efficiency*: promptitude, attendance, reliability, precision, adaptability, and economical disposition of resources[70]

EXHIBIT 2.27   Value-Based Productivity Form

Date	Class Title	Speaker	Hours Taught	No. of Participants	Value of Class	Cost to Participants
	Childbirth					
	Refreseher					
	Early Bird					
	C-Section					
	Repeat Childbirth					
	Children's Workshop					
	Diabetic Series					
	Coronary Artery Disease					
		Professional Community				
	Diabetic Workshop					
	Collaborative Nursing Practice					
	Medical Terminology					

Date	Patient's Name	Hours	No. of Partic.	Patient Education Cost

Source: C. R. Waterstadt and T. L. Phillips. "A Productivity System for a Hospital Education Department." *Journal of Nursing Staff Development* (May-June 1990): 143. Reprinted with permission.

Curtin and Zurlage acknowledge that human services such as nursing are difficult to test, return, or exchange if unsatisfactory. They propose a system for measuring nursing productivity that includes a nursing productivity ratio relating nursing productivity to hospital revenue, and a nursing productivity index.[71]

A nursing intensity index has been developed and tested in all departments at Johns Hopkins Hospital. First, a pilot study was done in which records of eight major services were examined. These records were scored by three raters, who reached an average agreement that varied from 82 to 95 percent. After modifications were made as a result of the pilot study, a full study was done using 784 records, each scored by two nurses. The results were as follows:

1. Nursing intensity levels varied widely within every clinical department and nursing unit.
2. The full study sample included 239 diagnostic-related groups. Of these, 64% consisted of only one level of nursing intensity, 31% contained two levels of nursing intensity, 4% contained three levels of nursing intensity, and 1% contained four levels of nursing intensity.
3. A weighted average coefficient of variation for total charges across all clinical departments was computed.
4. Average rating agreement across all clinical departments was 84%.
5. The nursing intensity index is both a valid and reliable instrument for patient classification.
6. The nursing intensity index correlates strongly (.61) with the severity of illness index.
7. It can be used to systematize cost allocation for nursing and do variable billing, establish sound nurse staffing systems, monitor quality of patient-care delivery, trace patient population trends, and do case mix analysis.[72]

Improving Nursing Productivity

Nursing productivity is being improved and the reported knowledge and skills are adding to the theory of nursing management. Rabin indicates that professionals can impose productivity values upon themselves. Managers should develop managerial goals and values toward a standard of performance for themselves. Professionals can commit themselves to fostering innovative attitudes and technologies, stimulating performance by commitment to constructive action and follow-ups, living up to standards of practice, keeping up to date, and being receptive to public review. Almost any profession can develop measurable standards of performance and productivity.[73]

Employers should measure nursing output objectively and pay for it accordingly in salary, benefits, and promotions. There has been some progress in nursing in the form of standards of practice, clinical ladders, and models of peer review. These gains need to be supported in the workplace, along with respect for the individual dignity of nurses, support for their personal commitment to professional goals, and support for the integrity of their professional judgments.[74]

Productivity can be managed and improved by

1. Planning that increases the variations between inputs and outputs:
   1.1 Increasing output and decreasing input
   1.2 Increasing output with input remaining constant
   1.3 Increasing output faster than input
   1.4 Having output remain constant with input decreasing
   1.5 Having output decrease more slowly than input
2. Soliciting staff's ideas and recommendations
3. Creating challenges
4. Managers showing interest in staff's achievement and concerns
5. Praising and rewarding good performances
6. Involving staff
7. Having a meaningful set or family of outcome measures for which data are available or easy to gather and over which workers have some control, and which are easily understood

8. Selecting measures compatible with white-collar functions and corporate measures
9. Monitoring workload changes in staffing requirements against established standards
10. Combining support of employees with understanding, motivation, and recognition
11. Increasing ratio of professional to nonprofessional staff
12. Placing admitted patients based on resource availability
13. Improving skill, energy, and motivation through staff development, books, tuition reimbursement, paid meals, yoga lessons, bonuses, vacation days, and other incentives
14. Implementing work simplification, work-flow analysis, and other approaches
15. Making an organizational diagnosis of problems, resources, and realities
16. Setting the climate for productivity by asking nurses what makes them productive and then implementing their suggestions (Measure before and after suggestions are put into effect.)
17. Decreasing waiting and stand-by time, and excessive coffee klatches, social breaks, and meal times
18. Stimulating nurse managers and clinical nurses to want to achieve excellence
19. Setting targets for increasing output on an annual basis without additional capital or employees
20. Having personnel keep and analyze time diaries to determine personal improvement actions
21. Setting personal objectives and measuring performance against them
22. Making a commitment to improved productivity, effectiveness (doing the right things), and efficiency (doing things right)
23. Seeking new products and services and new methods and ways of producing them
24. Seeking new and useful approaches to old problems
25. Improving quality of nursing products, emphasizing such ideas as consistency, longevity, riskiness, perfectibility, and value
26. Maintaining concern with the process and method of producing nursing care
27. Improving use of time
28. Reducing the cost of what nurses do by returning unused budgeted funds
29. Improving esthetics—the quality of work life and the pleasantness and beauty of the environment
30. Applying the ethical policy statements of professional nursing organizations
31. Gaining the confidence of peers
32. Recognizing the need to do better[75]

Personnel working in service areas can improve productivity by

1. Focusing on organizational strategy, customer service, mission, and results rather than methodology
2. Using self-directed work teams to break jobs into observable tasks and responsibilities (e.g., step-to-step, person-to-person, machine-to-person, unit-to-client or division and then to organization)
3. Observing, and then making changes or providing training to correct deficiencies
4. Watching for problems such as repetition, duplication, recurring delays, and waste of resources
5. Observing the outcome of a person's work by splitting the job into four main areas—managing self, managing resources, activities, and working with

others—and noting skills such as analytical thinking, ability to learn, adaptability, positive self-image, emphasis on results, time management, concern for standards, knowing how to influence others, and independence

6. Providing feedback that is specific, constructive, and frequent[76]

Case Study

At the Presbyterian Hospital of Dallas, a study revealed that more time was spent on clerical functions, telephone calls, and reporting patient conditions to other caregivers than on direct patient care. Actions were taken to change this and improved productivity greatly:

- A FAX machine network was instituted between nursing units and pharmacy, which reduced telephone calls and medication errors.
- A keyless narcotics system that included a personnel pass code was installed. The main control system was in pharmacy, but nurses could enter their personal pass codes at the narcotics cabinet. This reduced time wasted in searching for keys and produced an audit trail.
- A unit beeper system with eight beepers was purchased at a local store for $375. Beepers given to every staff member at the beginning of each shift made nursing assistants feel valued.[77]

Nursing Consumer Price Index

One good system for estimating future budgetary costs is to establish a consumer price index (CPI) for a nursing bread basket. This technique was presented at a Management Effectiveness Workshop for Nursing Service Facilitators by the American Nurses' Association.[78] The formula establishing the nursing CPI is

$$\text{Price index} = \frac{\Sigma\ (Pn \times Qo)}{\Sigma\ (Po \times Qo)} \times 100$$

Σ = sum of
Po = the price of a unit of the item in an initial period
Qo = the quantity or number of units of the item
Pn = the price of a unit of the item in any subsequent period

Example: Year 0

Item	Po	Qo	(Po × Qo)
RN	$4050/month	3	$ 12150
RN	$3125/month	2	$ 6250
RN	$2950/month	7	$ 20650
LPN	$1535/month	1	$ 1535
LPN	$1595/month	2	$ 3190
LPN	$1615/month	3	$ 4845
Nur. Asst.	$1210/month	6	$ 7260
Ward Clerk	$1000/month	1	$ 1000
			$ 56,880

The nursing CPI for the base period would be valued at 100. The nurse administrator or manager would include all items for the nursing CPI such as supplies and equipment, overtime, and fringe benefits. She or he would establish a period of time for pricing the items each year so as to use accurate data for budgeting purposes. This could be done by the calendar year if the budget is prepared for a fiscal year. After one year the items are again priced.

Example: Year 1

Item	P1	Qo	(P1 × Qo)
RN	$4150/month	3	$ 12450
RN	$3225/month	2	$ 6450
RN	$3050/month	7	$ 21350
LPN	$1585/month	1	$ 1585
LPN	$1645/month	2	$ 3290
LPN	$1665/month	3	$ 4995
Nur. Asst.	$1250/month	6	$ 7500
Ward Clerk	$1050/month	1	$ 1050
			$58,670

The market basket value of year 2 is divided by the market basket value of year 1:

$$\text{Nursing CPI2} = \frac{58,670.00}{56,880.00} \times 100 = 103.1$$

Year	NCPI Value
0	100
1	103

Salaries rose 3.1 percent between the base year (year 0) and the end of the first year (year 1). Using this system, nurse administrators can accurately predict budget requirements. If the CPI is computed monthly, the results can be compared with the same months of the preceding years. The objective is to establish an accurate picture of cost increases rather than guessing and thereby further inflating them.

Summary

Staffing and scheduling are major components of nursing management and are primary to the process of budgeting nursing personnel. Traditional patterns have been slavishly adhered to until recent years. A nursing division needs a practical and written philosophy that guides all staffing and scheduling activities and that is acceptable to the staff.

Studies can be used to determine staffing needs related to personnel skills, numbers of personnel, and time/workload requirements. Staffing can be planned by using computer models that calculate workload requirements from patient classification data or patient classification systems (PCSs). There are many modified approaches to nurse staffing and scheduling, including game theory, modified workweeks, team rotation, permanent shifts, and permanent weekends. Although some consultants advise against mixing modified workweeks, in practice they are frequently mixed.

Productivity, the unit of output of nursing, is a focus of increasing interest to nurse managers. It must include quality indicators of care that can be observed and measured. Productivity is commonly defined as the outputs of production divided by the inputs of production. Further research needs to be undertaken to determine the key to increased productivity by professional nurses. Is it money or some other aspect of job satisfaction? One theory is that a combination of work, environment, and rewards will maintain or increase productivity.

Experiential Exercises

1. (A) Based on the information below, use Exhibit 2.12, Formula for Estimating a Core Staff per Shift, to do the following exercise:
   - The average daily census (ADC) of a unit is 29 patients.
   - The basic average daily hours of care to be provided are 6 hours per patient per 24 hours.
   - The workday is 8 hours.
   (B) Determine the following:
   - The total hours of care needed on the average day to meet these standards.
   - The number of FTEs needed to staff the unit for 24 hours.
   - The number of 8-hour shifts needed per week.
   - The number of FTEs needed as basic staff for this unit.
   (C) Using the 12 Salt Lake City Community hospital's recommendations of staff mix, determine the mix of RNs to LPNs to aides.
   (D) Using Warsler's proportion for staffing shifts, determine the number of FTEs for days, evenings, and nights.
   (E) Make a table for basic staffing for this unit. Do not add complementary staff unless you give a rationale for it. Rationale may include allowances for vacations, holidays, sick leave, and other absences.
2. *Group Exercise*
   (A) Form groups of five to eight persons. This can be your permanent seminar group. You may want to consult a larger representative group of nursing personnel to gain their insights and ideas and to incorporate their beliefs and values into the staffing philosophy.
   (B) Elect a leader to move the group to completion.
   (C) Elect a recorder to write a record of the group's accomplishments.
   (D) Prepare to write a staffing philosophy. It should represent the beliefs of professional nurses about staffing and scheduling. Refer to an organization's mission, philosophy, vision and values, and objective statements.
   - List key words or statements that you believe should be addressed in a staffing philosophy.
   - Prepare an outline.
   - Write the staffing philosophy.

Remember that a hospital or other health-care institution exists to provide health care to people—to patients or clients. Also, an institution has to make a profit to stay in business. This applies as well to a not-for-profit institution, where any "profits" go to improving the facility and its human and material resources. Patients must be cared for 24 hours a day by nurses satisfied with their conditions of work. Prepare a rationale for your final document.

3. (A) Evaluate the staffing policies for the following areas of a health-care institution and state whether they need changing. If so, why?

vacations	use of "float" personnel
holidays	exchangeability of staff
sick leave	use of special abilities of individ-
weekends off	ual staff members
consecutive days off	exchanging hours
rotation to different shifts	requests of personnel
overtime	requests of management
part-time personnel	the workweek

(B) If policies do not exist, should they? An existing committee representing all levels of nursing personnel will tell you. Members of the committee will also tell you if policies are adequate. They will update or develop policies. Use a management plan. This activity may be done in your seminar group.

4. Identify the modified approaches to nurse staffing and scheduling in a division or a department of nursing in which you work. List the advantages and disadvantages. Get input from the staff.

5. Use Hanson's formula to determine productivity of each nursing unit for a division or department of nursing.

6. Identify at least 12 activities that can be done to improve productivity in the division or department of nursing in which you work.

7. Evaluate the Patient Classification System (PCS) of a major nursing organization by answering yes (circle Y) or no (circle N) to each of the following items.

(A) The PCS . . .

has a purpose including a unit of measure or time.	Y N
has a system for rating patients to differentiate intensity of care among definitive classes (4 or 5 categories).	Y N
has a system for translating ratings into staffing or FTEs by category (RNs, LPNs, NAs).	Y N
has a quality control or audit mechanism.	Y N
is understood by those who plan, schedule, and control the work.	Y N
is economical and convenient to audit and use.	Y N
is standardized as to procedures for accomplishing it.	Y N
is based on relative work sampling procedures.	Y N
is used.	Y N
reports required versus actual staffing.	Y N
provides for periodic updated training of raters.	Y N

(B) What needs to be done to improve the PCS? Make a management plan to accomplish it.

8. Use the items in question 7 to evaluate the staffing function in the institution in which you work.

9. Prepare a Consumer Price Index for a nursing unit for 2 years and include all personnel, supplies, and equipment.

Notes

1. L. R. Piper. "Basic Budgeting for ED Nursing Personnel." *Journal of Emergency Nursing* (Nov.-Dec. 1982):285-287.
2. Ibid.
3. E. Tzivides, V. Waterstraat, and W. Chamberlin. "Managing the Budget with a Fluctuating Census." *Nursing Management* (Mar. 1991):80B, 80F, 80H.

4. "Planning Your Replacement Budget." *Journal of Nursing Administration* (Nov. 1990): 3, 17, 24.

5. M. K. Aydelotte. *Nurse Staffing Methodology: A Review and Critique of Selected Literature* (Washington, DC: U.S. Government Printing Office, Jan. 1973):3.

6. Ibid., p. 26.

7. M. E. West. "Implementing Effective Nurse Staffing Systems in the Managed Hospital." *Topics in Health Care Financing* (Summer 1980):11-25.

8. J. N. Althaus, N. M. Hardyck, P. B. Pierce, and M. S. Rodgers. "Nurse Staffing in a Decentralized Organization: Part I." *The Journal of Nursing Administration* (Mar. 1982):34-39.

9. R. C. Minetti. "Computerized Nurse Staffing." *Hospitals* (July 16, 1983):90, 92; P. P. Shaheen. "Staffing and Scheduling: Reconcile Practical Means with the Real Goal." *Nursing Management* (Oct. 1985):64-69.

10. M. K. Aydelotte, op. cit., 26-31.

11. M. E. West, op. cit., 16.

12. M. E. West, op. cit., 17.

13. P. J. Schroder and K. L. McKeon. "What Is a Safe Staffing Pattern for Locked Long-Term and Acute Care Units for Adults?" *Journal of Psychosocial Nursing* 28, no. 12 (1990):36-37.

14. E. M. Price. *Staffing for Patient Care* (New York: Springer, 1970):12.

15. Ibid., 21-22.

16. "Study Questions All-RN Staffing." *RN* (Nov. 1983):15-16.

17. M. E. Warstler. "Some Management Techniques for Nursing Service Administrators." *Journal of Nursing Administration* (Nov.-Dec. 1972):25-34.

18. K. V. Rondeau. "Self-Scheduling Can Increase Job Satisfaction." *Medical Laboratory Observer* (Nov. 1990):22-24.

19. T. P. Herzog. "Productivity: Fighting the Battle of the Budget." *Nursing Management* (Jan. 1985):30-34; T. Porter-O'Grady. "Strategic Planning: Nursing Practice in the PPS." *Nursing Management* (Oct. 1985):53-56; K. Johnson. "A Practical Approach to Patient Classification." *Nursing Management* (June 1984):39-41, 44, 46; R. E. Schroeder, A. M. Rhodes, and R. E. Shields. "Nurse Acuity Systems: CASH vs. GRASP®." *Nursing Forum* (Feb. 1984):72-77; R. R. Alward. "Patient Classification Systems: The Ideal vs. Reality." *The Journal of Nursing Administration* (Feb. 1983):14-18; J. Nyberg and N. Wolff. "DRG Panic." *The Journal of Nursing Administration* (Apr. 1984):17-21.

20. E. J. Halloran and M. Kiley. "Case Mix Management." *Nursing Management* (Feb. 1984):39-41, 44-45.

21. R. E. Schroeder, A. M. Rhodes, and R. E. Shields, op. cit.

22. K. Johnson, op. cit.

23. Ibid., 41.

24. R. E. Schroeder, A. M. Rhodes, and R. E. Shields, op. cit.

25. R. R. Alward, op. cit.

26. J. A. Auger and V. Dee. "A Patient Classification System Based on the Behavioral System Model of Nursing: Part 1." *The Journal of Nursing Administration* (Apr. 1983):38-43.

27. V. Dee and J. A. Auger. "A Patient Classification System Based on the Behavioral System Model of Nursing: Part 2." *The Journal of Nursing Administration* (May 1983):18-23.

28. L. O'Brien-Pallas, P. Leatt, R. Deber, and J. Till. "A Comparison of Workload Estimates Using Three Methods of Patient Classification." *Canadian Journal of Nursing Administration* (Sep./Oct. 1989):16-23.

29. R. R. Alward, op. cit.

30. Ibid.

31. J. Nyberg and N. Wolff, op. cit.

32. T. E. Grazman. "Managing Unit Human Resources: A Microcomputer Model." *Nursing Management* (July 1983):18-22.

33. R. Adams and P. Duchene. "Computerization of Patient Acuity and Nursing Care Planning." *The Journal of Nursing Administration* (Apr. 1985):11-17.

34. P. Giovannetti and G. G. Mayer. "Building Confidence in Patient Classification Systems." *Nursing Management* (Aug. 1984):31-34; R. R. Alward, op. cit.

35. American Hospital Association. "Strategies: Flexible Scheduling." 1985, 12 pages.

36. Ibid.

37. J. A. Ricci. "10-Hour Night Shift: Cost vs. Savings." *Nursing Management* (Jan. 1984): 34-35, 38-42.

38. C. M. Fagin. "The Economic Value of Nursing Research." *American Journal of Nursing* (Dec. 1982):1844-1849.

39. A. G. Vic and R. C. McKay. "How Does the 12-Hour Shift Affect Patient Care?" *Journal of Nursing Administration* (Jan. 1982):12.

40. M. S. Washburn. "Fatigue and Critical Thinking on Eight- and Twelve-Hour Shifts." *Nursing Management* (Sep. 1991):80A-CC, 80D-CC, 80F-H-CC.

41. T. W. Lant and D. Gregory. "The Impact of 12-Hour Shift: An Analysis." *Nursing Management* (Oct. 1984):38A-38B, 38D-38F, 38H.

42. M. L. Metcalf. "The 12-Hour Weekend Plan—Does the Nursing Staff Really Like It? *The Journal of Nursing Administration* (Oct. 1982):16-19.

43. D. Froebe. "Scheduling: By Team or Individually." *Staffing: A Journal of Nursing Administration Reader* (Wakefield, Mass: Contemporary Publishing, 1975).

44. D. W. Fisher and E. Thomas. "A 'Premium Day' Approach to Weekend Nurse Staffing." *Staffing: A Journal of Nursing Administration Reader* (Wakefield, Mass: Contemporary Publishing, 1975).

45. S. I. Imig, J. A. Powell, K. Thorman. "Primary Nursing and Flexi-Staffing: Do They Mix?" *Nursing Management* (Aug. 1984):39-42.

46. K. O'Donnell. "A Flexible Role: Resource Acuity Nurse." *Nursing Management* (Mar. 1992):75-76.

47. K. B. Salwea. "Flexible Work Arrangements." *The Wall Street Journal* (Jan. 19, 1993):A1.

48. J. B. McGuire and J. R. Liro. "Flexible Work Schedules, Work Attitudes, and Perceptions of Productivity." *Public Personnel Management* (Spring 1986):65-73.

49. Ibid.

50. American Hospital Association, op. cit.; B. Arnold and E. Mills. "Care-12: Implementation of Flexible Scheduling." *The Journal of Nursing Administration* (Jul.-Aug. 1983):9-14; A. Mech, M. E. Mills, B. Arnold. "Wage and Hour Laws: Their Impact on 12-hour Scheduling." *The Journal of Nursing Administration* (Mar. 1984):24-25; M. L. Metcalf, op. cit.

51. P. Ancona. "Working Shifts Can Be Dangerous to Your Health, Experts Say." *San Antonio Express-News* (Feb. 19, 1994):1F-2F.

52. R. M. Kanter. *When Giants Learn to Dance* (New York, NY: Touchstone, 1989):302-314, 329; U.S. Bureau of the Census. *Statistical Abstract of the United States: 1995* 115th ed. (Washington, DC: USG PO, 1995):409.

53. J. Fierman. "The Contingency Work Force." *Fortune* (Jan. 24, 1994):30-34, 36.

54. A. Bruzzese. "Companies Turning to Temps to Fill Voids in Workplace." *San Antonio Express-News* (Apr. 19, 1994):1C, 7C.

55. M. Messmer. "Strategic Staffing." *Management Accounting* (Jun. 1992):28-30.

56. L. Hicks. "The Rise in Temps." *San Antonio Express-News* (Dec. 12, 1993):1H, 6H.

57. D. M. Tuttle. "A 'Transfer Fair' Approach to Staffing." *Nursing Management* (Dec. 1992):72-74.

58. B. Moores and A. Murphy. "Planning the Duty Rota, 1: Computerized Duty Rotas." *Nursing Times* (July 4, 1984):47-48; D. Canter. "Planning the Duty Rota, 2: Back to Basics." *Nursing Times* (July 4, 1984):49-50.

59. R. L. Hanson. "Applying Management Information Systems to Staffing." *The Journal of Nursing Administration* (Oct. 1982):5-9.

60. Ibid.

61. R. L. Hanson. "Staffing Statistics: Their Use and Usefulness." *Journal of Nursing Administration* (Nov. 1982):29-35.

62. D. S. Brown. "The Managerial Ethic and Productivity Improvement." *Public Productivity Review* (Sep. 1983):223-250.

63. R. L. Hanson. "Staffing Statistics: Their Use and Usefulness"; The formulas are Hanson's; applications here are the author's.

64. B. M. Artinian, F. D. O'Connor, and R. Brock. "Comparing Past and Present Nursing Productivity." *Nursing Management* (Oct. 1984):50-53.

65. D. L. Davis. "Assessing and Improving Productivity in the Operating Room." *AORN Journal* (Oct. 1984):630, 632, 634.

66. J. L. Smith, M. K. V. Mackey, and J. Markham. "Productivity Monitoring: A Recovery Room System for Economizing Operations." *Nursing Management* (May 1985): 34A-D, K-M.

67. C. B. Mailhot. "Setting OR's Course Toward Greater Productivity." *Nursing Management* (Oct. 1985):42I, J, L, M, P.

68. C. R. Waterstradt and T. L. Phillips. "A Productivity System for a Hospital Education Department." *Journal of Nursing Staff Development* (May-Jun. 1990):139-144.

69. S. A. W. Haas. "Sorting Out Nursing Productivity." *Nursing Management* (Apr. 1984): 37-40.

70. L. Curtin. "Reconciling Pay with Productivity." *Nursing Management* (Feb. 1984):7-8.

71. L. L. Curtin and C. L. Zurlage. "Nursing Productivity: From Data to Definition." *Nursing Management* (Jun. 1986):32-34, 38-41.

72. J. A. Reitz. "Toward a Comprehensive Nursing Intensity Index: Part 1, Development." *Nursing Management* (Aug. 1985):21-24, 26, 28-30; J. A. Reitz. "Toward a Comprehensive Intensity Index: Part 2, Testing." *Nursing Management* (Sep. 1985):31-32, 34, 36-40, 42.

73. J. Rabin. "Professionalism and Productivity." *Public Productivity Review* (Sep. 1983): 217-222.

74. L. Curtin, op. cit.

75. M. F. Fralic. "The Modern Professional and Productivity." Annual Meeting of the Alabama Society for Nursing Service Administrators, Huntsville, Ala, 1982; R. L. Hanson. "Managing Human Resources." *The Journal of Nursing Administration* (Dec. 1982):17-23; G. H. Kaye and J. Utenner. "Productivity: Managing for the Long Term." *Nursing Management* (Sep. 1985):12-13, 15; S. A. W. Haas, op. cit.; D. L. Davis, op. cit.; D. S. Brown, op. cit.

76. P. Ancona. "How to Measure Productivity and Improve Effectiveness among Workers." *San Antonio Express-News* (Jul. 24, 1993):1 B.

77. M. Gilliland, V. S. Crane, and D. G. Jones. "Productivity: Electronics Saves Steps—and Builds Networks." *Nursing Management* (Jul. 1991):56-59.

78. J. Bauer. "A Nursing Care Price Index." *American Journal of Nursing* (Jul. 1977):1150-1154.

References

Althaus, J. N., N. M. Hardyck, P. B. Pierce, and M. S. Rodgers. "Nurse Staffing in a Decentralized Organization: Part II." *The Journal of Nursing Administration* (Apr. 1982):18-22.

American Nurses' Association. *Standards of Nursing Administration Practice and a Statement on the Scope and Levels of Nursing Administration Practice and Qualifications of Nurse Administrators Across All Settings* (Washington, DC: 1988). In revision.

American Nurses' Association. *Standards of Clinical Nursing Practice* (Washington, DC: 1991).

Bermas, N. F., and A. Van Slyck. "Patient Classification Systems and the Nursing Department. *Hospitals* (Nov. 16, 1984):99-100.

Evans, C. L. S. "A Practical Staffing Calculator." *Nursing Management* (Apr. 1984):68-69.

Gebhardt, A. N. "Computers and Staff Allocation Made Easy." *Nursing Times* (Sep. 1982): 1471-1473.

Henney, C. R., and R. N. Bosworth. "A Computer-Based System for the Automatic Production of Nursing Workload Data." *Nursing Times* (July 10, 1980):1212-1217.

Jecmen, C., and N. M. Stuerke. "Computerization Helps Solve Staff Scheduling Problems." *Nursing Economics* (Nov.-Dec. 1983):209-211.

Jelinek, R. C., T. K. Zinn, and J. R. Brya. "Tell the Computer How Sick the Patients Are and It Will Tell How Many Nurses They Need." *Modern Hospital* (Dec. 1973):81-85.

Price, E. *Simplified Staffing: The Price Plan for Effective Scheduling*. Hospital Workshops, 30951 Cole Grade Road, Valley Center, Calif. 92082.

Stuerke, N. "Computers *Can* Advance Nursing Practice." *Nursing Management* (July 1984):27-28.

3

Supplies and Equipment, and Capital Budgets

A supplies and equipment budget and a capital equipment budget are developed separately although during the same budget calendar. The actual capital equipment budget may not be finalized until a dollar amount is established by administration.

Supplies and Equipment Budget

The supplies and equipment budget is part of the operating or cash budget. It includes all supplies and equipment used in provision of services, except capital equipment and supplies charged directly to patients. Examples of supplies to be budgeted include office supplies, medical and surgical supplies, pharmaceutical supplies, and others. Refer to Exhibits 1.5 and 1.6 in chapter 1.

Minor equipment includes such items as sphygmomanometers, otoscopes, and ophthalmoscopes. It is equipment that costs less than the base amount set for capital equipment. If the base amount is $500, all equipment under $500 appears as minor equipment in the supplies and equipment budget.

Generally, the director of materials management furnishes the total cost of supplies and equipment per cost center to the accounting office, and the accounting office generates a cost per patient day. This is used for budgeting purposes, increases for inflation being a decision of top management. Based on projected patient days and revenues, decisions can be made to increase or decrease the supplies and equipment budget.

Costs can be decreased by controlling the amounts of supplies and equipment kept in inventory. Nurse administrators should look at inventories they control and reduce them according to usage.

Factors that might influence the supply and equipment aspects of the budget include new program development in the institution, new physicians, and product upgrades. A product evaluation committee may be very cost effective.

Product Evaluation

Product Evaluation Committee

A product evaluation committee usually has as its members representatives of nursing, medical staff, central supply, and purchasing (see Exhibit 3.1). It is headed by a products and equipment specialist or medical materials manager, who can be a nurse. This committee is responsible for evaluation and purchase of supplies and equipment. Among its goals are

- standardization with all units using the same products,
- lower prices through higher volume,
- removal of contract negotiations between vendors and individual nursing units, allowing valuable time to be spent on nursing functions, and
- addition of a clinical perspective to purchases of all products; the purchasing department does not "just make changes" in products or purchases without appropriate assessment. All clinical implications are considered!

Thus systematic control of the introduction of patient-care products into the institution is achieved. See Exhibits 3.2 and 3.3 for a product information checklist and minutes of a product evaluation system.

The following is a suggested process for product evaluation by a committee:

1. Determine objectives of product evaluation.
2. Define use of the product with input from potential users.
3. Define objectives for each evaluation project.
4. Do initial review of various products: features, techniques for use, and prices.
5. Select products for evaluation, and evaluate techniques for use, staff acceptance, and problems.
6. Do in-service tests to use products.
7. Use simple closed-ended questions, open-ended questions, and rating scales to evaluate the product.
8. Compile and analyze data, including costs, cost savings, conversion cost, and reimbursement potential. The Deming theory of working with one supplier to improve products is noted in chapter 5.
9. Make decision for purchase.[1]

Capital Budget

A capital budget is usually separate from the operating budget (see Exhibit 3.4). A capital budget projects the planned costs of major purchases. Each item of a capital budget is defined in terms of dollar value and is an item of equipment that is reused over a period of time. The budget provides for depreciation of each item in the capital budget, sets aside the amount of depreciation in an escrow account, and uses this account to finance new capital budgets (see Exhibit 3.5). Depreciation records the declining value of a physical asset. In addition, department heads are required to justify and set priorities on capital budget items (see Exhibit 3.6). The exact definition as to what constitutes a capital budget item with regard to dollar amount and life expectancy varies among hospitals.

EXHIBIT 3.1   Product Evaluation and Standardization Committee

I. *Purpose*
1. To bring about cost containment in supply and equipment utilization through the review of the quality and cost of products utilized.
2. To review product utilization or special problems in order to maintain standards on the products throughout the hospital system and eliminate needless duplication.
3. To maintain communication among Hospitals, Nursing Service Departments, Medical Staff, and the Purchasing Department concerning product utilization and quality.
4. To evaluate items presented to Purchasing on which formal bids will be obtained.
5. To evaluate items not on bid as recommended by the Purchasing Department, a member of the committee, Administration, or individual departments through requests for evaluation or for addition to inventory.
6. To review performance of in-house products to determine if they fit present needs.

II. *Membership.* Membership of the committee shall consist of
1. Manager of Hospital Resource Analysis
2. Hospital Resource Analyst
3. Budget Director
4. Purchasing Agent
5. Nursing representative from each hospital
6. Ancillary representative from each hospital
   Nursing and Ancillary representatives from each hospital shall be appointed by the Administrator on a rotating basis. The infection control nurses will serve

in an ex-officio capacity when a product has infection control implications. Additional representatives from a facility will be used when a product is to be evaluated that has a distinctive group involved (e.g., OR representatives when OR equipment is involved).

III. *Operations/Meetings.* The Manager of Hospital Resource Analysis shall call and conduct the meeting and shall have voting privileges only in the case of a tie. The Committee shall meet on the third Friday of each month with the location rotating among the facilities. Meetings will usually be one hour long and shall not exceed two hours. A written agenda will be issued to each member prior to the meeting. The agenda will be strictly adhered to unless the committee votes to change it. The chairperson will provide time at the end of each meeting to discuss general information. If a problem arises, the Chairperson may appoint a subcommittee or member to investigate and resolve the problem and to report back to the committee at the next meeting.

Everyone will be given a chance to express his or her ideas before voting. The majority vote shall rule in all cases unless otherwise overridden by Administration. Visiting guests shall have no voting power.

Routine minutes shall be taken at each meeting and will be distributed at the following meeting.

Established July 1989, Policy 949-14, by authority of
_____.

Reviewed: July 1990, July 1992
Revised: August 1993, October 1994

Source: Courtesy of the University of South Alabama Medical Center, Mobile, Alabama.

Capital budgets also deal with maintenance, renovations, remodeling, improvements, expansion, land acquisition, and new buildings (see Exhibit 3.7). The financial manager for nursing is the nurse manager, who should evaluate past decisions and advise the nurse administrator whether they were good or bad.

All proposals for capital equipment must be fully evaluated for amount of use, method of payment, safety, replacement, and duplication of service, and every conceivable other factor, including the need for space, personnel, and renovation. The needs and desires of the medical staff should be considered. Their involvement in planning helps ensure wise purchases of capital equipment.

The capital budget must address increased forms of competition, dwindling financial resources, and regulatory constraints. Management should enhance conditions under which effective planning and capital budgeting increase the hospital's chance of long-term survival. Capital budgeting is a part of the overall budget planning process for the organization and not an entity unto itself.

EXHIBIT 3.2   Product Information and Justification Checklist

The goal of product evaluation is to provide optimal patient care while managing costs. Therefore, please provide all information requested on this checklist to the department of Hospital Resource Analysis for consideration by the Product Evaluation and Standardization Committee. This report must be reviewed and signed by your Assistant Adrninistrator before it can be evaluated by the committee.

1. Name and function of the product.
2. Is this a new product or a replacement?
3. How will the product be paid for (departmental budget, patient chargeable, etc.)?
4. Why is this product necessary or preferable to the current or other products, in your own words? Please discuss at least two other similar products.
5. What products are currently being used to perform this function in other departments and at all three hospitals?
6. What is the expected utilization of this product throughout the USA System?
7. What is the current utilization of the products that are performing this or a similar function throughout the USA System?
8. If this product is used to treat or prevent a specific ailment or range of ailments, what is the incidence of this ailment that is seen in the USA System?
9. What are the following costs, if applicable, for this product as compared to other similar products and how can these costs be justified?
   • purchase price
   • installation
   • training
   • personnel
   • support
   • maintenance (Also include who is responsible for maintenance.)
10. If cost savings are anticipated with the use of this product, how will those "savings" be utilized?
11. Who will control the use of the product?
12. If applicable, please provide a sample protocol for the use of this product that will be used to ensure proper use of this product.
13. What are the long-term implications of this product?

If you need assistance, please contact _____ or _____ at _____.

Source: Courtesy of the University of South Alabama Medical Center, Mobile, Alabama.

When each entry or item in the capital budget has been analyzed and reduced to the amount available, the budget is tabulated again. It is now ready to present to the board of directors (see Exhibit 3.4). With their approval, the list is distributed to cost-center managers who prepare requisitions for purchase. The purchasing department prepares bid specifications, with input from cost-center managers. Purchases are finalized based on results of bids submitted by vendors who meet the required specifications. Exhibit 3.8 is a status report of a capital budget in which all remaining dollars are commited. Purchases are finally entered into the depreciation budget schedule. The latter is published by the American Hospital Association and is considered the standard for the industry (see Exhibit 3.9).

Capital equipment accounts for approximately 10.4 percent of a hospital's annual expenditures.[2]

When evaluating capital equipment, evaluate similar products one at a time. When purchasing capital equipment, determine whether it can be upgraded or must be replaced when technology improves. Consider construction, durability, modularity, warranty, availability of parts, and service agreements as part of the total cost of equipment. Consider leasing versus buying.[3] According to

EXHIBIT 3.3   Product Evaluation and Standardization Committee Meeting

December 9, 1994
8:30 A.M., Board Room, USA Knollwood

Members Present
Chairman, Hospital Resource Analyst, USAMC
Director of Nursing, USAKPH
Director of Respiratory Therapy, USADH
Nurse Manager, Surgical Services, USADH
Director of Radiology, USAMC
SPD Supervisor, USAKPH
Nurse Manager, High Risk/Antenatal Obstetrics, USAMC
Director of Budgets, USAMC

Members Absent
Purchasing Agent, USAMC
Hospital Resource Analyst, USAMC

Guests
Trauma Coordinator, USAMC

PRODUCT EVALUATION

Closed Arterial Line System
The Director of Respiratory Therapy and the Trauma Coordinator presented their findings from the evaluation of the closed arterial line system. In their discussion with Nursing and Respiratory Care providers, there were many issues raised regarding the practicality of such a system. These issues revolved around tubing size, heparinization and sampling through the ports available on the SafeSite system. In general, they concluded that the issue of blood waste could be solved without purchasing such a system and that there was no documentation present which could prove that contamination with the current stopcock system was a problem. They therefore recommended that we not pursue this system any further at this time. However, they did recommend that we evaluate such systems again when it is time to bid our current system again.

The committee unanimously agreed to not recommend the addition of a Closed Arterial Line System.

OLD BUSINESS

Gloves
The data provided regarding glove usage was determined to have been helpful to managers in evaluating their departments. _____ requested that _____ provide comparable information for the current fiscal year to date. _____ addressed the quality issue with our current stock gloves. None of the other committee members have been made aware of a major quality problem with the gloves. It is unclear whether the problem has not been apparent in other departments or is just not being reported. _____ was not present at the meeting to answer how the company has responded to his inquiry regarding the quality issue.

After much discussion, it was decided that _____ would send a memo to all managers asking them to address specific quality issues to the committee representatives in their respective facilities.

Communication Issues
_____ brought up the problem that managers have in being informed of bid item changes in advance. Although it may not be possible to evaluate every item that is on bid, the committee determined that it would be helpful if the Purchasing Department could announce upcoming bids 3 to 6 months ahead of time. This would allow managers the opportunity to provide information regarding specific products. It was also suggested that bids be posted in all three facilities, rather than just at USAMC; this problem seems to be most apparent at USADH and USAKPH. _____ will discuss this with _____.

Presentation of Committee's Purpose to Managers
This presentation has not yet been accomplished. _____ agreed to have a proposal for this purpose ready for the January meeting. It was suggested that it might be helpful to have each facility's representatives make the presentation at their facility.

NEW BUSINESS

None.

The next regularly scheduled meeting will be held at USAMC on Friday, January 20, 199x at 8:30 A.M. in the USAMC Board Room.

The meeting was adjourned at 9:30 A.M.

Respectfully submitted,

Chairman

Source: Courtesy of the University of South Alabama Medical Center, Mobile, Alabama.

EXHIBIT 3.4   Capital Budget Requested FY 19xx–19xx: University of South Alabama Medical Center

Dept.	Item	Quantity	Amount
7th & 8th	Beds & misc. pat. furn.	85	$ 200,000.00
Admin	Pneumatic tube system	1	75,000.00
Anest	Capnograph-portable	1	4,200.00
Anest	Trans. Mon. - inc NIPB & O_2 Sat	1	9,200.00
Anest	Ventilators	2	5,050.00
Aero Med	Pro Pac 106	1	13,790.00
Bio Med	Safety tester	1	1,695.00
Blood Bk	Table top centrifuge	1	2,000.00
Blood Bk	Automated cell washer	1	6,250.00
Cath Lab	Pulse oximetry	1	2,600.00
Cath Lab	Dynamap	1	3,800.00
Clin. Lab	Miscellaneous equipment	1	250,000.00
Dialysis	Dialysis machine	1	25,000.00
Dietary	Refrigerator - bakery	1	3,500.00
Dietary	Refrigerator - bakery	1	6,950.00
Dietary	Refrigerator - cook area	1	3,500.00
Dietary	Refrigerator - PFS	1	3,100.00
Dietary	Meat slicer	1	3,500.00
ED	New monitoring system	1	160,000.00
ED	Propak monitor	1	3,500.00
Envir	High-speed burnisher	4	8,000.00
Envir	Slow-speed buffers	2	1,600.00
GI Lab	Video processor CV-100	1	20,000.00
HStation	Blood pressure monitor	1	4,500.00
HStation	Stress test system	1	20,000.00
HStation	ECG management system	1	70,000.00
MICU/CCU	Faceplates - central monitors	12	4,920.00
Nursing	Medication carts	17	25,000.00
Nutri	Computer & printer	1	2,011.00
OR	Laparoscopic video system	1	30,165.00
OR	Electrosurgical cautery	2	17,200.00
PACU	RR stretchers	10	20,000.00
Plant Op	4000-watt portable generator	1	1,495.00
Plant Op	8 ch. OPS card for telephone swi	1	1,337.00
Radio	Rebuilt film processor	1	12,000.00
Res. Th	Sterile pass-through drier	1	12,567.00
SPD	Washer decontaminator	1	75,000.00
Staff Dev	Overhead projector	1	700.00
Staff Dev	CPR mannikin	1	5,641.00
Total requested USA Medical Center			$1,114,771.00

Source: Courtesy of the University of South Alabama Medical Center, Mobile, Alabama.

EXHIBIT 3.5 Investment in Plant Assets for the Ten Months Ended July 31, 19xx

Plant assets consisting of land, buildings, and equipment are stated at cost or, if contributed, at fair market value at date of gift. No provision is made in the accounts for depreciation of plant assets. Investment in plant is reduced for disposal of plant assets.

All Hospital equipment purchases are funded by the renewals and replacements fund. The Hospital also uses plant assets purchased by the University. These assets are not presented in the Hospital's financial statements.

Depreciation expense is included in Medicare, Medicaid, and Blue Cross cost reports. This information is presented below.

	Cost	Depreciation Expense 07-31-xx	Accum. Depreciation 07-31-xx	Net Book Value 07-31-xx
Hospital-Designated Funds				
Land	$ 186,096	$ 0	$ 0	$ 186,096
Buildings	8,070,647	184,063	3,942,812	4,127,835
Fixed Equipment	10,386,318	605,671	5,878,008	4,508,310
Major Movable Equipment	15,079,892	1,235,052	8,971,493	6,108,399
Minor Equipment	186,757	0	186,757	0
Construction in Progress	762,874	0	0	762,874
Total	$34,672,584	$2,024,786	$18,979,070	$15,693,514
University-Designated Funds				
Buildings	$ 1,544,927	$ 39,481	$ 581,958	$ 962,969
Fixed Equipment	2,564,683	158,533	1,914,366	650,317
Major Movable Equipment	5,315,499	0	5,315,499	0
Total	$ 9,425,109	$ 198,014	$ 7,811,823	$ 1,613,286
Total equipment used for patient care	$44,097,693	$2,222,800	$26,790,893	$17,306,800

Source: Courtesy of the University of South Alabama Medical Center, Mobile, Alabama.

Wagner, hospitals in the United States spent $8.6 billion on capital equipment in 1989, which was 4.4 percent of their total expenditures.[4]

Part of the capital equipment budgeting process includes estimating the use of each item. For revenue budgeting purposes, a price or charge should be put on each item's use. The cost-center manager can then determine the break-even point at which the item will be paid for.

Summary

Major elements of nursing budgets include expenditures for supplies and equipment and for capital equipment. Generally equipment costing less than a fixed dollar amount is included in the supplies and equipment budget. A product evaluation committee helps to assure that supplies and equipment will promote effective and efficient patient care. The capital equipment budget includes equipment costing above a fixed dollar amount. It is separate from the supplies and equipment budget.

EXHIBIT 3.6   Capital Equipment Request Form

Hospital: USA Medical Center

Dept: Department of Nursing   **Dept no.**   60601

Equipment requested: 85 electric beds/7th-8th floor

Equipment description: Give a simple description of the device and its use.

85 electric beds with high-low features, ability for trendelenburg/reverse trendelenburg positions; instant CPR emergency lever; head of bed frame removable to facilitate cervical traction and emergency procedures; side arm control for patient use.

$210,000.00	**Equipment costs**	None	**Training costs**
Minimal	**Maintenance costs**	Incl in Equip.	**Shipping costs**
None	**Personnel costs**	None	**Supply costs**
None	**Installation/renovation costs**		

Expected useful life: 15   yrs

1	List priority (1-2-3-4) of equipment with regard to the requests submitted by your department
Yes	(Y/N) Will this item be a replacement for an existing piece of equipment? If "Y," what is to become of the existing equipment? Equipment to be evaluated by the Hospital Committee to determine.
No	(Y/N) Is this new technology or a new procedure? If "Y," how will the expense be recuperated (e.g., through revenue)?

Manager: _____

Assistant administrator: _____

Apr # _____

Source: Courtesy of the University of South Alabama Medical Center, Mobile, Alabama.

EXHIBIT 3.7 Statement of Changes in Fund Balance Renewals and Replacements Fund for the Ten Months Ended July 31, 19xx

Account Number	Description	Balances Prior Year	Funded Depreciation	Other Additions/ Deductions	Expended for Plant Facilities	Intrafund Transfers	Balances Current Year
79008	Unallocated—USAMC	$ 9,915,392.38	$2,222,800.29	$ 78,134.71	$ 0.00	$159,538.18-	$12,056,789.20
79030	Defects—Joint Commis	65,818.19	.00	.00	.00	65,818.19-	.00
79039	Information System	92,709.68	.00	.00	.00	.00	92,709.68
79050	Helicopter—USAMC	712,120.33	.00	127,667.94	.00	.00	839,788.27
79057	USAMC Emer Generator	48,562.09	.00	.00	.00	.00	48,562.09
79063	Donated Eq—Others	2,313.49	.00	153.00	1,928.70-	384.79-	153.00
79064	USAMC Aux Purch Eq	.00	.00	688.08-	538.08	150.00	.00
79068	Hosp Adm Purch Eq	.00	.00	33,809.52	33,809.52-	.00	.00
79075	HVAC System—Surgery	74,475.00	.00	.00	.00	74,475.00-	.00
79077	Labor Deliv Unit 3FL	291,990.72	.00	.00	.00	.00	291,990.72
79083	H.A.S. Telephone Sym	13,007.00	.00	.00	.00	13,007.00-	.00
79092	Capital Budget previous	364,110.78	.00	5,208.00-	334,654.47-	.00	24,248.31
79093	Xray Silver Recovery	49,944.03	.00	12,678.45	.00	.00	62,622.48
79095	Capital Exp <$10,000	75,414.38	.00	.00	146,864.18-	150,000.00	78,550.20
79097	Linear Accelerator	.00	.00	.00	45,994.26	45,994.26-	.00
79098	Mini Van	1,606.48	.00	2,847.51	.00	.00	4,453.99
79099	O/P Surg Cap Equip	161,720.27	.00	.00	225,718.54-	64,324.93	326.66
79101	O/P Surg Renov	37,425.00	.00	.00	1,316.60-	.00	36,108.40
79102	Angiograph Lab Eqmnt	1,000,000.00	.00	.00	189,259.00-	.00	810,741.00
79103	Nuclear Medical Eqmnt	284,000.00	.00	.00	246,035.68-	.00	37,964.32
79104	Telethon Purch Equip	.00	.00	40,185.00	40,185.00-	.00	.00
79105	Medical Rec Dict Sys	.00	.00	.00	.00	86,288.00	86,288.00
79106	Renal Transplant Prg	.00	.00	.00	.00	96,000.00	96,000.00
79110	ELENA-USAMC Damage	31,916.36	.00	5,629.15	.00	37,545.51-	.00
	Final Totals	$13,222,526.18	$2,222,800.29	$295,209.20	$1,173,239.35-	$ 0.00	$14,567,296.32

EXHIBIT 3.8 Capital Budget, as of June 30, 19xx

Department	Dept. No.	Item Description	Budget	Paid 06-30-xx	Encumbrances	Total Committed	Budget Balance
Nursing Services							
Nursing Services—Admin	60601	Software License	$ 0.00	$ 18,135.00	$2,000.00	$ 0.00	$ 0.00
		External Modem		527.12			
		Electric & Manual Beds–6		31,704.72			
		Cardio System Special Care Beds		13,725.00			
		Telemetry Monitoring System		113,080.12			
		COMPAQ Computer		9,842.70			
		Department Total	$189,014.66	$187,014.66	$2,000.00	$189,014.66	$ 0.00
Private U. 6th Floor	60609	Lifepack 7 Defibrillator		5,500.00			
		Facsimile Machine		1,600.00			
		Lifepack 7 Defibrillator		5,208.00			
		Department Total	$ 12,308.00	$ 12,308.00	0.00	$ 12,308.00	0.00
Coronary Care	60615	Lifepack 6 Defibrillator		7,621.32			
		Department Total	$ 7,621.32	$ 7,621.32	0.00	$ 7,621.32	0.00
5th Floor–Shared Supplies	60619	Facsimile Machine		1,550.00			
		Department Total	$ 1,550.00	$ 1,550.00	0.00	$ 1,550.00	0.00
5th Floor–North	60622	Lifepack 7 Defibrillator		5,500.00			
		Department Total	$ 5,500.00	$ 5,500.00	0.00	$ 5,500.00	0.00
CCU	60626	Telemetry Transmitters		3,300.00			
		Department Total	$ 3,300.00	$ 3,300.00	0.00	$ 3,300.00	0.00
Pediatric Unit	60630	Lifepack 7 Defibrillator		5,500.00			
		Facsimile Machine		1,550.00			
		Department Total	$ 7,050.00	$ 7,050.00	$ 0.00	$ 7,050.00	$ 0.00

Source: Courtesy of the University of South Alabama Medical Center, Mobile, Alabama.

EXHIBIT 3.9 Composite Estimated Useful Lives
of Depreciable Hospital Assets

Item	Years
Building Components, Buildings, and Fixed Equipment	
Boiler house	15–25
Masonry building, reinforced concrete frame	25–30
Masonry building, steel frame	
Fireproofed	25–30
Not fireproofed	20–25
Masonry building, wood frame	20–25
Multilevel parking structure, masonry	20–25
Reinforced concrete building, common design	25–30
Residence	
Masonry	20–25
Wood frame	15–20
Storage building	
Masonry	20–25
Wood frame	15–20
Movable Equipment	
Major movable equipment	7–12
Minor movable equipment	2–5

Source: Reproduced with permission from *Estimated Useful Lives of Depreciable Hospital Assets,* published by American Hospital Publishing Inc., copyright © 1993. All rights reserved.

Experiential Exercises

1. Prepare a supplies and equipment budget using the format below or use one from the institution in which you work or are assigned for clinical experience. You may also refer to exhibits in chapter 1.

Supplies and Expense Budget

Account Number	Department	Qty.	Description of Equipment	Cost

2. Examine a health-care business's capital budget for the previous year. What was the total dollar amount requested? Approved? What process was used to produce the capital budget? What was the degree of participation by nurses?
3. Prepare a capital equipment budget request using the format of Exhibit 3.6 or use one from the institution in which you work or are assigned for clinical experience.

Notes

1. M. Dickerson. "Product Evaluation: A Strategy for Controlling a Supply and Equipment Budget." In *Patients and Purse Strings*. J. C. Scherubel, ed., NLN Publication #20-2192, 2 (New York: National League for Nursing, 1988):465-468.
2. C. Tokarsi. "Creative Proposal Plays to Tough Crowd." *Modern Health Care* (Mar. 4, 1991):53-56.
3. B. Aronsohn and N. Deal. "Navigating the Maze of Capital Equipment Acquisition." *Nursing Management* (Nov. 1992):46-48.
4. M. Wagner. "The Many Reasons Why Hospitals Buy Technology." *Modern Health Care* (Aug. 6, 1990):21-23.

Reference

Vracin, R. A. "Capital Budgeting." In *Handbook of Health Care Accounting and Finance*. W. O. Cleverly, Ed. (Gaithersburg, Md: Aspen, 1982):323-351.

4

Computers, Information Systems, and Nursing Management

Richard J. Swansburg, B.S.N., M.S.C.I.S, R.N.

> The process of computerization is moving through our world with the power
> of its own momentum, transforming our experiences of life and culture.[1]

As the year 2000 approaches it is time we all face the fact that the technorevolution is firmly upon us. Wherever we turn in our lives, we encounter products of the computer age: watches, automatic teller machines, credit and debit cards, televisions and VCRs, home appliances, FAX machines, home computers, computers in the workplace, among others. We must come to terms with the problems and opportunities computers in our society present.[2]

The challenge of embracing and utilizing computers will be critical for the management of health care in transition. Nurse managers will have to assimilate the knowledge and gain the expertise to understand and interact with this constantly changing technology, and then they must be capable of teaching and impressing it upon others. Any barriers to assimilation and conveyance will need to be overcome and removed.

Ethical and legal issues need to be advanced in scope to address new and changing technology. Concepts of privacy, confidentiality, and security should be instilled in nursing personnel, not only in terms of operational guidelines (data and physical security, policies and procedures), but in terms of professionalism and responsibility. Control of information needs to be taught as a management issue, not a technical one.

Computer interaction may be further complicated by exposure to multiple hardware and software platforms. There is a new focus towards the integration of these distributed and often highly differentiated environments. The problems of computer phobia may be lessened with the implementation of graphical user interfaces (GUI, a visual system by which the user interacts with the computer)

and pointing devices. The tools used by managers should also be representative of these changes as interactive multimedia becomes commonplace.

As computers are brought into the home and are increasingly used in elementary, middle, and high school education, they are being incorporated into our nursing curriculums at advanced levels as well. They are being merged into all facets of professional nursing. This explosive growth of computer use in health care, the complexity and cost of different computer systems, and rapid changes in hospital computer technologies place nurse managers and educators in critical positions. They must have knowledge of computers and information systems in general and an understanding of the key issues involved in automation in order to make computer tools useful in nursing practice.[3]

Finally, speculation is the name of the game when trying to predict technological trends and how they might be used in health care.

The State of the Art

State of the art is one of those phrases that, in the beginning, meant a set of circumstances characterizing a craft or its principles, or a branch of learning.[4] Now it tends to be a cliché commonly used by salespeople and consultants to impress upon one the idea that something is as advanced as is technologically possible. Even Nursing Information Systems Specialists use the cliché.

Examples of its usage have emerged in publications. In discussing the preparation of nurses for information systems, Romano states, "to prepare nurses to practice in the increasingly technological environments of the future, and to direct and control the impact of technology on nursing are no small challenges. An awareness and involvement with the state of the art of computers and technology in health can be that awesome first step."[5] And in describing computing resources to support nursing informatics, Heller, Romano, Moray, and Gassert state, "in addition to existing computing resources available in the school of nursing and throughout the campus, a state-of-the-art microcomputer laboratory was dedicated to support the specialization in Nursing Informatics."[6]

The problem with the state of the art is that the development cycle for a new generation of a technological product, such as a microprocessor, is now approximately 18 months.[7] This means that what is state of the art today is often old technology in a year and a half. With this in mind, this chapter presents a scenario of what today's environment could be like if current technology were used.

Hardware

Even in this era of downsizing many companies may view their mainframes as the center of a large, corporate-wide network. The mainframe is a hub connecting distributed minicomputers and PC/LAN (Personal Computer/Local Area Network) clusters. It serves as information reservoirs, siphoning data to PCs, workstations, and minicomputers.[8] A minicomputer can be used to handle the needs of a large nursing department, and can also serve as a hub connecting workstations and microcomputer-based LANs.

A LAN cluster is the focus of hardware for each nursing department. Workstations and microcomputers act as point-of-care technology centers at

the patients' bedsides. These computers can integrate computerized patient-monitoring systems that measure ECG, arterial blood pressure, pulmonary artery pressure, temperature, chest drainage, urine output, cardiac output, respiratory cycle pulse, tidal volume, peak airway pressure, blood I/O, and fluid I/O.[9]

These point-of-care computers have color displays and are capable of three-dimensional (3-D) graphics and full-motion video. Interaction is via a pointing device—your finger, a mouse, or a light pen. A camera supplies the capability of video interaction and monitoring. Finally, stacks of compact disk drives are attached to provide access to a never-ending electronic library.

Software

State-of-the-art software centers around an open-systems model and a multi-tasking operating system. The open-systems approach seeks to integrate many software environments, regardless of their hardware platforms. A multitasking operating system provides greater computing power and efficiency for the end user than a single tasking one like DOS. The workplace is managed through a graphical user interface, and diverse automated systems are integrated and presented via interactive multimedia.

Interactive multimedia combines full-motion video, narration, art and animation, text, and stereo music. It allows people the ability to interact with information from multiple sources in new ways. The same information may be expressed simultaneously from many points of view. It is the medium that will soon replace paper and printed information as we know them.[10]

Nursing Management Concerns

Due to increasing economic pressure and government regulation, nursing-care delivery systems have been created with important implications for nursing management. In an effort to streamline operations and improve efficiency, nursing personnel are being cross-trained and are being increasingly exposed to computers and information systems. Cross-training prepares professionals to function effectively in multiple areas; faced with increased patient acuity, changing technology, and specialization, nurses have to accurately coordinate clinical information to deliver quality nursing care. They use relevant information logically, systematically, and cost-effectively to make sound decisions.[11]

Nurse managers must work with nurse educators to confront the challenge of developing effective and efficient training programs for nursing staff who may be working with a variety of computers and information systems.[12] They must address such issues as barriers to computerization and learning; ethical, legal and security concerns; and the recruitment and retention of highly effective professionals.

Barriers to Computerization

The first barrier to overcome in dealing with computers is computer phobia. A general fear of change seems to exist within us all, and for some, being forced to

work with computers elicits common reactions of apprehension and anxiety. Following are some tips for conquering computer phobia:

- Do not procrastinate.
- Seek a nonthreatening environment, one in which everyone will feel comfortable.
- Maintain a positive attitude that learning will take place. Fear of not learning is a problem.
- Encourage hands-on opportunities.
- Indicate that knowing how to type is helpful but not essential.
- Do not allow the use of computer jargon. Use words that everyone understands.
- Insist that learning sessions last less than two hours and not cover too many subjects.
- Encourage note taking.
- Do not allow interruptions.
- Encourage assertiveness and requests for help.
- Encourage practice.
- Everyone relax![13]

Other elements of computer phobia are the fear of making mistakes and erasing data, and the fear of losing a job. Computer phobia can be overcome through proper management, education, and hands-on training.

Another barrier centers around the perception of cost versus benefit. The Health and Human Services Secretary's Commission on Nursing projected that health-care institutions allocate approximately 2.5 percent of their operating budgets for information technology. In contrast, other service industries such as banking and insurance allocate from 7 to 10 percent. The inappropriateness of this low allocation of revenues is that health care is more information-intensive than the figures imply.[14]

Often administrators and nurses have a hard time believing that computer technology can enhance productivity and improve quality. Although some studies appear to show that computerized information systems save time, nurses may circumvent the information system, thus defeating its time savings. Even if time is saved from paperwork, there is concern that nurses will not use this time to focus on patient care.[15] Managers should become involved by researching information technology, installed or planned, and determining if it is beneficial to nursing. Finding it so, they should inform others about its positive effects and advantages.

A final barrier relates to a system whose capabilities do not meet the organization's needs. Nurses who feel that the information system does not promote their clinical decision making and that it will detract from the amount of time spent doing patient care, will not use it. This is usually due to not involving staff nurses in the decision-making process from beginning to end. The solution seems to be to involve the staff in any decisions related to automation. Staff should be allowed to develop the system and fit it to the organization.

Ethical, Legal, and Security Issues

Ethical means conforming to professional standards of conduct. "Privacy means control over exposure of self or information about oneself and freedom from intrusion. Privacy denotes the right of an individual to decide how much personal information to share. It includes a right to secrecy of information and protection against the misuse or release of this information."[16] *Confidentiality* means

being entrusted with the privacy of others. The relationship of the three can be expressed as a patient entrusting his or her privacy to a professional who has an ethical responsibility to maintain the confidentiality of that privacy.

Legal issues associated with automation involve the confidentiality of patient information, and the risk associated with clinical decision making based on computerized information. One method of addressing these issues is by maintaining professional standards. Information systems should be designed, developed, and implemented to validate patient outcomes and support professional nursing standards. This means that computer technology for nursing use needs to be based on nursing input from start to finish. This requires the use of expert nurses who have sufficient clinical, theoretical, educational, research, and management expertise to adequately represent professional standards. It also requires a unified nursing profession that can specify clear design criteria and professional standards.[17]

Nurses should also be capable of assessing and managing the legal risks associated with automated information management. Computer data should be examined, analyzed, interpreted, and appraised. Forced selections and unclear logic should be questioned. Nurses should not hold as fact the belief that clinical decision making based on the use of technology results in better patient care.

The American Nurses' Association, the American Medical Records Association, and the Canadian Nurses' Association offer guidelines and strategies for minimizing legal risks associated with automated charting:

- Never give your computer password to anyone.
- Do not leave a computer terminal unattended after you've logged on.
- Follow procedure for modifying mistakes. Computer entries are part of the permanent record and cannot be deleted.
- Do not leave patient information displayed on a screen for others to see. Also, keep track of printed information about patients, and dispose of it appropriately when it is no longer needed.
- Follow your institution's confidentiality policies and procedures.[18]

Security means the level to which hardware, software, and information is safe from abuse and unauthorized use or access, whether accidental or intentional. From a management standpoint, professionals need to be aware that security must be overseen from physical, operational, and ethical viewpoints.

Physical security deals with the control of access to hardware, the assessment and determination of environmental threats, and the prevention of loss. Operational security deals with the threats to information. It includes the assessment and prevention of unauthorized access or use of information, the policies and procedures governing the management of information, and the procedures required for recovery from loss of information whether deleted, stolen, or leaked. Ethical security deals with the individual's ability to conform to professional standards of conduct. This means that nurses have to respect the privacy of information. They must accept and enforce all guidelines imposed for the maintenance of physical and operational security of computer systems.

Nurse managers should be aware of various security measures built into information systems. One of the first things that should be present is the ability to perform auditing. This means leaving a trail of who did what, where, and when. Logs can record who, when, and where the system is accessed. This same

information can be captured when vital information is created, modified, or deleted. Once this information is captured, standard procedures should be in place for the routine auditing of this information.

A significant amount of security may be associated with an individual's computer identification (ID). Every individual should be assigned his or her own personal ID. This ID should have the person's name, title, department, security level, and menu linked to it. There should be a password that protects the ID and is known only by the user. Procedures should be in place to force users to change their passwords every 30 to 90 days, and allow them to change them on their own as desired. Also, a number of each user's old passwords should be stored for comparison purposes, and the user should not be allowed to reuse passwords. The security level should be implemented in a hierarchical manner from administrator to nursing assistant. It can be a range of numbers from largest to smallest which can be tested to determine who can perform particular functions. Menus that determine the capability to interact with the system should be developed and assigned based on departmental and job requirements.

Recruitment and Retention

Strategies that promote nursing satisfaction are paramount, considering the investment in recruiting, training, developing, and retaining qualified nurses.[19] The reasons that nurses select an employer include location, salary and benefits, and flexibility of scheduling. The reasons that nurses remain in their jobs include peer and medical staff support, open communication to management and input into decision making, model for professional practice, and reimbursement of tuition.[20]

It is time to also consider the use of technology to create an environment to promote nursing satisfaction. Technology can be the building block to develop positive and attractive work surroundings. The use of point-of-care information systems, telecommunications, and automated skill-mix and resource scheduling will help recruit and retain nursing professionals.[21]

The activities related to recruitment and retention are important enough that the development of an automated recruitment program may be warranted. The objectives would be to provide accurate and timely tracking and monitoring of recruitment activities and costs.[22]

General-Purpose Microcomputer Software

Today's nursing management should be prepared to support increasing use of automation in all areas of nursing. Part of this support includes a greater interaction with microcomputers. Many nursing professionals come in contact with microcomputers on a daily basis. Nurses use microcomputers for patient care documentation, budgeting, policy and procedure documentation, personnel records, patient and staff education, and inventory control, among others.

Nursing managers should be using microcomputers and general-purpose software as tools for increasing their own productivity. General-purpose software can afford nurse managers the opportunity to develop and use their own applications. Such applications often are identified when managers recognize

that some repetitive task they are performing can be simplified by automation.[23] Some of the general-purpose programs available for nurse managers include spreadsheet programs, word processing and desktop publishing programs, database management programs, graphics programs, communications programs, and integrated programs.

Spreadsheets

A *spreadsheet* is a tool used to record and manipulate numbers. Originally spreadsheets were paper ledgers used for business accounting, such as the recording of debits and credits. With the coming of the microcomputer, electronic spreadsheets were developed. An electronic spreadsheet is a software package that turns a microcomputer into a highly sophisticated calculator. Huge quantities of numbers can be recorded, manipulated, and stored quite simply and easily. Nurse managers could use spreadsheets to maintain statistics, create graphics, and plan budgets. For examples, see Exhibits 4.1 and 4.2.

A spreadsheet is made up of columns and rows of memory cells. These cells can be variable in size to allow for small or very large numbers. In addition to numbers, cells can store text and formulas. Text is used for titles, column and row headers, comments, and instructions. Formulas are used to perform the actual mathematical manipulation of memory cells and their numbers, such as addition, subtraction, multiplication, division, and even special math functions such as averages and standard deviations. Formulas are what really make a spreadsheet a powerful number-crunching tool. Spreadsheets also have functions for copying, moving, inserting, and deleting cells. One of the most important spreadsheet functions is graphing, which allows numbers to be displayed in a graphic form. See Exhibits 4.3 through 4.5 for examples of pie, line, and bar graphs.

Spreadsheets are the best tool to use in situations that require the management of a lot of numbers. For this reason, they are particularly pertinent to financial management, where they speed up the processes of budgeting, forecasting, developing tables and schedules, and so on.

Word Processing and Desktop Publishing

Word processing is the manipulation of words and special characters to produce a printed document. *Desktop publishing* is the manipulation of text and graphics to produce documents of publication quality. Five years ago the difference between the two was vast. Today each has incorporated aspects of the other. Examples of documents produced from both are memorandums, letters, policies and procedures, forms, labels, instruction sheets, manuals, signs, books, and others. See Exhibits 4.6 through 4.8 for examples.

Advantages to word processing and desktop publishing are:

- A document can be visualized on a computer display screen exactly as it will look when printed.
- A document can be modified or changed very quickly and easily without having to entirely redo it.
- A document can be printed numerous times with the same material presented in different formats.

EXHIBIT 4.1 Example of Statistics for New Hires and Terminations

| | Nursing Orientation Statistics | | | | | | | | | | | | |
	Jan	Feb	Mar	Apr	May	Jun	Jul	Aug	Sep	Oct	Nov	Dec	Totals
Hires													
RNs	10	6	8	5	7	27	11	8	13	3	3	5	106
LPNs	3	3	6	1	2	11	5	2	7	4	2	1	47
USs	0	0	0	0	2	1	0	0	2	0	1	0	6
NAs	1	0	0	3	0	2	0	1	1	1	1	0	10
Terminations													
RNs	11	4	10	6	3	17	8	11	9	5	1	1	86
LPNs	2	5	4	1	3	8	3	5	3	5	1	1	41
USs	0	0	0	1	1	1	0	0	2	0	1	0	6
NAs	1	0	1	2	0	2	0	1	1	1	1	0	10

Source: Courtesy of the University of South Alabama Medical Center, Mobile, Alabama.

EXHIBIT 4.2 Example of a Budget

Hospital Information Systems Budget
October 19xx–September 19xx

Sub Code	Description	Original Budget	Balance Available	Percent Used	Oct 'xx Current	Year	Nov 'xx Current	Year	Dec 'xx Current	Year	Jan 'xx Current	Year
1600	Student Wages	$12,000	$ (514)	104%	$373	$373	$ 786	$1,160	$1,612	$2,771	$1,121	$3,892
1660	Accrued Salaries	0	(567)	0	214	214	229	443	183	626	(314)	312
	Salaries	12,000	(1,081)	109	587	587	1,015	1,603	1,795	3,397	807	4,204
2110	Medical/Surgical Supplies	100	54	46		0		0		0		0
2130	Drugs	0	(8)	0	2	2		2		2		2
2320	Medical/Surgical Supplies	100	46	54	2	2		2		2		2
2330	Office Supplies	500	291	42	35	35	3	38	23	61	6	67
2340	Copying and Binding	200	97	51	14	14	3	17	6	23	43	66
	Printing	0	(64)	0		0		0	1	1		1
2400	Housekeeping Supplies	0	(7)	0		0		0		0		0
2500	Maintenance Supplies	100	100	0		0		0		0		0
2700	Food Expense	0	0	0		0		0		0		0
	General Supplies	800	418	48	49	49	6	55	30	85	49	134
3110	Travel	0	(220)	0		0		0		0		0
3140	Local Travel	0	(245)	0	18	18	34	52	4	56	13	70
3160	Workshop and Training	0	(68)	0		0		0	68	68		68
	Travel/Entertainment	0	(533)	0	18	18	34	52	72	124	13	138
3230	Contract Labor	0	0	0		0		0		0		0
3290	Computer Software	700	340	51		0	279	279		279		279
3360	Equipment Maintenance/Repair	500	160	68		0		0		0		0
3370	Maintenance Contracts	1,560	312	80		0		0		0		0
3410	Equipment Rental	0	(70)	0		0		0		0		0
3650	Telephone Base	100	64	36		0	31	31	5	36		36
3660	Telephone—Long Distance	0	(4)	0		0		0		0		0
3720	Books and Subscriptions	0	(60)	0		0		0		0		0
	Other Expenses	2,860	742	74	0	0	310	310	5	315	0	315
5050	Minor Equipment (<$500)	1,500	707	53	0	0	450	450	139	589	(139)	450
	Minor Equipment Expenses	1,500	707	53	0	0	450	450	139	589	(139)	450
	Total Expenses	$17,260	$ 298	98%	$657	$657	$1,815	$2,472	$2,041	$4,513	$ 730	$5,243

(Continued)

131

EXHIBIT 4.2 Example of a Budget (*Continued*)

Hospital Information Systems Budget
October 19xx–September 19xx

Sub Code	Description	Original Budget	Balance Available	Percent Used	Feb 'xx Current	Year	Mar 'xx Current	Year	Apr 'xx Current	Year	May 'xx Current	Year
1600	Student Wages	$12,000	$ (514)	104%	$1,087	$4,979	$ 984	$5,963	$1,046	$ 7,010	$1,103	$ 8,113
1660	Accrued Salaries	0	(567)	0	21	333	76	409	(20)	389	247	636
	Salaries	12,000	(1,081)	109	1,108	5,312	1,060	6,372	1,026	7,399	1,350	8,749
2110	Medical/Surgical Supplies	100	54	46	2	2		2	2	4	5	8
2130	Drugs	0	(8)	0	2	2		2	2	2	1	3
	Medical/Surgical Supplies	100	46	54	2	4	0	4	2	6	6	12
2320	Office Supplies	500	291	42	3	70	141	211	17	228	16	244
2330	Copying and Binding	200	97	51	10	76		76		76	21	97
2340	Printing	0	(64)	0	39	40		40		40	6	46
2400	Housekeeping Supplies	0	(7)	0	2	2		2	2	4		4
2500	Maintenance Supplies	100	100	0		0		0		0		0
2700	Food Expense	0	0	0		0		0		0		0
	General Supplies	800	418	48	53	188	141	329	19	348	43	391
3110	Travel	0	(220)	0		0		0	220	220		220
3140	Local Travel	0	(245)	0		70	53	122		122	39	162
3160	Workshop and Training	0	(68)	0		68		68		68		68
	Travel/Entertainment	0	(533)	0	0	138	53	190	220	411	39	450
3230	Contract Labor	0	0	0	0	0		0		0		0
3290	Computer Software	700	340	51	279	279		279		279	102	381
3360	Equipment Maintenance/Repair	500	160	68		0	8	8	68	76		76
3370	Maintenance Contracts	1,560	312	80	1,644	1,644	84	1,728		1,728	(891)	838
3410	Equipment Rental	0	(70)	0		0		0		0		0
3650	Telephone Base	100	64	36	36	36		36		36	36	36
3660	Telephone–Long Distance	0	(4)	0		0		0	4	4		4
3720	Books and Subscriptions	0	(60)	0		0	60	60		60		60
	Other Expenses	2,860	742	74	1,644	1,959	152	2,111	72	2,183	(788)	1,395
5050	Minor Equipment (<$500)	1,500	707	53	15	465	119	584	0	584	0	584
	Minor Equipment Expenses	1,500	707	53	15	465	119	584	0	584	0	584
	Total Expenses	$17,260	$ 298	98%	$2,822	$8,065	$1,525	$9,591	$1,340	$10,931	$ 650	$11,581

132

Hospital Information Systems Budget
October 19xx–September 19xx

Sub Code	Description	Original Budget	Balance Available	Percent Used	Jun 'xx Current	Year	Jul 'xx Current	Year	Aug 'xx Current	Year	Sep 'xx Current	Year
1600	Student Wages	$12,000	$ (514)	104%	$1,019	$9,132	$1,818	$10,950	$1,564	$12,514	$ 0	$12,514
1660	Accrued Salaries	0	(567)	0	(57)	579	(325)	254	313	567		567
	Salaries	12,000	(1,081)	109	962	9,711	1,493	11,204	1,877	13,081	0	13,081
2110	Medical/Surgical Supplies	100	54	46	20	29	5	34	13	46		46
2130	Drugs	0	(8)	0	5	8		8		8		8
	Medical/Surgical Supplies	100	46	54	25	37	5	42	13	54	0	54
2320	Office Supplies	500	291	42	(54)	191	16	207	2	209		209
2330	Copying and Binding	200	97	51		97	3	100	3	103		103
2340	Printing	0	(64)	0		46	18	64		64		64
2400	Housekeeping Supplies	0	(7)	0	2	6		6	1	7		7
2500	Maintenance Supplies	100	100	0		0		0		0		0
2700	Food Expense	0	0	0		0		0		0		0
	General Supplies	800	418	48	(52)	339	37	376	6	382	0	382
3110	Travel	0	(220)	0		220		220		220		220
3140	Local Travel	0	(245)	0		162	59	220	25	245		245
3160	Workshop and Training	0	(68)	0		68		68		68		68
	Travel	0	(533)	0	0	450	59	508	25	533	0	533
3230	Travel/Entertainment	0	0	0		0		0		0	0	0
3290	Contract Labor	0	0	0		0		0		0		0
3360	Computer Software	700	340	51	75	456		456	(97)	360		360
3370	Equipment Maintenance/Repair	500	160	68	64	140		140	200	340		340
3410	Maintenance Contracts	1,560	312	80	137	975	137	1,112	137	1,249		1,249
	Equipment Rental	0	(70)	0	70	70		70		70		70
3650	Telephone Base	100	64	36		36		36		36		36
3660	Telephone—Long Distance	0	(4)	0		4		4		4		4
3720	Books and Subscriptions	0	(60)	0		60		60		60		60
	Other Expenses	2,860	742	74	346	1,741	137	1,878	240	2,118	0	2,118
5050	Minor Equipment (<$500)	1,500	707	53	209	793	0	793	0	793	0	793
	Minor Equipment Expenses	1,500	707	53	209	793	0	793	0	793	0	793
	Total Expenses	$17,260	$ 298	98%	$1,490	$13,071	$1,730	$14,801	$2,161	$16,962	$ 0	$16,962

Source: Courtesy of the University of South Alabama Medical Center, Mobile, Alabama.

EXHIBIT 4.3   Example of a Pie Graph

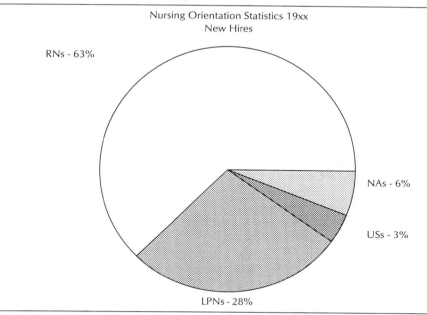

Nursing Orientation Statistics 19xx
New Hires

RNs - 63%

NAs - 6%

USs - 3%

LPNs - 28%

- Special graphics can be incorporated to enhance or highlight the content of a document.
- Document management is simplified with the linking of chapters and the automatic generation of a table of contents and index.
- Multiple documents (upwards of 750 typed pages) can be stored as compressed electronic files on a removable and transportable magnetic disk as small as 3½ inches square by 2 millimeters deep.

Word processing and desktop publishing programs have facilities for the management of multiple document styles. Styles contain formatting codes that are grouped under a single structure. When applied to a section of text or an entire document, they can save time and ensure consistency.[24] A library of styles can be created and used among different documents. Styles can establish

- font type, size, and style, such as Courier 10-point normal, *Times Roman* 12-point italic, or **Helvetica** 14-point bold
- spacing between lines and paragraphs
- margins and tabs
- page headers and footers
- footnote or outline formats
- paper size and type

Other tools often included in these programs are a spell checker, a thesaurus, and a grammar checker. The spell checker contains a dictionary to which the text can be compared; words not in the dictionary can be added to a supplement. Words spelled correctly but used incorrectly are not identified (e.g., there/their). When the dictionary is invoked, words that are not recognized are highlighted. A list of alternative words is generated along with options to replace, edit, or add the word to the supplement. The thesaurus

EXHIBIT 4.4 Example of a Bar Graph

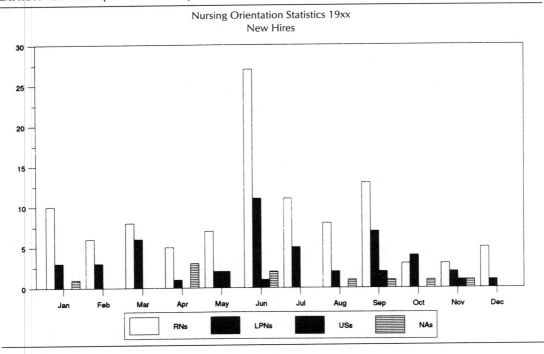

EXHIBIT 4.5 Example of a Line Graph

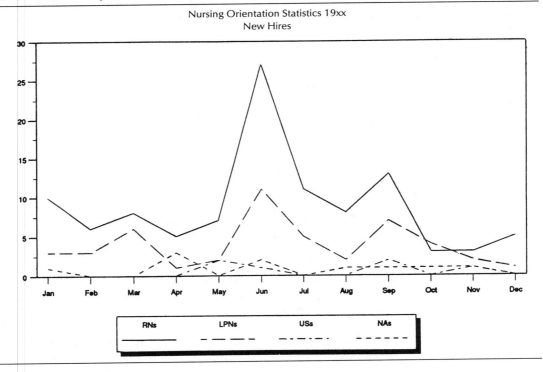

EXHIBIT 4.6   Example of a Memorandum

UNIVERSITY OF SOUTH ALABAMA
MEDICAL CENTER

HOSPITAL
INFORMATION
SYSTEMS

2451 FILLINGIM STREET
MOBILE, AL 36617
205 471 7679

September 13, 19XX

TO :   Mr. Charles Jones
               Manager, Systems Programming

FROM :   Richard J. Swansburg
               Management Systems Specialist

SUBJECT :   Changes to Microcomputer Definition on 3745 Token-Ring

Please change the information related to Mr. Sanders' host connection via the 3745 Token-Ring
network at USAMC. The old information is as follows:

Machine	Operating System	3270 Emulation	Token-Ring Address	Node I.D.	Logical Unit	Term I.D.	Home Printer	System Accesses
IBM 8590	OS/2	Communications Manager	400004012590	B1011	H47LU02	AM6G	DPPG	CICS, HOSCICS, TSO

The new information is as follows:

Machine	Operating System	3270 Emulation	Token-Ring Address	Node I.D.	Logical Unit	Term I.D.	Home Printer	System Accesses
IBM 9552	DOS	PC3270	400004012552	B1011	H47LU02	AM6G	DPPG	CICS, HOSCICS, TSO

If you have any questions, please call.

Thank you.

Source: Courtesy of the University of South Alabama Medical Center, Mobile, Alabama.

generates a list of synonyms and antonyms that can be used in place of selected words. The grammar checker is used to check the document for simple
errors of grammar and style. It will interpret the presentation of the subject
and make recommendations for improvement.

Other utilities are available for performing block functions that operate on
words, sentences, paragraphs, or pages within a document. These functions
include copying, moving, deleting, bolding, underlining, and case conversion.
Searching for and replacing particular words or phrases can be done by a simple
request. Text can be justified and words hyphenated within set margins automatically. Pages can be defined and numbered automatically also.

EXHIBIT 4.7 Example of a Policy Statement

UNIVERSITY OF SOUTH ALABAMA MEDICAL CENTER Hospital Information Systems	Approved by: Date: October 9, 19xx Page: 1 of 1

SUBJECT: Eating

Departmental employees will be allowed to eat within the department as long as the following guidelines are followed:

- All food and liquids will be consumed away from any computer equipment.
- No dishes, glasses, cups, silverware, trays, etc. will be brought out of the cafeteria. All dishes and silverware brought from home will be taken home in a timely manner.
- An appropriate trash container will be identified for the placement of all food and utensil waste disposal.
- Departmental personnel will be responsible for emptying the trash container as needed and at the end of each day.

Source: Courtesy of the University of South Alabama Medical Center, Mobile, Alabama.

Shell documents can be created where the main content of a document never changes, but some areas are reserved for text that will change each time a new document is created from it. The best examples of this are memorandums and letters, where the same memo or letter goes to many different destinations. The document and a list of variable information (e.g., dates, addressees, addresses) can actually be created separately and merged at printing time.

In nursing management there are many documents that can be managed efficiently by word processing and desktop publishing programs.

Database Management

A computer database is the electronic counterpart to the standard file cabinet and its contents. It is used to store data and can be manipulated for information much like paper files. Nurse managers could use a microcomputer and a database management program in place of a manual filing system to handle many of their information and record-keeping needs. Examples include personnel records, education records, equipment inventory, and budget management.

A microcomputer database program allows databases to be created by defining their record layouts and data fields. When a data field is defined, its length is set and the type of data that can be stored in it established. Data types can be character (allowing letters, numbers, and special symbols), numeric (allowing only numbers), logical (allowing only yes or no; true or false), or date (allowing only numbers in a date format.) See Exhibit 4.9 for an example of data fields and Exhibit 4.10 for an example of actual data entry.

Once a database is created, procedures can be established to

- create information
- modify information
- display information
- delete information
- generate printed reports

Menus can also be created to allow easy access to and execution of the procedures; see Exhibit 4.11 for an example. Most database tools have application generators that will lead the user through a series of steps to define a database, its procedures, and its menus. The greatest advantage to database management

EXHIBIT 4.8 Example of a Computer-Generated Form

19XX

SICK LEAVE

E U B

Oct
Nov
Dec
Jan
Feb
Mar
Apr
May
Jun
Jul
Aug
Sep

TOTAL TIME

Reg | OT | Sick | Spec | Code

8 Present (Enter Hrs Worked)
A Absent (No Pay)
(A) Absent on Hospital Business
S Sick (No Pay)
(S) Sick (Sick Leave Paid)
V Vacation
DO Day Off
H Holiday

HOLIDAYS

NY	MG	4TH	LD	TG	CH	PH1	PH2	PH3

VACATION

Remarks

Name ___ Last ___ First ___ Middle ___ Job Title

Address

Department | Perm/Temp | Scheduled Hrs | Department # | Social Security # | Employment Date

138

EXHIBIT 4.9   Example of Data Fields

TABLE=EMPLOYEE
******* COLUMNS *******

Column Name	Type	Length	Attributes
EMP_NAME	Character (Fixed)	30	Data required, Text
EMP_SSN	Character (Fixed)	9	Data required, Text
EMP_JOB_CODE	Character (Fixed)	1	Text
EMP_ASSIGN_NUM	Character (Fixed)	3	Text
EMP_POS_NUM	Character (Fixed)	6	Data required, Text
EMP_CLASS_CODE	Character (Fixed)	4	Text
EMP_CLASS_TITLE	Character (Fixed)	30	Text
EMP_JOB_STATUS	Character (Fixed)	2	Text
EMP_HIRE_DATE	Date		
EMP_TERM_DATE	Date		
EMP_PAY_ID	Character (Fixed)	1	Text
EMP_LIC_NO	Character (Fixed)	14	Text
EMP_LIC_REN_NO	Character (Fixed)	14	Text
EMP_LIC_DATE	Date		
EMP_LIC_EXP	Date		
EMP_LIAB_INS	Numeric	10	Integer
EMP_UNIT	Character (Fixed)	10	Text
EMP_SHIFT	Character (Fixed)	10	Text
EMP_ADDRESS_1	Character (Fixed)	30	Text
EMP_ADDRESS_2	Character (Fixed)	30	Text
EMP_CITY	Character (Fixed)	20	Text
EMP_STATE	Character (Fixed)	2	Text
EMP_ZIP	Character (Fixed)	10	Text
EMP_PHONE	Character (Fixed)	12	Text

Index Name:	EMPLOYEE
Duplicates allowed:	No
Column Name	Order

EMP_NAME	Ascending
EMP_POS_NUM	Ascending

is the ease in maintaining information and the timely retrieval of this information in report format, as illustrated in Exhibit 4.12.

Graphics

Nurse managers can realize another valuable tool through the use of graphics programs. These programs can produce graphics for presentations, illustrations, and teaching. Graphics can be printed, displayed to a monitor, or projected on to a screen for viewing by large numbers of people. They can also be converted to overhead transparencies, videotapes, slides, and other presentation aids.

In the past, graphics programs focused on the visual display of numerical data in the form of bar, line, and pie graphs. This relates to the early use of graphics by business and management. Marks emphasizes this point when listing the following advantages of computer graphics for nursing management:

- They can illustrate the whole picture concisely.
- They can display trends.
- They can summarize analysis for planning.

EXHIBIT 4.10   Example of Data Entry

Change Employee Records	

```
                Name : Swansburg, Richard J.                    SSN : 454567654
            Job Code : P              Assignment # : 008         Position # : 00132
          Class Code : 3187           Class Title : Management Systems Spec II
          Job Status : 11             Hire Date : 06-04-1979     Pay Code : A
             Address : 1110 Abilene Drive West
                       –

                City : Mobile             State : AL                  Zip : 36695
               Phone : 205 633 9172
```

EXHIBIT 4.11   Example of Database Menu

```
                              Employee Menu

          ***  Select option with mouse or type letter for underlined option.  ***
                              [Add Employee]
                         [Change/Display Employee]
                  [Change/Display Employee and Pay Period]
                             [Delete Employee]
                          [Print Employee Listing]
                     [Print Employee Pay Periods Listing]
                      [Print Selected Pay Period Listing]
```

- They can show relationships among factors.
- They can provide control information for decision making by quickly providing facts.[25]

Today graphics systems can be used in a multitude of ways to illustrate almost anything. Features have been incorporated to display graphics like a slide show or with animation. This capability can be very helpful to the nurse manager trying to present information related to various clinical subjects. See Exhibits 4.13 and 4.14 for examples.

There are a number of ways graphics can be created. They can be created as part of the program in association with some numerical data; they can be scanned by a hand-held or full-page scanner; they can be created free-hand by the user; or they can be purchased as an add-on to the graphics program.

Communications

Communications software permits nurse managers to access other computers for a variety of purposes. This may be in a dedicated manner (the link is maintained even when it is not in use) or it can be in a nondedicated manner (the link is only maintained while being used). Dedicated links can be associated with access to the organization's information systems, or with access to resources on a local area network (LAN). Nondedicated links can be associated with access to various on-line services such as bulletin boards, support services, and remote information systems.

Communications software can allow the nurse manager to support staff nurses in their interactions with information systems. The manager, when contacted about a problem, can access the system and mirror what the staff member

EXHIBIT 4.12 Example of Database Report

Employee Pay Periods Listing
Fiscal Year: 19xx–19xx

Employee Name: Swansburg, Richard J.

Pay Pd	Begin Date	Reg	OT	Hol	Vac	Sick	Other	Other	Other	Other	Vac Bal	Sick Bal	Comp Earned	Comp Taken	Comp Bal
01	09-20-19xx	78.25	–	–	–	1.75	– –	– –	– –	– –	172.58	828.39	3.00	–	78.50
02	10-04-19xx	31.00	–	–	48.00	–	1.00 181	– –	– –	– –	–	834.02	–	–	–
03	10-18-19xx	64.00	–	–	8.00	–	8.00 181	– –	– –	– –	183.04	836.72	–	–	–
04	11-01-19xx	80.00	–	–	–	–	– –	– –	– –	– –	140.28	836.10	–	–	74.50
06	11-29-19xx	80.00	–	–	–	–	8.00 181	– –	– –	– –	142.74	849.37	–	–	–
10	01-24-19xx	72.00	–	–	–	–	8.00 181	– –	– –	– –	163.66	853.89	3.00	–	–
11	02-07-19xx	80.00	–	–	–	–	– –	– –	– –	– –	168.89	848.75	–	–	81.50
12	02-21-19xx	72.00	–	8.00	–	–	– –	– –	– –	– –	174.12	852.44	–	–	–
13	03-07-19xx	80.00	–	–	–	–	– –	– –	– –	– –	179.35	856.13	–	–	81.00
14	03-21-19xx	63.50	–	–	16.00	0.50	– –	– –	– –	– –	184.58	859.82	–	–	–
15	04-04-19xx	75.50	–	–	–	3.00	1.50 181	– –	– –	– –	189.81	863.01	3.00	0.50	–
16	04-18-19xx	40.00	–	–	–	–	40.00 181	– –	– –	– –	179.04	–	–	–	81.00
17	05-02-19xx	24.00	–	–	56.00	–	– –	– –	– –	– –	–	839.40	–	–	81.00
18	05-16-19xx	72.00	–	–	8.00	–	– –	– –	– –	– –	173.51	843.09	–	–	81.00
19	05-30-19xx	80.00	–	–	–	–	– –	– –	– –	– –	122.74	846.78	–	–	–
20	06-13-19xx	56.00	–	–	24.00	–	– –	– –	– –	– –	119.97	850.47	–	–	–
21	06-27-19xx	70.00	–	8.00	–	–	2.00 181	– –	– –	– –	125.20	854.16	–	–	84.00
22	07-11-19xx	66.00	–	–	–	14.00	– –	– –	– –	– –	106.43	–	–	–	–
23	07-25-19xx	80.00	–	–	–	–	– –	– –	– –	– –	–	845.55	–	–	–
24	08-08-19xx	64.00	–	–	–	–	16.00 181	– –	– –	– –	116.90	849.24	–	–	–
25	08-22-19xx	80.00	–	–	–	–	– –	– –	– –	– –	122.13	836.93	–	–	–
26	09-05-19xx	56.00	–	8.00	16.00	–	– –	– –	– –	– –	127.37	–	–	–	–

141

EXHIBIT 4.13   Example of Presentation Graphics to Discuss the Anatomy of the Ear

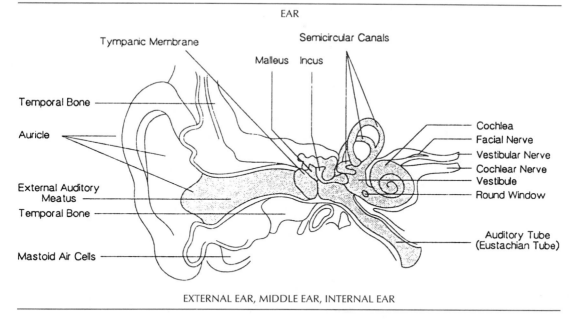

EXTERNAL EAR, MIDDLE EAR, INTERNAL EAR

is doing. The nurse manager can also use communications software to move information in the form of a file transfer. This might be to transfer data to and from the host system (mainframe or minicomputer), across a LAN, or to another microcomputer at home.

Integrated Software

Integrated programs seek to combine word processing, spreadsheets, database management, graphics, and communications. This integration allows information to be readily moved among the components. A report being created in the word processor can draw a table of numbers from the spreadsheet, a graph from the graphics component, and other information from a database.[26] This document can then be sent to another location via the communications component.

This integration can simplify preparation and analysis of information. However, these programs tend to lack the full functionality of programs in the individual components' domains. The standard programs of today also provide excellent import and export facilities to most of the popular software in other areas.

Information Systems

Nurse managers are beginning to find that the demands of working with automation in nursing can be great. Managers may be asked to interact with specialized and generalized nursing information systems, as well as hospital information systems.

EXHIBIT 4.14   Example of Presentation Graphics to Discuss the Anatomy of the Eye

EYE

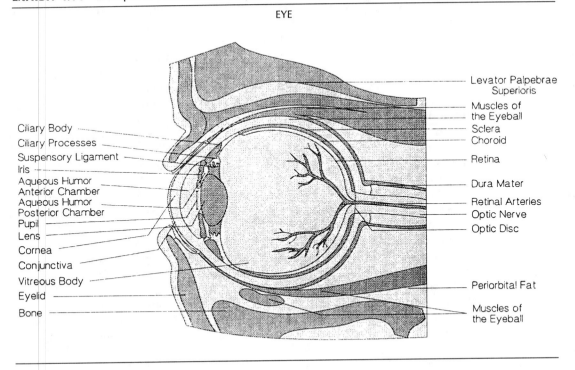

Nursing Information Systems

Nursing information systems are software packages developed specifically to serve the needs of nursing. These programs may be explicit to a particular area of nursing application, or they may be general to the support of the nursing services division. Examples of nursing areas that benefit from unique information systems support include mental health, neonatology, acute care, urology, enterostomal therapy, oncology, maternity, operating room, and infection control.

General nursing information systems have multiple programs, or modules, which are used to perform various clinical, educational, and managerial functions. Most nursing information systems have modules for patient classification, staffing, scheduling, personnel management, and report generation. Other modules may be included such as budget development, resource allocation and cost control, case mix and DRG analysis, quality management, staff development, modeling and simulation for decision making, strategic planning, short-term demands for forecasting and work planning, and program evaluation.

Modules for patient classification, staffing, scheduling, personnel management, and report generation are often interrelated. Patients are classified according to established acuity criteria. The patient-classification information is input to the staffing module, and staffing levels are calculated according to various workload formulas. Also, actual staffing is input and a comparison of census, patient acuity, needed staffing, and actual staffing can be made. Schedules are then prepared using the information from the staffing and personnel records modules.

Quality management and DRG analysis are done to associate patient acuity, quality of care, and DRG. This is helpful for establishing future guidelines and care needs for patients according to their DRGs. The budget is also supported by the census, patient acuity, and needed staffing patterns. This information is invaluable to support requests for additional full- and part-time employees. The report generation module allows all of the stored information to be retrieved and output in a timely and presentable manner.

Nursing information systems can be used to make patient care more effective and economical. Clinical components include patient history and assessment, nursing care plans, nursing progress notes and charting, patient monitoring, order entry and results reporting, patient education, and discharge planning. This can all be done at the nurse's station or, with more progressive systems, from the patient's bedside.

Clinical nurses can use the nursing information system to replace manual systems of data recording. This may reduce costs while permitting improved quality of care as well as quality of work life. Clinical nurses can collect and input clinical data and use the computer to analyze it to formulate treatment plans. They can use quantitative decision analysis to support clinical judgements. Automated consultation can be applied to screen for adverse drug reactions, interactions, and preparation of correct dosages. Computers can be programmed to reject orders that could cause problems in these and other areas, thus preventing errors.[27]

Curtin reminds nurses to provide "high touch" in this inhuman "high-tech" world. Technology, computers, and information systems provide the knowledge to save lives or prolong them. Nurses can return control over their lives to patients and families who have lost their freedom of action or become unable to understand. Nurses can keep control of cybernetics through the exercise of human compassion.[28] High-tech includes the new scientific knowledge of microelectronics, computers, sensors, processors, displays, and education. Its object is the solution of society's total problems, not just those of health care including nursing.[29] Helping nurses provide high touch while using high-tech should be a primary goal of nurse managers.

Hospital Information Systems

Hospital information systems are large, complex computer systems designed to help communicate and manage the information needs of a hospital. They are tools for interdepartmental and intradepartmental use. A hospital information system usually has applications for admissions, medical records, accounting, business services, nursing, laboratory, radiology, pharmacy, central supply, nutrition services, personnel, and payroll. Numerous other applications can exist for any department and for practically any purpose.

Admissions applications include patient scheduling, preadmission, admissions, discharges, transfers, and census procedures. Some medical records applications include master patient-index maintenance, abstracting (diagnosis/procedure/DRG coding), transcription and correspondence, and medical record locator procedures. Business and accounting procedures include patient insurance verification, billing, billing follow-up, billing inquiry, accounts payable, accounts receivable, cash processing, and service master and third-party maintenance.

EXHIBIT 4.15 Management Plan Worksheet

OBJECTIVE: Implement an information system

Activities	Target Dates	Person(s) Responsible	Accomplishments

Assessment
  Make strategic plan
  including a budget
	Sept. 1–15	Swansburg and other
		team members	

Planning	Oct. 1–Nov. 15	Swansburg and other team members	
Implementation	Jan. 1 _____	Swansburg and key users	
Evaluation (simultaneous)	Jan. 1 _____	Swansburg and key users	

Applications in other areas such as nursing (the nursing information system), laboratory, radiology, pharmacy, and central supply may be so voluminous and complex that they have their own information systems. These systems stand alone and run independently of the hospital information system, but are usually interfaced for information transfer.

Hospital information systems tend to be developed with mainframe and minicomputers in mind, although the trend today seems to be towards downsizing and distributed data networks. The advantages and disadvantages of each strategy should be weighed prior to implementation of an information system. Selection, development, and implementation of information systems can take years. This time varies depending on the system and the complexity of its applications. It may actually be a continuous process. The initial cost can be millions of dollars for the hardware and software. Continued yearly maintenance is required and can cost hundreds of thousands or even millions of dollars.

Implementation of Information Systems

Nurse managers should be involved in the implementation and development of information systems and the direction of their users. Implementation of an information system requires preparation of a management plan. See Exhibit 4.15. The first step is to form an implementation committee to assess the current system and what is wanted out of the proposed system. This assessment should lead to a strategic plan, which is necessary because acquiring an information system requires expenditure of a large amount of human, material, and financial resources. It includes provision for continuous updates, a characteristic of a service economy in the information age.

Assessment

The study team that makes the assessment should include information systems personnel, nurse mangers, nurse educators, clinical nurses, human resource personnel, and ancillary personnel from other departments who will be exposed to the system. They can use many references and techniques to gather data for assessment. Sources of data include liaison with the information systems department, visits to businesses, industries, and other nursing

departments, professional consultants, in-house resources, and phone banks, conferences, and seminars.[30]

Information systems have to be modeled for the organization and the personnel who will use them. When nurses are not involved in developing these systems, then the systems do not make a major impact on clinical decision making nor do they meet nursing's needs. Therefore, each phase of the development process benefits from nursing input.[31]

The assessment team must work within the capital investment policies and procedures of the institution, because procurement of hardware falls within the realm of the capital budget. Thus, time schedules and budget procedures are important. The team looks at the management style of the organization because the information system they recommend or purchase will reflect centralization or decentralization of control. If there is a desire to increase decentralization and participatory management, development of the information system can be used to facilitate these processes.

Availability of space for hardware, personnel, and supplies is determined. Determination of external environmental influences is assessed. Does the information systems department or higher corporate entity affect information systems development? In one hospital the mainframe computer was physically located and controlled by the university's computer center, thus placing many restrictions on the information systems. The assessment team analyzes types of systems available, including hardware and software.

Once a thorough assessment is completed, the formal findings are presented to top management and interested others for analysis and approval. The assessment team can be converted to a planning team or a new one can be formed. There should be some uniformity. This is achieved in many organizations by a full-time nursing information systems specialist whose job is to coordinate the activities of nursing information systems.

Planning

The second major step in implementing an information system is development of the specific management plan. The plan should include objectives, resources needed, communication strategy, a phase-in schedule, a budget that includes operating costs, identification of savings, benefits, and possible revenues, and an evaluation plan. The management plan should be concrete and in writing.

To support the information system's objectives, the team identifies the system requirements. They can obtain and evaluate sample requests for proposals (RFPs) from vendors. Criteria for a specific system are recommended.

Security should be considered during this phase. Provision must be made for confidentiality of records. An aspect often overlooked is the protection of software copyright. In this information age we transact intangible property as opposed to tangible property—information business versus manufacturing business. It is difficult to retain control of the property of computer information. As McKenzie-Sanders foresaw, some software is now safeguarded by law; other programs are given away as a promotion, thus eliminating the need for safeguards.[32]

The information systems plan should provide for computer downtime. How will critical functions be managed when the computer is down? Procedures and

forms need to be developed to capture and manipulate information during periods of downtime. Also, this information will have to be input to the computer when it is up and running again.

The completed plan is presented to top management for approval. They will coordinate it with the policies and procedures required for approval of capital expenditures, which usually includes action by the board of trustees. With final approval the information system is selected and purchased, sometimes through a bidding system that may keep the cost down. Another option proposes that the system be totally developed in-house. Careful planning of the system avoids waste; information systems are expensive.

Implementation

The nursing information systems specialist coordinates the implementation of the information system with involvement of nurse users throughout the total project. This process builds users' trust and confidence. This person works with the implementation team, which includes the key users. The team should keep track of nurses' attitudes toward implementation of computer systems.

Nurse managers can work with nurse educators and the nursing information systems specialist to develop a curriculum for educating nurses in computer use. The organization provides a comfortable setting for nurses to make the best use of computers.[33]

Implementation of the information system can be done using the principles of planned change. The nursing information systems specialist can be the change agent. Peers influence others to learn. A teaching plan should be developed. Audiovisuals, computer terminals, and a system-specific manual are used for training. Formal teaching sessions should be provided, with the staff being allowed to leave their stations for uninterrupted training. A pilot unit can be selected and used. Resource personnel (to include staff development educators, nurse managers, staff nurses, etc.) should be available on all shifts for assistance.[34]

Vendors frequently provide training in use of hardware and software. In addition, there are self-directed training programs.

Evaluation

A predetermined evaluation plan that includes Gantt charts or a similar controlling process is best for keeping the plan on target. Questionnaires, surveys, interviews, observations, and quality circles can be used to evaluate user acceptance and achievement of objectives. Feedback from these sources can be used to modify the information system.

Even after the initial implementation of an information system, education is a continuous need. New capabilities are developed and added and staff turn over. This educational need requires dedicated resources, including a special classroom designed to include the computer hardware that mimics what is used in the work environments. Hardware may be computer terminals, microcomputers, and printers. It should also include a big-screen projector.

Software should include a training system that mirrors the real system—complete with nursing stations, patients, and physicians.[35] Some type of multimedia software should also be available for presentation to the big screen. Last but not

least, there is a requirement for resource personnel. For larger institutions there should be at least two nurse liaisons for automation. It has been advocated that all management and staff development personnel be cross-trained for this area because automation affects all areas of nursing. The overall coordinator for computer direction should be the nursing information systems specialist.

Nurse managers and staff development educators must develop effective and efficient training programs for a diverse nursing staff using diverse information systems. As Axford states,

> Established principles of teaching and learning are as applicable to computer training as to any other teaching–learning setting. Specifically, effective computer training will accommodate individual variation in learning styles. Sound computer training addresses the cognitive, affective, and psychomotor aspects of the learning tasks. Adult learning principles are as important in computer training as they are in any continuing professional education endeavor.[36]

Applications for Nursing Management

There are many applications for nurse managers. In addition to those associated with the use of general-purpose microcomputer software, other applications include a calendar of events, an employee database management system, and the use of interactive multimedia for staff and employee education.

A calendar can be useful in supplying clinical staff with dates and times of staff meetings, committee meetings, and educational events. See Exhibit 4.16 for an example. Educational events would include continuing education, annual reviews, and patient education. Information for the calendar can even be provided from the employee database.

An employee database management system can be an effective method of collecting and reporting nursing staff credentialing, special skills, and educational development. See Exhibits 4.9 and 4.17 for examples of database field definitions. Access to this information can identify employees' participation in education and those with special skills or credentials. It can also identify employees facing deadlines for credentialing renewal and those who need additional training. See Exhibit 4.18 for an example of an employee education report. This information can also meet the reporting needs of the institution as to the requirements of the state board of nursing and the Joint Commission on Accreditation of Healthcare Organizations. Education components may include

- new employee orientation
- clinical specialty courses
- continuing education offerings
- competency validation of skills
- nursing station in-service education
- annual required reviews[37]

The development and implementation of this employee information system can follow the assessment, planning, implementation, and evaluation cycle.

Interactive multimedia is the educational media of tomorrow. It has the capability to solve the problems related to education today.[38] It mixes multiple media sources to provide interaction with the user. This method of instruction

EXHIBIT 4.16 Example of a Staff Development Calendar

Staff Development Calendar
October 19XX

Monday	Tuesday	Wednesday	Thursday	Friday
				1
4 Nursing Orientation Begins 8:00 AM Room 324 Nursing Assistant Course Intake/Output 7:30 - 8:30 AM 7:30 - 8:30 PM Room 334	**5** RN's and LPN's Understanding ECGs 7:30 - 8:30 AM 7:30 - 8:30 PM Room 334	**6** Diabetes Management Class 2:30 - 3:30 PM Room 334	**7** Diabetes Nutrition Class 2:30 - 3:30 PM Room 334	**8** RN's and LPN's Antibiotic Therapy 7:30 - 8:30 AM 7:30 - 8:30 PM Room 334
11 Nursing Assistant Course Body Mechanics 7:30 - 8:30 AM 7:30 - 8:30 PM Room 334	**12** RN's and LPN's Basic Genetics 7:30 - 8:30 AM 7:30 - 8:30 PM Room 334	**13**	**14**	**15** RN's and LPN's Understanding ECGs 7:30 - 8:30 AM 7:30 - 8:30 PM Room 334
18 ACLS Class Begins 8:00 AM Room 324 Nursing Assistant Course Intake/Output 7:30 - 8:30 AM 7:30 - 8:30 PM Room 334	**19** Annual Education Day Fire and Safety 8:00 - 11:30 AM Room 344 CPR 1:00 - 3:30 PM Room 354	**20** Diabetes Management Class 2:30 - 3:30 PM Room 334	**21** RN's and LPN's Antibiotic Therapy 7:30 - 8:30 AM 7:30 - 8:30 PM Room 334 Diabetes Nutrition Class 2:30 - 3:30 PM Room 334	**22**
25 Nursing Assistant Course Body Mechanics 7:30 - 8:30 AM 7:30 - 8:30 PM Room 334	**26**	**27** RN's and LPN's Basic Genetics 7:30 - 8:30 AM 7:30 - 8:30 PM Room 334	**28**	**29**

Source: Courtesy of the University of South Alabama Medical Center, Mobile, Alabama.

EXHIBIT 4.17   Example of Educational Course Data Fields

TABLE=EDCOURSE

****** COLUMNS ******

Column Name	Type	Length	Attributes
EDCOU_CODE	Character (Fixed)	6	Data required, Text
EDCOU_DESC	Character (Fixed)	35	Data required, Text
EDCOU_TYPE	Character (Fixed)	6	Data required, Text
EDCOU_CLAS_HRS	Numeric	5	Integer
EDCOU_CLIN_HRS	Numeric	5	Integer
EDCOU_CONT_HRS	Numeric	5	Integer

Index Name:	EDTYPE
Duplicates allowed:	No
Column Name	Order

EDCO_TYPE	Ascending
EDCO_CODE	Ascending

TABLE=EMCOURSE

******COLUMNS******

Column Name	Type	Length	Attributes
EMCOU_CODE	Character (Fixed)	6	Data required, Text
EMCOU_POS_NUM	Character (Fixed)	6	Data required, Text
EMCOU_COMP_DATE	Date		
EMCOU_EVAL_CODE	Character (Fixed)	2	Text

Index Name:	EMPOS
Duplicates Allowed:	No
Column Name	Order

EMCOU_POS_NUM	Ascending

provides flexibility, independence for learners, reinforcement, and feedback. Students are able to control the presentation of content. They can work the program in any order, and segments can be selected and repeated as desired. The program provides students immediate, individualized feedback based on their answers to the program's questions.[39]

The development and authoring of an interactive program involves a number of steps, the first of which is the determination of the content of the instructional program. The second relates to the preparation of a script for the video components of the program. Next a flowchart is constructed to direct the authoring process. See Exhibit 4.19 for an example flowchart. Finally, the computer programming is done using a software package developed specifically for interaction.[40] These programs are commonly called *authoring systems*.

The implications for applications using this technology appear to be unlimited.

Curriculum and Careers

It would appear that the time to start educating nurses about automation is while they are in school, beginning at the undergraduate level by integrating

EXHIBIT 4.18   Example of Employee Education Record

EMPLOYEE EDUCATION RECORD

Employee Name : Jones, Mary L
Position Number : 353367
Nursing Unit : Med/Surg

Course Type	Description	Date Complete	Eval Code	Class Hours	Clinical Hours	Contact Hours
C	Antibiotic Therapy	10/08/9x	S			1.0
	Basic Genetics	10/12/9x	S			1.0
	Subtotal Continuing Education					2.0
I	Patient Monitoring	10/06/9x	S	4.0		
	Infusion Pumps	10/06/9x	S	1.0		
	Subtotal Inservice Education			5.0		
O	Personnel	10/04/9x	S	2.0		
	Fire and Safety	10/04/9x	S	3.0		
	Infection Control	10/04/9x	S	3.0		
	Legal Issues	10/05/9x	S	4.0		
	CPR	10/05/9x	S	4.0		
	Information Systems	10/07/9x	S	8.0		
	Unit Orientation	11/05/9x	S		136.0	
	Subtotal Orientation			24.0	136.0	
S	IV Certification	10/08/9x	S	3.0		
	Subtotal Skills Competency			3.0		
	Totals			32.0	136.0	2.0

Source: Courtesy of the University of South Alabama Medical Center, Mobile, Alabama.

informatics into the curriculum. Student nurses could take an introductory course in computer fundamentals, a course in the use of microcomputers and general-purpose software for enhancing personal productivity. There will be advanced incorporation of the computer into clinical education. These two courses could be integrated into nursing courses and clinical experience.

A practical environment can be created with bedside terminals linked to a hospital's or vendor's training system. The desire is to create a realistic effect by simulating an automated nursing station like those in hospitals today. Students can use the system to practice order entry, nursing assessments, care planning, and charting. They can learn how to combine "high-touch" care with high-tech efficiency.[41]

This curriculum can even be taken a step further by collecting, analyzing, and organizing actual patient data into a clinical nursing abstract. Students can be taught nursing content based on information from actual practice. For a particular diagnosis, students can study its interventions and outcomes. Assessment data can be accessed to examine etiologies, signs, symptoms, related medical diagnoses, and medical therapies.[42]

Today there are several graduate programs with curriculums for advanced degrees in nursing informatics. They are designed to provide specialized education to nurses interested in pursuing careers as nurse engineers, nursing information systems specialists, or systems nurses. These curriculums should

EXHIBIT 4.19   Example of a Flowchart

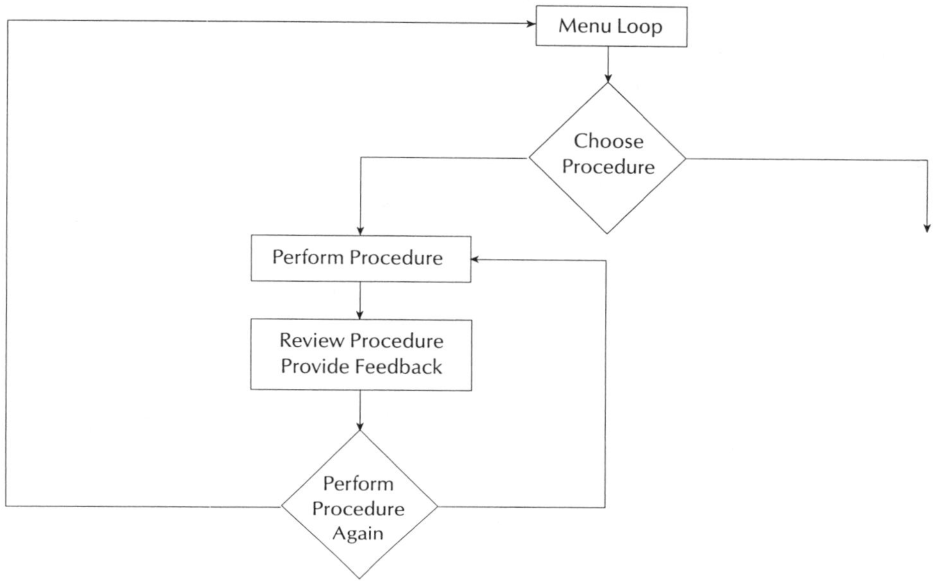

Source: Courtesy of the University of South Alabama Medical Center, Mobile, Alabama.

utilize an interdisciplinary approach. Courses would combine the study of nursing with theoretical and practical foundations of management and information sciences.[43]

A Human Resources Information System

The management of human resources can be a formidable task for today's health-care organizations. The collection and manipulation of information associated with this management can require significant time and personnel in itself. The development and implementation of a human resources information system can be a blessing to the organization and the professionals who manage these resources. See Exhibit 4.20 for an example of a human resources system model.

A couple of front-end systems can be established to analyze information related to all of the job applicants who apply to the organization, and to analyze information related to the advertising and recruitment of these applicants. Some information needs to be retained about everyone who applies for any employment position. This information can be useful for understanding the professional market. There are also concerns about equal opportunity regardless of race, disability, sex, age, creed, and such. The applications analysis system can show how many people apply for a position by these indicators. See Exhibit 4.21 for an example report. The advertising analysis system can provide recruitment information related to the method and placement of advertisements. See Exhibit 4.22 for an example report.

EXHIBIT 4.20   A Human Resources Information System Model

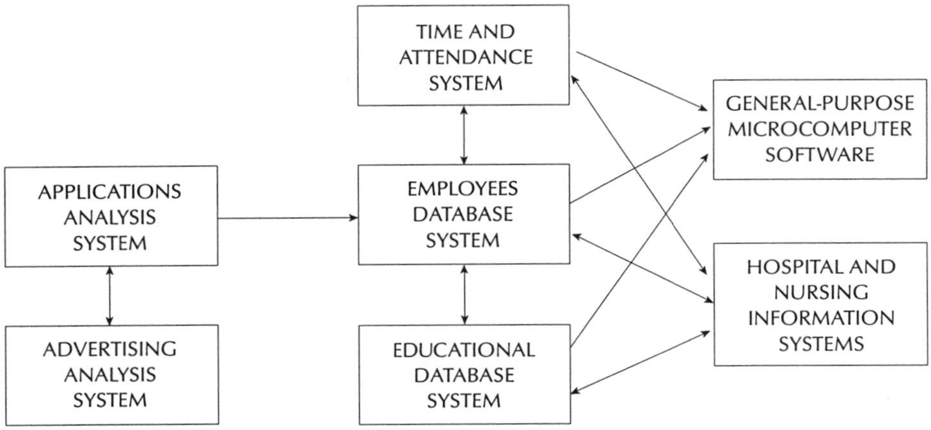

Source: Courtesy of the University of South Alabama Medical Center, Mobile, Alabama.

The central foundation of the human resources system is the employees database system. Information about applicants who are hired can be pulled from the applications analysis system and added to the employees system. This system maintains all of the relevant information related to employees and their positions from the moment they are hired until they are terminated. See Exhibit 4.23 for an example of information placed on an ID card, and Exhibit 4.24 for an example of a termination list. This part of the human resources system will be the basis for integrating additional components such as an educational database system and a time and attendance system.

The educational system maintains all of the information associated with the education of employees. See Exhibit 4.18 for an example. The time and attendance system maintains the information associated with employees' work, vacation, holiday, and sick time. The information here produces timesheets. See Exhibit 4.25 for an example. From these systems information can be exported and imported to the hospital and nursing information systems. It can also be exported to general-purpose microcomputer software for various purposes.

Forecasting

Forecasting in its broadest meaning tries to describe the probable future, anticipating the impact of present decisions or actions on future activities of nursing. Forecasting uses simple techniques such as graphs and hand calculators. It also uses complicated mathematical models that can be developed using desktop computer software packages. Development of mathematical equations that can be used to fit and balance relationships between and among variables is termed *modeling*. Forecasting uses models. Managers decide which variables

EXHIBIT 4.21 An Applications Analysis Report

Applications Analysis Report
for the month of
August 19xx

	POSITION	F	M	AM	AS	BA	CA	HI	PI	DIS	VET	DIS VET
01412	REGISTERED NURSE	3	0	0	0	2	1	0	0	0	0	0
02456	REGISTERED NURSE	2	0	0	0	1	1	0	0	0	0	0
02457	REGISTERED NURSE	6	2	0	1	2	4	1	0	0	0	0
11923	LICENSED PRACTICAL NURSE	7	0	0	0	5	2	0	0	0	0	0
15934	ASSISTANT ADMINISTRATOR	3	12	0	0	0	15	0	0	0	0	0
22921	UNIT SECRETARY	11	1	0	1	8	3	0	0	1	0	0
23110	EDUCATION SPECIALIST	5	2	0	0	2	5	0	0	0	1	0

Source: Courtesy of the University of South Alabama Medical Center, Mobile, Alabama.

EXHIBIT 4.22 An Advertisement Analysis Report

Advertisement Analysis Report
for the month of
August 19xx

ADD NUM	PLACEMENT	DATE	RN	LPN	PHR	PT	RT	CLK	MGR	OTH
1622	CHANNELS 4, 11	08/06/xx	3	2	0	0	1	0	0	5
1734	NEWSPAPER	08/08/xx	1	1	1	0	0	1	0	3
1622	CHANNELS 4, 11	08/13/xx	0	3	0	1	0	1	1	1
1734	NEWSPAPER	08/15/xx	5	0	0	0	1	3	0	2
1432	NEWSPAPER	08/15/xx	0	0	2	0	0	0	0	0
1622	CHANNELS 4, 11	08/20/xx	3	3	0	0	0	2	0	7
1734	NEWSPAPER	08/22/xx	8	3	0	2	3	0	1	3
1622	CHANNELS 4, 11	08/27/xx	0	1	1	0	0	1	0	1
1734	NEWSPAPER	08/29/xx	3	5	0	0	2	8	2	3

Source: Courtesy of the University of South Alabama Medical Center, Mobile, Alabama.

EXHIBIT 4.23 An Employee ID Badge

9/XX
Expiration Date

RICHARD J. SWANSBURG
Name

MGMT SYSTEMS SPECIALIST
Title

HOSPITAL INFO SYSTEMS
Department

SWANSBURG, RICHARD J.

to include and the form of models. In management there are budget models, inventory models, production process models, cash-flow models, models for workforce planning, models of distribution systems, linear programming resource allocation models, and many others.

Trends extrapolation forecasting describes the probable future by projecting the systematic pattern of change (increase or decrease) using the prevailing tendencies of a time series. *Trend impact analysis* is a method of analyzing the impact or consequences of the pattern of change (increase or decrease) over time. An example would be the effect of an increased acuity level of patients over a one-year period of operational costs, use of resources, cash flow, and other elements of budgeting.

In budgeting, forecasting is the predicting or estimating of the revenue and expenses of a cost center or group of cost centers. One could say budgeting is one form of forecasting. Forecasting is expressed in units of some kind such as cases or time. It requires the data of historical trends, changes in provider staff (particularly physicians), and new or deleted programs.[44]

Spreadsheets and databases are the tools of forecasting. Although spreadsheets are excellent for calculating numbers, databases are more efficient for manipulating data containing numerous logical relationships. Databases allow the user to add or edit information by filling in blank fields or changing existing information.[45]

Many internal and external factors affect forecasting including demographics, government policies, technology, and changes in care modalities. Cumulative data improves the accuracy of forecasting.[46]

EXHIBIT 4.24   An Employee Termination List

| | | Employee Termination List
for the month of
August 19xx | | |
POSITION	NAME	TITLE	DATE	REASON
00356	Burkett, Mary J.	Registered Nurse	08/26/xx	Q
10234	Walker, Helen M.	Licensed Practical Nurse	08/08/xx	Q
16212	McGaw, Janet K.	Registered Nurse	08/13/xx	F
17335	Fox, Donald M.	Registered Nurse	08/05/xx	Q
17336	Rios, Carolyn S.	Registered Nurse	08/22/xx	R
18549	Crouse, Melanie J.	Unit Secretary	08/01/xx	Q
18675	Felan, Marcus K.	Respiratory Therapist	08/29/xx	Q

Source: Courtesy of the University of South Alabama Medical Center, Mobile, Alabama.

Variance

Variance is a statistical term used to indicate the difference between expected results and actual results. In budgeting variance tells the manager that results are greater or less than predicted. Variance is expressed in raw numbers, percentages, and formulas. Variances can be programmed into the spreadsheet so as to be automatically reported. For each subcode of Exhibit 1.10 a formula that subtracts the percentage used from the percentage of fiscal year elapsed is the variance percentage. A similar formula could be used for the totals of the subcode groups so that subtracting the actual fiscal year amounts from the revised budgets amounts would provide the various amounts in dollars. Similarly forecasting models could be developed to predict revenue and expense by months and then provide the variances as they occur. Thus historical data is provided to revise forecasts and budgets. Similar data could be derived to compare monthly variances due to seasonal fluctuations of the budget. This kind of forecasting and use of variance leads to more precise budgeting and provides managers the information to make better decisions.

In budgeting variance occurs in the workload or volume, examples being more or fewer procedures, cases, tests, and other outputs. Price variances occur in purchases of supplies and equipment as well as utilities and other costs of doing business. Quantity variances relate to the numbers of resources required to perform a procedure or test, or to do a case. The resources may be supplies, equipment, utilities, and other items.[47]

Variances are categorized as acuity-volume, price-rate, and quality-use variances. A model for the acuity-volume variance would indicate the average dollar amount of supplies (or personnel or other) per category of patient. Differences between the average or predicted and the actual are variances.[48]

Profits are a positive variance; losses a negative one. Both can be expressed in dollars or percentages. Properly programmed computers process huge amounts of data quickly and economically, which leads to more accurate forecasting as well as to better modeling.[49]

Spreadsheets must be programmed to provide a specific model or template. One can be designed to calculate all budgeting activities including flexible budget variances. They can be converted into tables and graphics for visual display.[50]

EXHIBIT 4.25 An Employee Timesheet

Employee Timesheet Report
10/04/xx 07:40

Employee : 424345543 Cole, Mary   Department : 51134 Medical/Surgical

DAY	DATE	IN	OUT	HOURS	DEPT	SCHED	REG	OT	HOL	VAC	SIC	OTHER	BREAK	TOT
SUN	09/19/xx	0700	1535	8.58		1	8.00						.50	8.00
MON	09/20/xx	0703	1537	8.57		1	8.00						.50	8.00
TUE	09/21/xx													
WED	09/22/xx	0659	1531	8.53		1	8.00						.50	8.00
THU	09/23/xx	0701	1523	8.37		1	8.00						.50	8.00
FRI	09/24/xx	0707	1528	8.35		1	8.00						.50	8.00
SAT	09/25/xx													
SUN	09/26/xx													
MON	09/27/xx	0655	1537	8.70		1	8.00						.50	8.00
TUE	09/28/xx	0706	1529	8.38		1	8.00						.50	8.00
WED	09/29/xx	0659	1529	8.50		1	8.00						.50	8.00
THU	09/30/xx	0701	1525	8.40		1	8.00						.50	8.00
FRI	10/01/xx													
SAT	10/02/xx	0707	1535	8.47		1	8.00						.50	8.00
	Totals						80.00	0.00	0.00	0.00	0.00	0.00	5.00	80.00

Source: Courtesy of the University of South Alabama Medical Center, Mobile, Alabama.

Future Trends

Trends for the future include totally automated medical records, voice interaction, expert systems, artificial intelligence, and the increased use of optical disks and robotics. The thought of a paperless medical record or budget sounds interesting and is probably possible today. It would allow immediate and complete access to patient information from many locations. The use of voice interaction will eliminate the barriers associated with data entry.[51] Expert systems and artificial intelligence will enhance the process of clinical decision making. Robotics are already being used in surgery for the positioning of surgical instruments, in labs for the transport and placement of samples, and in nursing for the delivery of supplies and medications. These trends will continue.

Other trends indicate information technology that is becoming easier to use and with greater end-user responsibility. Software is fast becoming more graphical and user friendly. Almost all software today has on-line help and is menu-driven. This means users only have to select what they want to do from a list of items on the screen, and if a problem is encountered help is only a keystroke or mouse click away. Many software development programs have instructions that are almost English-like. What used to take weeks and months to program can now be done in days or weeks.

Users are becoming more involved in designing applications and handling most things themselves. Expanded user involvement will occur as users become more knowledgeable about computer hardware and software. Software will continue to become easier for users to manipulate, and software vendors will provide greater technical support. The best examples are already evident in laboratory, pharmacy, central supply, and nursing information systems, where very little help is involved from information systems personnel.

Robotics

Robots will assist nurses in performing numerous tasks. The most practical use of robotics is in electronic carts, which are used to store and transport drugs, linens, and other supplies. These carts can be remote-controlled and can actually follow predefined routes along the floor. Another example is robotic arms, which can do heavy lifting. Robotics seems destined for procedures that humans are unable to perform such as delicate, microscopic eye, brain, or spinal surgeries; or procedures where direct contact is contraindicated due to health hazards, such as a patient with no immune system or exposure to toxic chemicals or radioactive elements.

Voice Communication and Optical Disks

Voice communication will allow nurses to talk to their computers. Keyboards and bar code readers will not be needed to enter or retrieve information. The computer will be requested to retrieve information or to record it by voice command. Optical disks will revolutionize information storage with their ability to store many times as much information in the same space as on current storage media. Microcomputers today use removable floppy diskettes for limited information storage and nonremovable hard disks for volume

information storage. New optical laser disks will be removable and the same size as floppy diskettes, but will store many times as much information as a hard disk.

Conversant computers are widely used in industry. They tell airline baggage handlers which conveyor to put bags on and bank customers their account balances. Conversant computers can identify product deficiencies during manufacturing. They can maintain supply inventories, recording the voice print and processing a spoken reply. They are used to move cameras on spacecraft and to turn on lights and roll up windows on cars. With use of conversant computers, productivity on assembly lines has increased by 25 to 40 percent. Speaker-dependent machines use voice prints, so they must be programmed with the user's voice. Speaker-independent machines can understand any speaker. At present, voice communication is not 100 percent accurate. Even though computers have hardware to support voice technology, there is still little software available. Users have not responded well to computer-synthesized voices.[52]

Expert Systems and Artificial Intelligence

Other future trends in software are expert systems and artificial intelligence (AI). Expert systems exist today. Nurses have access to a huge quantity of information that can assist them in making everyday decisions. With expert systems, the nurse identifies the problem, the criteria defining the problem, and objectives for handling the situation. The expert system evaluates the information and provides a list of alternative ways to manage the situation. The nurse then evaluates the alternatives and makes decisions.

Expert systems encode the relevant knowledge and experience of experts to make it available to less knowledgeable and less experienced persons. An example would be to take the total knowledge and experience of clinical nurse specialists in neuroscience nursing, encode it in a computer program, and make it available to clinical nurses working in the neuroscience area. They would consult it to solve nursing-care problems. Similarly, expert systems can be developed for nursing budgeting.

Expert systems encode specialized knowledge including rules and product descriptions to solve difficult problems by supporting human reasoning. They use symbolic reasoning and perform above the level of competence of nonexpert humans. They use heuristic techniques rather than algorithms to provide good answers, but they do not always reach the optimum ones. Heuristic programs use rules of thumb to search through alternative solutions to problems.[53]

Expert systems are software products that combine sophisticated representational and computing techniques with expert knowledge. Eventually they will support nursing decision making. Although they are not widely used, their use will increase as regional computer systems are established with extensive nursing and medical databases to link clinical nurse specialists, educators, managers, and researchers.

An example of a nursing expert system is MANAGER. It is being applied to planning and control of the nursing staff at a regional hospital in Toulouse, France. MANAGER uses three categories of managerial activities as a decision

taxonomy: strategic planning, management control, and operational control. This expert system "provides decision makers with an ordered set of plausible solutions." Twelve rules are used to control possible nurse transfers among departments. This is one activity of the expert system MANAGER applied to nursing management.[54]

Expert support systems are a further development of expert systems. They are software programs using specialized symbolic reasoning to help nurses solve difficult problems. These support systems pair humans with expert systems.[55]

With artificial intelligence the machine is actually capable of "thinking" and acting on its own. The difference between artificial intelligence and an expert system is the fact that the machine with artificial intelligence would proceed to make the decision for handling the situation. In nurse staffing, for example, with an expert system the nurse manager would describe the situation and the machine would supply alternatives for handling the staff. With artificial intelligence, the machine could continuously monitor the patients' needs and manage staffing without human intervention. Some individuals do not believe artificial intelligence is possible and at best it appears to be some years away.

Artificial intelligence attempts to develop ideas into computer operations duplicating human intelligence. Such systems use quantitative and qualitative data. Artificial intelligence is being used in robotics, the understanding of natural language, and expert systems.[56]

The industry is now capable of building computerized information systems to appeal simultaneously to the right and left sides of the brain. People share many judgements or assumptions and few symbolic numbers (symbols representing numbers and having a widely perceived meaning) and beliefs. They store facts, use them with a conceptual framework to connect them, and then identify them with a particular problem. The conceptual framework is called a *schema, cognitive map,* or *conceptual model.*

Conceptual models are compared to external physical representations by individuals such as artists or engineers. They change perceived differences in one or both. People compare their conceptual models by sending them to others. Each influences the other.

Conceptual models are created to solve organizational problems by identifying root causes. Market forces determine prices and quality of service. The Advocate Conceptualization/Communication/Creativity Support System can be used as a technological tool to manage communications and satisfy stakeholders. This concept will accelerate the corporate change to a systems worldview. It will provide the linking corporate language. Ultimately health care will use these systems.[57]

Summary

Nursing can expect almost anything from computers, but should not expect everything. There should not be concern that somebody else is using state-of-the-art equipment and software, because if it really is state of the art and beneficial, everyone will soon be using it.

The intent of this chapter is to provide an overview of nursing and computers. The computer is a necessary information-handling tool, and most people feel the impact of it on their daily lives. In fact, the computer is now a necessity in managing the complex financial structure of today's health care.

Computers are used to support and run highly complex information systems that have tremendous capabilities for manipulation and storage of information. Almost any nursing application can be implemented through an information system. There are systems that assist nursing in patient-care documentation, order processing, clinical decision making, and patient and professional education.

Other general-purpose microcomputer software is also available to enhance personal productivity. Nurses have needs for document preparation, number crunching, and record keeping. Nurse managers should find graphics, multimedia, and communications software invaluable tools for presentations and educational support.

In the future more and more will be accomplished through computers. All nurses will have to be able to interact with these machines. Nurse managers are finding themselves in crucial positions. Nursing schools are incorporating the use of the computer into the nursing curriculum. New positions are being developed for nurses in computer education and support.

The computer has come of age. These machines are tools that already assist most of us in performing numerous tasks. They are excellent for the management of all types of information.

Experiential Exercises

1. Do a survey to identify the computer applications used during each of the three phases of budgeting.
   - Which applications originate in the business office?
   - Which applications originate at nursing division level?
   - Which applications originate at nursing unit level?
   - Which of the computer applications supply information to users? How is the information used?
2. Do a literature search to identify the status of expert systems in nursing management.
3. Identify the availability of software systems applicable to budgeting including those for staffing, scheduling, productivity, and management of human resources, supplies, and equipment.

Notes

1. F. R. Vlasses. "Computerized Documentation Systems: Blessings or Curse?" *Orthopaedic Nursing* (Jan.-Feb. 1993):51-52.
2. S. W. White. "The Universal Computer." *National Forum* (Summer 1991):2.
3. R. L. Axford. "Implementation of Nursing Computer Systems, A New Challenge for Staff Development Departments." *Journal of Nursing Staff Development* (Summer 1988):125-130.
4. *Webster's New World Dictionary of the American Language* (New York, NY: Simon and Schuster, 1979).

5. C. A. Romano. "Preparing Nurses for the Development and Implementation of Information Systems." NLN Publication 14-2234 (New York: National League for Nursing, 1988):83-92.

6. B. R. Heller, C. A. Romano, L. R. Moray, and C. A. Gassert. "The Implementation of the First Graduate Program in Nursing Informatics." *Computers in Nursing* (Sep.-Oct. 1989):209-213.

7. B. Nadel. "The Cyrix Plan: Catch Up, Then Lead." *PC Magazine* (Apr. 27, 1993):126.

8. J. Rothfeder. "Is Big Iron Good for You." *Beyond Computing* (May-June 1993):24-27.

9. K. Andreoli and L. A. Musser. "Computers in Nursing Care: The State of the Art." *Nursing Outlook* (Jan.-Feb. 1985):16-25.

10. "Swords Speak in First Interactive Multimedia Novel." *San Antonio Light* (Oct. 19, 1992):E8.

11. C. M. Boston. "Justifying Costs for Continuing Education Departments." *Nursing Economics* (Mar.-Apr. 1986):83-85.

12. R. L. Axford, op. cit.

13. C. Buszta. "Conquering Computer Phobia: Advice from Someone Who Did It." *RN* (Dec. 1989):57.

14. C. T. Barry and L. K. Gibbons. "Information Systems Technology: Barriers and Challenges to Implementation." *The Journal of Nursing Administration* (Feb. 1990):40-42.

15. K. Abbott. "Student Nurses' Conceptions of Computer Use in Hospitals." *Computers in Nursing* (Mar.-Apr. 1993):78-89.

16. C. A. Romano. "Privacy, Confidentiality, and Security of Computerized Systems." *Computers in Nursing* (May-June 1987):99–104.

17. L. K. Woolery. "Professional Standards and Ethical Dilemmas in Nursing Information Systems." *The Journal of Nursing Administration* (Oct. 1990):50-53.

18. P. Iyer. "Computer Charting: Minimizing Legal Risks." *Nursing* (May 1993):86.

19. E. A. Sorrentino. "Overcoming Barriers to Automation." *Nursing Forum* (Mar. 1991):21-23.

20. R. Spitzer-Lehmann. "Recruitment and Retention of Our Greatest Asset." *Nursing Administration Quarterly* (Summer 1990):66-69.

21. M. G. Adamski and B. R. Hagen. "Using Technology to Create a Professional Environment for Recruitment and Retention." *Nursing Administration Quarterly* (Summer 1990):32-37.

22. P. P. Garre. "A Computerized Recruitment Program." *The Journal of Nursing Administration* (Jan. 1990):24-27.

23. M. J. Schank and L. D. Doney. "General-Purpose Microcomputer Software: New Tools for Nursing Professionals." *Nursing Management* (July 1987):26-28.

24. *WordPerfect Version 5.2 Reference.* (Orem, Utah: WordPerfect Corporation, 1993):541.

25. F. E. Marks. "Computer Graphics for Nursing Managers." *Nursing Management* (July 1984):19-20, 22-23, 25-26.

26. S. A. Finkler. "Microcomputers in Nursing Administration, A Software Overview." *The Journal of Nursing Administration* (Apr. 1985):18-23.

27. H. W. Gottinger. "Computers in Hospital Care: A Qualitative Assessment." *Human Systems Management* (Fall 1984):324-345.

28. L. Curtin. "Nursing: High Touch in a High-Tech World." *Nursing Management* (July 1984):7-8.

29. P. McKenzie-Sanders. "The Central Focus of the Information Age." *Business Quarterly* (Winter 1983):87-91.

30. L. J. McCarthy. "Taking Charge of Computerization." *Nursing Management* (July 1985):35-36, 38, 40.

31. M. F. Hendrickson. "The Nurse Engineer: A Way to Better Nursing Information Systems." *Computers in Nursing* (Mar.-Apr. 1993):67-71.

32. P. McKenzie-Sanders, op. cit.

33. S. Krampf and S. Robinson. "Managing Nurses' Attitudes Toward Computers." *Nursing Management* (July 1984):29, 32-34.
34. C. Hanson, C. R. Menkiena, and E. Meterko. "Successful Implementation of an Automated Nurse-Information System, Staff Development's Role." *Journal of Nursing Staff Development* (Sep.-Oct. 1990):229-232.
35. P. Boykin and C. Romano. "Decision: Education." *Computers in Nursing* (Mar.-Apr. 1985):70-73.
36. R. L. Axford, op. cit.
37. J. E. Robinette and P. S. Weitzel. "Design and Development of a Computerized Education Records System." *The Journal of Continuing Education in Nursing* (July-Aug. 1989):174-182.
38. M. Rogers. "MTV, IBM, Tennyson and You." *Newsweek Special Issue* (Fall-Winter 1990):50-52.
39. A. R. Redland and C. Kilmon. "Interactive Video, Rational and Practicalities of One Experience." *Computers in Nursing* (Mar.-Apr 1986):68–72.
40. M. A. Sweeney and C. Gulino. "From Variables to Videodiscs, Interactive Video in the Clinical Setting." *Computers in Nursing* (Aug. 1988):157-163.
41. R. L. Simpson. "Closing the Gap between School and Service." *Nursing Management* (Nov. 1990):16-17.
42. J. C. McCloskey. "The Nursing Minimum Data Set: Benefits and Implications for Nurse Educators." NLN Publication 41-2199 (New York: National League for Nursing, 1988):119-126.
43. C. A. Romano and B. R. Heller. "Nursing Informatics: A Model Curriculum for an Emerging Role." *Nurse Educator* (Mar.-Apr. 1990):16-19.
44. S. Klann. "Mastering the OR Budgeting Process Is Key to Success." *OR Manager* (Oct. 1989):10-11.
45. S. F. Schrader. "Labor Budgeting." *AORN Journal* (Apr. 1993):925-927.
46. M. C. Corley and B. E. Satterwhite. "Forecasting Ambulatory Clinic Workload to Facilitate Budgeting." *Nursing Economics* (Mar.-Apr. 1993):77-81, 114.
47. G. R. Whitman. "Analyzing and Forecasting Budgets." In *Management Issues in Critical Care*, C. Birdsall (St. Louis, Mo: Mosby, 1991):287-308.
48. P. D. Francisco. "Flexible Budgeting and Variance Analysis." *Nursing Management* (Nov. 1989):40-43.
49. H. Koontz and H. Weihrich. *Essentials of Management* 5th. ed. (New York: McGraw-Hill, 1990):428-433.
50. S. A. Finkler. "Variance Analysis Part II, Use of Computers." *Journal of Nursing Administration* (Sep. 1991):9-15.
51. L. Lancaster. "Nursing Information Systems in the Year 2000: Another Perspective." *Computers in Nursing* (Jan.-Feb. 1993):3-5.
52. N. Madlin. "Conversant Computers." *Management Review* (Apr. 1986):59-60.
53. F. L. Luconi, T. W. Malone, and M. S. Scott Morton. "Expert Systems: The Next Challenge for Managers." *Sloan Management Review* (Summer 1986):3-14.
54. C. J. Ernst. "A Relational Expert System for Nursing Management Control." *Human Systems Management* (Fall 1984):286-293.
55. F. L. Luconi, T. W. Malone, and M. S. Scott Morton, op. cit.
56. Ibid.
57. L. C. Charalambides. "Systematic Organizational Communications." *Human Systems Management* (Apr. 1985):309-321.

Appendix 4.1   Glossary of Computer Terms

ABEND: Abnormal end of task.

Algorithm: A prescribed set of rules for the solution of a problem in a finite number of steps.

Artificial intelligence: The capability of a machine to proceed or perform functions that are normally concerned with human intelligence, such as learning, adapting, reasoning, self-correction, automatic improvement.

Authoring: A structured approach to combining all the media elements in an interactive production.

Authoring systems: Software that integrates the multimedia components of an interactive production. To include the computer, CD-ROM, sound, and so on.

Bar code reader: An optical scanning unit that can read documents encoded in a special bar code. A laser scanner.

Batch processing: A systems approach to processing that calls for similar input items to be grouped for processing during the same machine run.

Binary: (1) The number system based on the number 2, and (2) pertaining to a choice or condition where there are two possibilities.

Bit: The smallest unit of data, a binary digit of 0 or 1.

Buffer: Intermediate storage, used in input/output operations to temporarily hold information.

Bug: A mistake or error in a computer program.

Byte: A set of eight adjoining bits thought of as a unit.

Cache: A storage buffer that contains frequently accessed instructions and data.

Central processing unit (CPU): The part of the computer that contains the circuits that calculate and perform logical decisions based on a set of instructions.

Character: A letter, digit, or other symbol used as part of the representation of data. A byte.

Compact disk (CD): A type of disk storage that uses magnetic optical recording and lasers.

CRT (cathode ray tube): Cathode ray terminal. A display terminal used as an input/output station.

Data: Representation of information in a form suitable for processing.

Database: A collection of files or tables.

Disk: A round, flat medium that is rotated in order to read or write data.

DOS: Disk operating system.

Downtime: The elapsed time when a computer is not available for use, may be scheduled for maintenance, or unscheduled because of machine or program problems.

Expert systems: Systems that rely on large amounts of information to provide assistance in decision making.

Field: A unit of information within a record.

File: A collection of related data with a given structure.

Forecasting: Describing the possible future, anticipating the impact of present decisions or actions on future activities of nursing. Forecasting uses simple techniques, such as graphs and hand calculators, and complicated mathematical models that can be developed using desktop computer software packages.

GUI (graphical user interface): Graphical software that allows you to interact with and perform operations on a computer.

Hard copy: Printed computer output: reports, lists, documents.

Hardware: The physical computer equipment.

Hospital Information System (HIS): A system designed to facilitate the day-to-day needs of a hospital; a system that stores and manipulates information for interhospital communication and support.

Input/Output (I/O): The transfer of data between an external source and internal storage.

Interface: The point at which independent systems or computers interact.

Key field: A field within a record that makes that record unique with respect to other records in a file.

Kilobyte: 1,024 bytes or characters.

Laser scanner: A type of device that uses a laser to recognize and receive input.

Local area network (LAN): Two or more computers connected for local resource sharing.

Mainframe computer: A large computer capable of being used and interacted with by hundreds of users seemingly simultaneously.

Management Information System (MIS): A system designed to manipulate information to assist in management decision making.

Megabyte (MB): Approximately 1,000,000 bytes.

Microcomputer: A small computer built around a microprocessor.

Minicomputer: A medium-sized computer, smaller than a mainframe but larger than a microcomputer.

Modeling: Development of mathematical equations that can be used to fit and balance relationships

between or among variables. Forecasting uses models. Managers decide which variables to include and the form of the model. In management there are budget models, inventory models, production process models, cash-flow models, models for workforce planning, models of distribution systems, linear programming resource allocation models, and many others.

Modem: A device that converts digital data from a computer to an analog signal that can be transmitted on a telecommunications line and that converts received analog transmissions to digital data.

Multimedia: The combination of different elements of media such as text, graphics, audio, video, animation, and sound.

Multitasking: A mode of operation that provides for concurrent performance of two or more tasks.

Number crunching: A process of taking numbers and performing mathematical functions on them.

Nursing Management Information System (NMIS): A type of information system geared towards assisting nurse managers in performing their management functions.

On-line processing: A form of input processing whereby information is input and updated at that time.

Operating system: An organized collection of techniques and procedures combined into programs that direct a computer's operation.

Optical disk: A compact disk.

Printer: A terminal or peripheral that produces hard copy or printed output.

Program: A set of computer instructions directing the computer to perform some operation.

Random access: A storage technique whereby a record can be addressed and accessed directly at its location in the file.

Record: A group of related fields of information treated as a unit.

Robotics: Machines that work automatically and perform physical movements.

Scenario projection: Use of a scenario, or set of planning assumptions, to describe and plan for the possible future state of the environment at a point in time and considering the economic, political, social, technological, and natural effects. Scenario projections use trends and trend analysis.

Sequential access: A storage technique whereby a record can be addressed and accessed only after all those before it have been.

Simulation forecasting: Risk analysis, a procedure that mimics possible or probable business conditions to describe the possible future of each. Simulations stress model structure.

Software: A program or set of programs written to tell the computer hardware how to do something.

Spreadsheet: A specialized type of software for manipulation of numbers.

Table: A collection of related data with a given structure.

Trend: Systematic pattern of change (increase or decrease) over time based on history or a particular theory. *Example:* an increase in the acuity level of patients over a one-year period.

Trend impact analysis: Analysis of the impact or consequences of the pattern of change (increase or decrease) over time. *Example:* How will the increased acuity level of patients over a one-year period affect operational costs, use of resources, cash flow, and so on?

Trend line: A straight line fitted to a graph plotting trends in a time series. It shows the pattern of change (increase or decrease) over time.

Trends extrapolation forecasting: Describing the possible future by projecting the systematic pattern of change (increase or decrease) using the prevailing tendencies of a time series.

User-friendly (software): Easy to use because of menus and help facilities.

Voice communication: Interaction with a computer by its recognition of human voice.

Word processing: The manipulation of words within documents by a computer.

Word processor: A specialized type of software for manipulation of printed material.

5

Variance Analysis

Linda Roussel, R.N., D.S.N.

> *Improve quality (and) you automatically improve productivity. You capture the market with lower price and better quality. You stay in business and you provide jobs. It's so simple.*
>
> W. Edwards Deming[1]

Budgeting involves establishing a financial plan for operating a unit, department, and organization. Such a plan is formalized and quantified. The budget makes tangible the organization's mission, purpose, and service objectives. As a management tool, the budget generally compares expected revenues to expected expenses in order to determine the organization's expected financial results. Such a tool uses quantified plans to control operations, otherwise the process becomes an act in futility.

Sophisticated budgets have become cornerstones to organizational management because the need to control costs is critical to sound financial management. Controlling costs has become a directive secondary to limited governmental resources, continuation of quality services, and in many cases survival of the organization. Budgeting affords the nurse manager the ability to plan for the resources needed to run a quality operation. Should a budget not provide such a framework to control costs during the year, resources may be squandered and quality diminished. Budgeting provides one tool, one plan in which limited resources and quality standards form the backdrop for the organization's continued financial success and quality improvement. Analyzing and investigating deviations or variances from the expected financial outcomes to the actual results yields essential data. Specifically, such comparative data allow the nurse manager the opportunity to determine causative factors of the variances. It is through the process of variance analysis

and discovery that changes can be made and growth becomes possible. With quality management as a framework and variance analysis as a statistical tool, improvement may be realized.

What Is Variance Analysis?

Variance analysis is the aspect of the budgeting process by which actual financial results are compared to anticipated budgetary outcomes. An investigation generally follows to determine causative factors relative to the variances.[2] A variance describes the difference between the experienced result and the planned result, that is, the quantified result that varies from the budget. Variance analysis is an integral component of budgeting and the quality management process.

Joiner and Gaudard describe variation as a central theme in Deming's work. Variances in data, figures, performance, and outcomes alert the manager to recognizing, analyzing, and responding to such variations. Basics about variation include the following: (1) all variation is caused; (2) common, special, tampering, and structural are four main types of causes; (3) understanding each type of cause is essential to appropriate managerial action; (4) timely data is imperative to intervening when special causes occur; (5) common cause variations are more complex and require in-depth knowledge of the process or system being improved; basic statistical tools such as flowcharts, cause-and-effect diagrams, stratification analysis, and Pareto analysis are cornerstones of this understanding; (6) a system is said to be in statistical control when all variation is due to common causes; and (7) statistical calculations on process data determine the degree of system variation present within an organization.[3]

The Language Is Statistics

Variation

Deming advocated the use of the language of statistics to identify which problems are caused by workers and which by the system. The most used statistical tool is that of variation. The results indicate when an activity is in statistical control or the degree of variation. Statistics are used to control variation by teaching workers to work more intelligently. The common language of statistics stimulates discussion between workers and bosses at quality circle meetings.[4] Variation is the concept that distinguishes normal routine changes in a process from unusual, abnormal changes that can be attributed to specific causes. Variations in performance are mostly attributable to the system. Deming, in examples, found 400 percent variation in performance attributable to the system.[5]

According to Deming, Shewhart, and others, there are chance causes and special or assigned causes of variation. Chance causes are common causes that are the fault of the system. Chance or common causes are ever-present system variations, such as process input or conditions. They cause small, random shifts

in output daily. They occur in 85 to 90 percent of cases and require fundamental system change by managers who must search them out. Chance causes are controlled causes. A system in which variation is totally influenced by controlled or common (chance) causes is said to be in statistical control.

In budgeting, an example of a controlled variation resulting from a common or chance cause could be selection of a product that costs less than anticipated due to a low bid being accepted by management. As a result of the product turning out to be inferior, thus increasing waste, personnel use more and increase costs to a point above the upper limits of variation.

A special or assigned cause is specific to a group of workers, an area, or a machine. It is uncontrolled variation due to assignable causes or sources. Special causes occur in 10 to 15 percent of cases. They require finding the source and then preventive action by the local workforce. Special causes require obtaining timely data to effect changes that will prevent bad causes and keep good causes happening. An example of an uncontrolled variation in budgeting resulting from a special cause could be decreased costs due to personnel modifying procedures and eliminating wastage of supplies. The resultant variance is below the lower limits of variation. In this instance variation and its causes are both good. See Exhibit 5.1.

Management by action uses the Deming (Shewhart) cycle. See Exhibit 5.2. It should be kept in constant motion and used at all levels of the organization. Reports should conform to the new system.[6] Training in statistical process control (SPC) takes the guesswork out of what is really happening in the operation. SPC aims to prevent errors by identifying where they occur. The process is then tightened to improve the outcome. In looking at safety systems, Smith indicated that 85 to 90 percent of problems have common causes (system) while only 10 to 15 percent of problems have special causes (employees). Using control charts to determine whether the causes of accidents are common or special leads to development of methods to prevent accidents. Employees can then set goals to reduce the special causes.[7]

Variation is a part of everything—of the supplies used by nurses, of employee performance, and of many other activities. In addition to common and special causes, there are others. One is tampering or making unnecessary adjustments to compensate for common cause variation. Another is structural variation caused by seasonal patterns and long-term trends.[8]

Deming purports that improving quality increases productivity and can be accomplished through statistical process control (SPC) techniques. Such techniques use statistical analyses to monitor process performance with the goal of anticipating and preventing quality problems. A basic principle of SPC is that processes produce variation in output. Using SPC techniques, the nurse manager determines whether the variation is due to normal or abnormal causes. Once statistically controlled, managers are able to shift the process average closer to the desired level. Control charts for attributes and variables are developed and alert the manager of times to intervene and remove abnormal causes and times to leave the process alone. Budgets that are out of control, that have abnormal variances, indicate possible problems with quality or productivity or both. Understanding variance analysis gives the nurse manager an essential tool for financial planning and operational management.

EXHIBIT 5.1   Assigning Responsibility for Variation

Type of Variation	Frequency of Occurrence	Characteristic	Action Needed	Responsibility
Common cause	High (> 90%)	Fault of the system	Fundamental system change	Management
Special cause	Low (< 10%)	Traceable to an assignable cause	Find the source and take preventive measures	Local workforce

Source: Reprinted with permission from A. E. Francis and J. M. Gerwels. "Building a Better Budget." *Quality Progress* (October 1989):71.

Uses and Justification

Finkler and Kovner describe three principal reasons for calculating variance: improving accuracy in future budgeting, eliminating unfavorable variances over the coming months, and determining performance evaluation of units or departments and their managers.[9]

Basic to variance analysis in the budgeting process is understanding the costs of quality. Kirk contends that avoidable costs of quality are the losses experienced when a quality product or service is not delivered and the organization continues to pay the price. Such costs may include rework, lost business or reputation, and malpractice. Necessary costs of quality include the dollars spent to design and implement a good system and include continuous quality assurance, quality control, and quality improvement. Kirk further purports that systematic support is essential to a total quality organization. Systematic methods ensure conformity to desired standards or norms. "Organization-wide systems must support this effort: the strategic planning system, performance management system, measurement system, budgetary system, and management information system. Otherwise, we will work against ourselves."[10]

Variance reports are often given to nurse managers for justification. The focus from this perspective is on the evaluative role of variance analysis instead of on planning and control. Such requirements set up a defensive posture instead of trying to understand the reasons for the variance and thus preventing more problems. Analyzing or investigating the variance is the goal in explaining why the variance occurred. Variances can illuminate actual costs in excess of budget, however, they cannot determine if such resulted from quality-of-care improvements or ineffective work practices. For example, if variances arose as a result of defective equipment, a system error, then the process of providing cost-effective care although in statistical control may create variance of increased costs if not identified and corrected immediately. By discovering the downtime of such equipment, actions can be taken to eliminate these occurrences and bring the process back under cost control. Future costs will be lower if the investigation led to replacing or repairing the defective equipment, thereby alerting personnel to the need for equipment that consistently works. Additionally, such information may lead to further understanding of vendor relationships, purchasing responsibilities, employees' decision-making abilities in repairing or replacing faulty equipment, and other such occurrences in the process. Improvement comes from using the information to control outcomes. Placing blame on others who failed to control results becomes futile in the quality management process when managers understand variance analysis.[11]

EXHIBIT 5.2 The Deming (Shewhart) Cycle

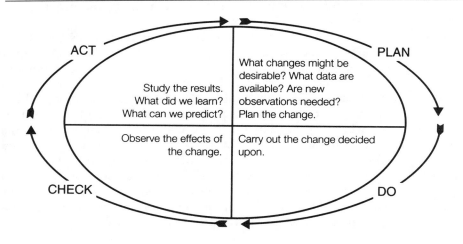

Source: Reprinted with permission from A. E. Francis and J. M. Gerwels. "Building a Better Budget." *Quality Progress* (October 1989):73.

Causes of Variances

Internal or external causes may contribute to variances within an organization. Internal causes include technological advances, organizational policy, changes in quality-of-care standards, shifts in regulatory or licensure standards, and inefficient health-care practices. Variances attributable to external causes may include unexpected shifts in availability of staff, limitations in supplies and equipment, and price changes for products.[12]

Deming's point 4 of his quality management model purports eliminating the variance relative to suppliers. In essence, Deming believes that ending the practice of awarding business on price tag alone is critical; total cost can be minimized by working with a single supplier. Two primary motivating factors behind this principle include quality improvement and cost reduction. Specifically, variation in purchasing costs results from downtime, service, warranty, process adjustment to accommodate incoming product variability, scrap and rework, administration, and damage to an organization's reputation with its customers due to unsatisfactory performance of the product. Key potential benefits of adhering to point 4 include single sourcing, reduced supplier base, and longer-term relationships.[13] Eliminating variance at any and all levels of organizational operation is key to quality control and effective financial management.

Application in Quality Management

Quality Improvement—Deming's Model

W. Edwards Deming is considered by many to be the pioneer in quality management. Overall philosophy of management and specific statistical techniques

to evaluate and improve quality are major aspects of Deming's approach. The overarching goals are to improve productivity and provide a quality product or service.[14]

Deming's theory of management includes 14 points. See Exhibit 5.3. Deming's model outlines seven deadly diseases, which he believes decrease productivity and profitability along with destroying employee morale. See Exhibit 5.4. Deming insists on quantitative data reporting which indicates that quality and productivity can only be assessed, controlled, and improved by the appropriate use of statistical techniques. Understanding and pinpointing problems can only be ascertained by the interpretation of objective data via statistical methods. Deming perceives a systems approach in which people, methods, material, and equipment together produce the product or service. Additionally, Deming supports going beyond the organization to include suppliers, dealers, engineers, marketing and sales people, and managers as vital links to the organization's increased productivity and success. Deming envisions SPC application at any stage in the process, or to the entire process.[15]

Variation from a Quality Management Perspective

Sustained improvement in productivity cannot be achieved without consideration of management theory and statistical processes. Quantitative data are necessary and can only be assessed, controlled, and improved by appropriate use of statistical methodology. Deming conveys two major sources of variations both in tangible products and services: normal and abnormal. Normal variations are a myriad of naturally occurring, extraneous, and unsystematic factors existing in the system. Such variations are considered normal causes or chance happenings often occurring randomly in the process. Mainstone and Levi describe a partial list of such factors in the output that include inconsistency in raw materials, poorly trained staff, unreliable equipment, and poor product design.[16]

Abnormal variations refer to the occurrence of unusual, nonrandom factors that alter the system's performance and outcomes. Such unusual, episodic incidents cause significant deviations from the modal outcome. "Abnormal variation generally arises on an irregular basis and influences only some of the product. A broken tool or an inappropriate adjustment are examples of factors that produce abnormal variations."[17] In most cases, abnormal variations can be corrected in order to bring the process back into statistical control. Identifying the reasons for such occurrences and eliminating them are methods used to put the system back in order.

Normal causes of variation do not disrupt the normal distribution curve; the system remains statistically in control. "Statistical control is not a natural condition for a process. It must be achieved by eliminating the special causes in the process."[18] Eliminating common causes allows for the random, yet predictable variations. Statistical control is a major goal of managers because an unstable process cannot be improved. Systematic control affords the manager opportunities to shift the process average closer to the desired level, or reduce the amount of normal variation in the system.[19]

EXHIBIT 5.3 Deming's 14 Points

1. Create constancy of purpose toward improvement of product and service. Everyone should have a clear goal every day, month after month. Satisfy the customer and reduce variation so all employees do not have to constantly shift their priorities.
2. Adopt a new philosophy by learning how to improve systems in the presence of variation, thus reducing variation in materials, people, processes, and products. End tampering and overreacting to variation.
3. Cease dependence on inspection to achieve quality by thoroughly understanding the sources of variation in processes and working to reduce variation.
4. End the practice of awarding business on the basis of price tag alone. Instead, minimize total cost by working with a single supplier.
5. Improve constantly and forever every process for planning, production, and service. Everyone uses PDCA (plan-do-check-act) cycle.
6. Institute training on the job. Know methods of performing tasks and standardize training. Accommodate variation in ways people learn.
7. Adopt and institute leadership. Work to help employees do their jobs better and with less effort. Learn which employees are within the system and which are not. Support company goals, focus on internal and external customers, coach, and nurture pride in workmanship.

8. Drive out fear, including fear of reprisal, fear of failure, fear of providing information, fear of not knowing, fear of giving up control, and fear of change. Fear makes accurate data nonexistent.
9. Break down barriers among staff areas, between departments. Promote cooperation. What is the constant, common goal?
10. Eliminate slogans, exhortations, and targets for the workforce. Improvement requires changed methods and processes. Leaders change the system.
11. Eliminate numerical quotas for the workforce and numerical goals for management. All people do not work at the same level of speed. There will be variation. Use realistic production standards. Eliminate management by objectives and use a system that rewards people's efforts toward improvement.
12. Remove barriers that rob people of pride of workmanship. Eliminate the annual rating or merit system.
13. Institute a vigorous program of education and self-improvement for everyone. This can be any education that improves self-esteem and potential to contribute to improvements in existing processes and advances in technology.
14. Put everyone in the company to work to accomplish the transformation.

Note: Deming rejected the concept of TQM, saying it was undefined.

Source: Reprinted from *Out of the Crisis* by W. Edwards Deming by permission of MIT and The W. Edwards Deming Institute. Published by MIT, Center for Advanced Engineering Study, Cambridge, Mass. 02139. Copyright © 1986 by The W. Edwards Deming Institute.

Mainstone and Levi describe the deleterious consequences of failing to distinguish normal from abnormal variations. Tampering with normal, random causes of variation often leads to increased variability, higher costs, and increased frustration as employees and managers continue to unsuccessfully "fix" the system. Second, random occurrences may be attributed to the worker rather than the factors built into the system; the employee may be erroneously reprimanded or rewarded for outcomes beyond his or her control. Behavior is thereby reinforced by action that is both unfair and self-defeating.[20] Thus performance appraisal systems based on Deming's logic would include three ratings: within the system, outside the system on the high side, and outside the system on the low side.[21] See Exhibit 5.5. This method of appraisal makes the assumption that almost all employees are in the system. Dissatisfaction with the average level of performance or spread of distribution requires that managers remove performance barriers and change the system. Distinguishing normal from abnormal variations in the budgetary system has much to do with performance systems, management systems, and financial systems.

EXHIBIT 5.4   Deming's Seven Deadly Diseases

1. Lack of constancy of purpose
2. Emphasis on short-term profits
3. Evaluation of performance, merit rating, or annual review
4. Management by use of only visible figures
5. Mobility of management
6. Excessive medical costs
7. Excessive costs of liability

Source: Reprinted from *Out of the Crisis* by W. Edwards Deming by permission of MIT and The W. Edwards Deming Institute. Published by MIT, Center for Advanced Engineering Study, Cambridge, Mass. 02139. Copyright © 1986 by The W. Edwards Deming Institute.

Control Charts

Data Analysis

Quality is not just another passing fad. Just as business and industry have the high quality to compete in international markets, the U.S. health-care industry's institution of quality management (QM) at every level of the process will support its expansion to provide at least an affordable safety net for all citizens. Deming states that quality must be defined and employees trained to deliver quality products and services. According to Deming we should "measure the variations in a process in order to pinpoint the causes of poor quality and then how to gradually reduce those variations."[22]

Quality control should be on-line rather than end-line. This is achieved by sampling products during the process to determine the right course to correct variations if the product deviates from the acceptable range. Quality improves as variability decreases.[23]

Statistical charts are used to plot variations from the ideal in the production process and determine the right course to correct identified variations.

Pareto charts are one example of control charts. The Pareto principle states that most effects come from relatively few causes. Eighty percent of rework costs due to quality come from 20 percent of the possible causes. The Pareto principle is one of the most powerful decision tools available. Among the data that can be plotted on Pareto charts for nursing services are wasted time, number of jobs that have to be redone, customer inquiries, and number of errors, accidents, incidents, infections, and complications.[24] See Exhibit 5.6.

When constructing a Pareto diagram, place the most frequent cause on the left and arrange in descending order of occurrence. The impact on the system becomes obvious, as does the priority for fixing it. A double Pareto diagram can be used to contrast two areas; an example would be the use of flexible work shifts for before and after improvement. One must recognize which data are useful. Group consensus should be taken to identify important causes and problems. Nominal group technique may be used:

1. Give each person ten 3" × 5" cards.
2. Have each person write problems and causes on cards, one for each card.

EXHIBIT 5.5 Distribution of Employee Skills

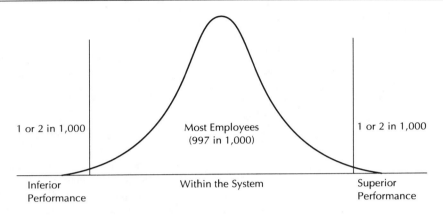

Source: Gitlow, H. S., and Gitlow, S. H. *The Deming Guide to Quality and Competitive Position.* © 1987, p. 123. Reprinted by permission of Prentice-Hall, Upper Saddle River, New Jersey.

3. Have each person rate causes by importance (from 10 = most important to 1 = least important)
4. Compile numbers for each cause.
5. Construct a Pareto chart.[25]

Pareto charts can be used to plot reasons that nurses leave an agency. Reasons can be constructed using the National Commission on Nursing report or a career book, and exit interviews.

Calculating system variations on process data allows control limits to be set, with variations being expected in the process due to aggregate common causes. Data can be plotted on a graph to show upper control limits (UCL) and lower control limits (LCL). If all points fall within these lines, and variations are due to common causes, one should not tamper. See Exhibit 5.7.

It is common but wrong to treat all causes of variance as special and to tamper. Plot all data on control charts, including performance appraisals. Performance appraisals are often based on a system of common cause variation. Plotting data reveals who performs at a level outside the system—above (UCL) or below (LCL) the control limits. Learn what causes an employee to perform outside the system (below) and correct the cause by fixing the system. Dispense with praise and blame sessions. Study the performance appraisal system, find the special causes, and prevent them from recurring. If all causes are common causes, study ways to improve the variation in the system so that all employees improve. Remember to remove such barriers to pride of work as annual or merit ratings. Instead, provide leadership to reduce upstream variation.[26]

Cohen describes seven basic teamwork tools used in quality function development (QFD) at Digital Equipment Corporation (DEC) as a structural method for planning. They are

1. scatter diagram
2. histogram
3. check sheet

EXHIBIT 5.6   Generalized Pareto Diagram

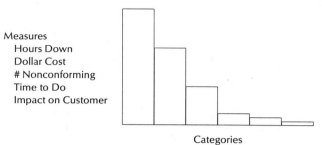

Measures
    Hours Down
    Dollar Cost
    # Nonconforming
    Time to Do
    Impact on Customer

Categories
Causes, products, manufacturing lines, operators,
administrative areas, equipment, cost centers

Source: J. T. Burr. Center for Quality and Applied Statistics, Rochester
Institute of Technology, One Lomb Memorial Dr., P. O. Box 9887,
Rochester, NY 14623-0887. Reprinted with permission.

4. Pareto diagram
5. run chart
6. control chart
7. cause-and-effect diagram

These are problem-solving tools as contrasted to physical tools. Teams use
them to solve problems of past events through data analysis, cause-and-effect
analysis, and process management. In nursing, QFD could prepare a structured
list of a patient's needs (nursing diagnosis) and evaluate each proposed service
and function (nursing prescription) according to the impact it has in meeting
this patient's needs. Physical tools are technology-based. They include spreadsheet programs, electronic calculators, telephones, word-processing software,
and all the materials needed to give nursing care to patients. Physical tools do
not solve problems.[27]

Fishbone analysis is also used in conjunction with Pareto analysis, although
they may be used separately. It has been successfully used at the Rotor Clip
Company of Somerset, New Jersey, as a problem-solving technique as follows:

1. Involve all employees having knowledge of the problem/product/service.
2. Express the problem in the simplest terms possible.
3. Divide the problem into potential problem areas. Draw a fishbone structure.
   See Exhibit 5.8.
4. Use brainstorming technique to identify reasons for the problem. Assign
   reasons to appropriate problem areas.
5. Review all the causes and decide on and test the solution(s).[28]

Application in Budgeting

A budget provides objective, quantifiable data for trending cost of personnel,
supplies, equipment, and capital items. Volume, price or rate, and quantity or

EXHIBIT 5.7 Statistical Control Chart: All Points Falling within Control Limits

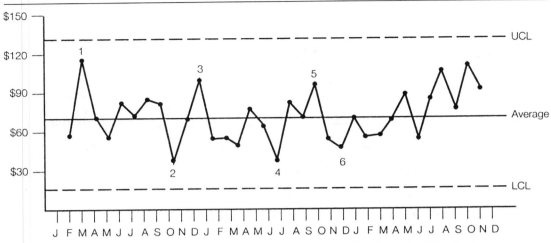

use variances are important to understanding variance analysis in the flexible budgeting process.

The *volume variance* can be defined as the amount of variance in any line item that is related to changes of workload level. For example, if an operating room is budgeted for 2500 cases when actually there were 3500 cases, additional expenses would be expected. One would expect variable costs to rise in proportion to increased workload. Such costs would constitute a volume variance. "Higher volume demands higher costs. If the higher volume was not budgeted for, there will be spending in excess of budget."[29] Nurse managers are held accountable for cost containment and control, however increased revenues are not generally attributed to excellent management of resources.

Price or *rate variance* refers to the portion of the total variance attributed to spending more or less per unit for a service or product than had been initially expected. Rate variance refers to labor resources for which the average hourly rate has varied from anticipated wages. Price variance is considered in the anticipated price of supplies. An example would be the cost per package of dressing sponges. The terms *price* and *rate variance* are often used interchangeably in practice. The nurse manager may have control of rate variance particularly as it relates to hiring nursing staff or requesting temporary agency personnel. In order to get the best rates, did the nurse manager consider qualifications of the nursing staff in meeting the unit's/patients' needs? Did she or he shop around for the best temporary agency rates? Such variances would be under the control and responsibility of the nurse manager. Price variance may be the responsibility of central supply or the purchasing department. Should such be the case, the responsible department predicts all prices for supplies and is thereby accountable for paying higher prices than originally predicted.[30]

A third type of variance is the *quantity* or *use variance*. Quantity or use variance refers to the use of more or less of a resource than expected for a given

EXHIBIT 5.8   A Fishbone Diagram

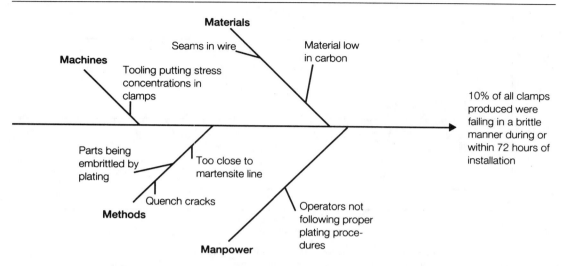

Note: The fishbone diagram shown here helped Rotor Clip isolate the cause of defective parts. Seams in the wire turned out to be the culprit.

Source: B. Rudin. "Simple Tools Solve Complex Problems." *Quality* (April 1990):50. Reprinted with permission from *Quality*, a publication of Hitchcock/Chilton Publishing, a Capital Cities/ABC, Inc., Company.

workload level. It focuses on how much of the resource has been used. The terms *quantity* and *use variance* are often used interchangeably, however there is a slight difference. For example, quantity of supplies would be factored into cost per patient day. If more supplies are used per patient day than anticipated based on workload level, quantity variance would exceed expected outcomes. With regards to use variance, use refers to actual use of particular supplies. For example, the actual usage of IV tubings would be factored into the care of the patient receiving total parenteral nutrition. Such would take into consideration the number of tubing changes required by infection-control standards and patient acuity. If usage exceeded protocol standards, a use variance would be identified requiring justification for the abnormal variance.[31]

The Deming (Shewhart) cycle illustrated in Exhibit 5.2 provides the nurse manager with a conceptual model for building a better budget.[32] Flexible budgeting and variance analysis are proposed for improving the basic components of the business. Flexible budgeting, as compared to classical budgeting techniques, affords the nurse manager more opportunities to make sense of variances.

The classical budgeting process generally monitors budget variations from month to month or on a quarterly basis; seeking explanation for unfavorable results is also a part of the process. Sorting out common causes or special causes is not a part of the process and in essence treats all variances as special causes. System improvements are not built into the budget and are not accounted for by variance. Such an evaluation from a classical budgeting perspective is fragmented, incomplete, and often deleterious to the organization. Historical data from budget numbers are used to make judgments for future events; such data

EXHIBIT 5.9   A Flowchart for an Improved Business Management Process

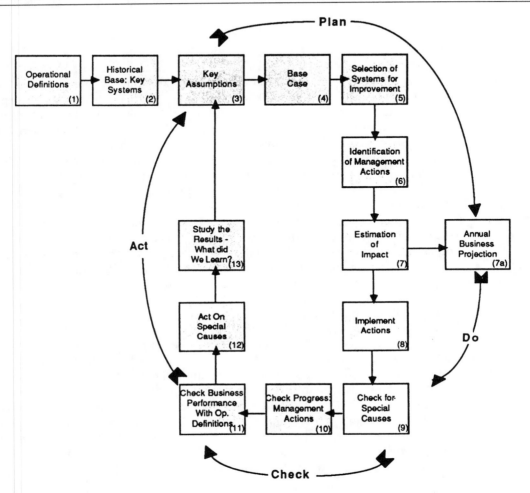

Source: A. E. Francis and J. M. Gerwels. "Building a Better Budget." *Quality Progress* (Oct. 1989):74. Reprinted with permission.

is not rigorously examined and lacks specificity with regards to true variance within the system. Applying the Deming (Shewhart) cycle to the budgeting process, Francis and Gerwels describe a flowchart for improved business management processes including budgeting.[33] See Exhibit 5.9.

Applying this flowchart to the nursing budget, nurse managers would:

1. Define, operationally, what is important to the business, how to measure it, and the agreed-upon test. Examine the strategic plan for clues.
2. Define key elements of the nursing business. They could be human resource systems, supply systems, equipment systems, policy and procedure systems, and nursing products, and others such as physical plant and support systems. Prepare a chart of special causes for each system for the past 3 years.

3. Identify key assumptions such as inflation, and organizational and plant restructuring.
4. Use all data to determine a base care or outcome for each system.[34]

The remaining steps are evident in Exhibit 5.9.

Of particular importance is the plotting of expected or common cause variances as compared to special or abnormal variances. Such a special cause chart would be a cornerstone of the plan-do-check-act (PDCA) cycle. "The manager operating the system should be primarily concerned with identifying and acting on special causes. The more senior manager should be primarily concerned with helping the organization improve these systems."[35] See Exhibit 5.10 for an actual budget formed using this process. Using such a model, variance analysis of personnel, supplies and equipment, and capital budgets can be identified, understood, and appropriately acted upon to improve financial management and productivity.

Variance has long been used as a statistical or mathematical concept. As such variance explains differences between projected or expected and actual outcomes. During the execution stage of budgeting, variance is a technique used to control or evaluate the financial aspects of budgeting. Variances are reported in monthly account statements for each cost center and enterprise. Monthly reports show transactions for a current month and cumulative data for the year to date. These reports may show variances for personnel expenses, supplies and equipment expenses, capital expenses, revenues, and for numerous activities that influence productivity such as performance appraisal, total quality management, achievement of objectives, staffing, human resource management, pay for performance, and numerous activities within each of these categories. An example of variance analysis extracted from Exhibit 5.11 follows.

Exhibit 5.11 (on page 182) is a cumulative account statement for the final month of the fiscal year ending September 30. It is for salaries, fringe benefits, and supplies and equipment expenses of the medical intensive care, coronary care, coronary care II cost center 60680. To summarize the expense variances, one looks at the last column, "percent used." These variances are:

Code	Revised Original Budget	Actual FY Expenses	Variances	Percent Variance
Salaries				
1000	$2,100,193.00	$2,227,196.22	$127,003.22–	(–6%)
Employee Benefits				
1700	387,276.00	398,449.84	11,173.84–	(–2%)
Med/Surg Supplies				
2000	316,465.00	357,984.72	41,726.73–	(–13%)
General Supplies				
2330–2700	9,550.00	10,095.49	565.39–	(–5%)
Travel and Entertainment				
3000	2,260.00	1,218.05	1,041.95	(+47%)
Other Expenses				
3200	96,752.00	80,041.43	16,352.28	(+17%)
Minor Equipment				
5050	9,000.00	6,480.28	2,519.72	(+28%)
9000	75,000.00		75,000.00	(100%)
Total	$2,996,496.00	$3,081,466.03	$085,555.23–	(–2%)

EXHIBIT 5.10   Budget Formation Using Special Cause Charts

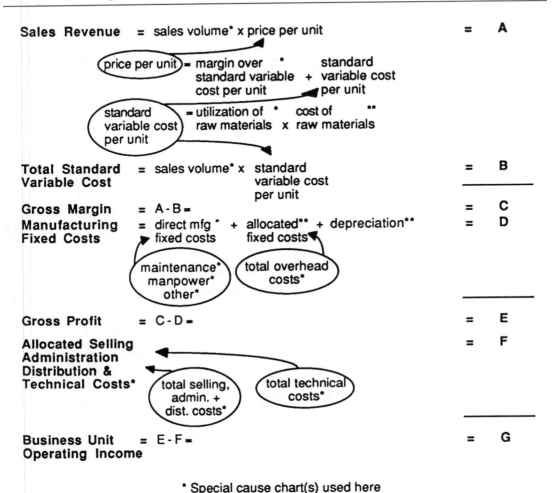

Sales Revenue   = sales volume* x price per unit   =   **A**

(price per unit)= margin over   *   standard
                standard variable + variable cost
                cost per unit   per unit

standard   = utilization of *   cost of   **
variable cost   raw materials   x raw materials
per unit

Total Standard   = sales volume* x standard   =   **B**
Variable Cost   variable cost
                                      per unit

Gross Margin   = A - B =   =   **C**
Manufacturing   = direct mfg *   + allocated** + depreciation**   =   **D**
Fixed Costs   fixed costs   fixed costs

maintenance*   total overhead
manpower*   costs*
other*

Gross Profit   = C - D =   =   **E**

Allocated Selling   =   **F**
Administration
Distribution &
Technical Costs*   total selling,   total technical
                      admin. +   costs*
                      dist. costs*

Business Unit   = E - F =   =   **G**
Operating Income

* Special cause chart(s) used here
** Assumption used here

Source: A. E. Francis and J. M. Gerwels. "Building a Better Budget." *Quality Progress* (Oct. 1989):75. Reprinted with permission.

The variance is a debit of the actual FY expense minus the revised original budget. The variance percent is obtained by dividing $127,003.22 by the original budget of $2,100,193.00. It is also the difference between the 100% of the fiscal year elapsed and the 106% of the budget used. The cumulative losses were less because of a revision adding $75,000.00 (code 9000) to the budget and reducing the variance to $85,555.23 or –2%.

During the fiscal year the cost-center manager would review the monthly account statements to determine the causes of the negative variances in salaries, employee benefits, and supplies. The causes could be increased census (patient days), higher patient acuities, and increased employee absences, among

EXHIBIT 5.11 Cumulative Account Statement

University of South Alabama
Financial Records System
Medical Intensive Care/Coronary Care/Coronary Care II Expenses

Obj Code	Description	Budgets		Actuals		Open Commitments	Balance Available	Percent Used
		Original	Revised	Current Month	Fiscal Year			
1000	Salaries	$2,106,248.00	$2,100,193.00	$195,732.19	$2,227,196.22		$127,003.22−	106%
1700	Employee Benefits	421,250.00	387,276.00	26,467.09	398,449.84		11,173.84−	102
2000	Med/Surg Supplies	338,813.00	316,465.00	22,690.25	357,984.72	$207.01	41,726.73−	113
2330 to 2700	General Supplies	9,550.00	9,550.00	1,363.76	10,095.49	19.90	565.39−	105
3000	Travel/Entertainment	2,260.00	2,260.00	55.00	1,218.05		1,041.95	53
3200	Other Expenses	21,752.00	96,752.00	6,497.79	80,041.43	358.29	16,352.28	83
5050	Hos. Minor EQ (< $500)	9,000.00	9,000.00	2,138.28	6,480.28		2,519.72	72
9000		75,000.00					75,000.00	0
	Account Totals	$2,903,873.00	$2,996,496.00	$254,944.36	$3,081,466.03	$585.20	$ 85,555.25−	102%

Source: Courtesy of the University of South Alabama Medical Center, Mobile, Alabama.

others. The cost-center manager looks at the revenue reports to determine if actual revenues are exceeding budgeted revenues.

Exhibit 5.12 depicts cumulative revenues for overall nursing cost centers through August 31 of the fiscal year (11 months). Variances are shown in the columns "balance available" and "perc used." Negative balances represent revenues needed to meet the projected annual budget, for example anesthesiology and chemotherapy. Positive balances represent revenues that exceeded the projected annual budget such as enterostomal therapy and 5th floor north. Since total revenues are at 94 percent and approximately 92 percent of the fiscal year has lapsed, revenues are ahead of budget.

Financial reports provide cost-center managers with variance data on projected or budgeted versus actual bed occupancy, and budgeted versus actual revenues from bad debt recovery, snack bar, telephones, sale of supplies, state appropriation, and insurance companies. All of these variances can be incorporated in Pareto charts or other tools described in this chapter and its references. Causes are then determined to be fixed by managers if common, by workforce if special.

Variance as a Controlling Technique

Variance shows or tells how things differ from an established norm or standard. A negative variance or outcome indicates that an institution can improve management of a service, program, or product. A positive variance or outcome indicates that an institution is performing above the expected norm or standard. In the case management system, CareMaps® (Center for Case Management, South Natick, Massachusetts) represent the norm or standard. See Exhibits 5.13 and 5.14 for an explanation and an example of CareMaps®.

Case Management

Case management is more than a modality of nursing. It has been described as

> A clinical system that focuses on the accountability of an identified individual or group for conditioning a patient's care (or care for a group of patients) across a continuum of care; ensuring and facilitating the achievement of quality, and clinical and cost outcomes; negotiating, procuring, and coordinating services and resources needed by the patient/family; intervening at busy points (and/or when significant variance occurs) for individual patients; addressing and resolving patterns in aggregate variances that have a negative quality-cost impact; and creating opportunities and systems to enhance outcomes.[36]

"Simply stated, case management is a process of coordinating services and the case manager is the person who does the coordinating."[37]

The New England Medical Center Hospital's model of case management was designed as a clinical one. The underlying assumption was that caregivers of each discipline needed to have management skills, better patient-care management tools, and more responsible administrative support to create quality clinical outcomes in a new cost-conscious milieu. The organizational structure is flat, with attending-level physician and "selected primary-care nurses expanded into case

EXHIBIT 5.12 Cumulative Revenue Statement

Financial Records System
Responsibility Roll-Up Report as of 08/31/xx

Cost-Center   9-82301
Reports To   9-81000

To: USAMC–Administration

Responsibility Units	Budgets Original	Budgets Revised A	Revenue Current Month	Revenue Actual Fiscal Year	Revenue Project Year B	Open Commitments C	Balance Available A-B-C	Perc Used (B+C)
Anesthesiology	$ 4,203,755-	$ 4,203,755-	$ 470,412-	$ 3,906,857-	$ 3,906,857-		$ 296,899-	93%
Revenue–Enter Thpy	106,456-	106,456-	9,515-	133,313-	133,313-		26,857	125
Chemothrapy–O/P Revn	231,521-	231,521-	15,571-	185,018-	185,018-		46,503-	79
Orthopedic Cast Room	126,016-	126,016-	9,656-	114,280-	114,280-		11,737-	91
5th Floor North/Reve	32,564-	32,564-	1,404-	33,320-	33,320-		756	102
5th Floor South/Reve	6,056,267-	6,056,267-	503,351-	5,482,415-	5,482,415-		573,852-	91
8th Flr Medical/Reve	1,139,047-	1,139,047-	121,441-	1,180,773-	1,180,773-		41,726	104
Med Interm Care Unit	562,259-	562,259-	57,553-	606,869-	606,869-		44,610	108
Medical ICU/Revenue	3,819,082-	3,819,082-	351,690-	3,571,803-	3,571,803-		247,279-	93
Coronary Care/Revenu	3,900,258-	3,900,258-	350,270-	3,800,021-	3,800,021-		100,237-	97
6th Flr Surgical/Rev	2,763,898-	2,763,898-	177,984-	2,267,255-	2,267,255-		496,643-	82
Burn Center/Revenue	3,294,420-	3,294,420-	327,518-	3,085,763-	3,085,763-		208,657-	93
9th Flr Surgical/Rev	2,937,940-	2,937,940-	250,444-	2,625,102-	2,625,102-		312,838-	89
Surg Intrm Care Unit	555,408-	555,408-	58,805-	686,725-	686,725-		131,317	123
Surgical ICU/Revenue	3,745,078-	3,745,078-	355,160-	3,584,463-	3,584,463-		160,615-	95
Neuro/Trauma ICU/Rev	1,663,253-	1,663,253-	153,300-	1,686,600-	1,686,600-		23,347	101
Dialysis Unit/Revenu	402,438-	402,438-	97,350-	917,848-	917,848-		515,410	228
Newborn Nursery/Reve	1,539,834-	1,226,458-	114,840-	1,134,625-	1,134,625-		91,833-	92
Premature Nursy/Reve	1,180,526-	1,493,902-	135,844-	1,099,352-	1,099,352-		394,551-	73
Neonatal Nursy/Reven	9,654,616-	9,906,764-	947,802-	9,634,428-	9,634,428-		272,337-	97
Obstetric Unit/Reven	2,122,726-	2,122,726-	214,110-	1,970,452-	1,970,452-		152,275-	92
Obstetric Unit/Reven	1,788,453-	1,788,453-	212,351-	1,768,709-	1,768,709-		19,744-	98
Pediatric ICU/Revenu				1,300	1,300		1,300-	

184

							%
Delivery Room/Reven	7,309,607–	7,309,607–	699,301–	6,740,034–	6,740,034–	569,573–	92
Operating Room	10,151,408–	10,151,408–	1,095,651–	9,634,221–	9,634,221–	517,188–	94
Recovery Room/EAU	1,517,090–	1,517,090–	119,411–	1,518,057–	1,518,057–	966	100
EAU	151,366–	151,366–	9,100–	213,410–	213,410–	62,044	140
Emergency Room	4,814,903–	4,814,903–	530,790–	4,749,627–	4,749,627–	65,276–	98
OR-Outpatint Surg-ER	2,191,032–	2,191,032–	106,004–	1,892,242–	1,892,242–	298,790–	86
OR-O/P Surgy Shac	412,369–	412,369–	40,663–	335,542–	335,542–	76,827–	81
**Total	$78,373,590–	$78,625,738–	$7,537,291–	$74,557,824–	$74,557,824–	$4,067,921–	94
Rev/Exp By Fund							
Operating Revenues	78,373,590–	78,625,738–	7,537,291–	74,557,824–	74,557,824–	4,067,921–	94
**Total	$78,373,590–	$78,625,738–	$7,537,291–	$74,557,824–	$74,557,824–	$4,067,921–	94
Rev/Exp By Type							
Revenues	78,373,590	78,625,738	7,537,291	74,557,824	74,557,824	4.067,921	94
Expenses							
Salaries							
Employee Benefits							
Med/Sur Supply							
Office/Other Suply							
Travel/Entertain							
Other Expenses							
Rev/Exp By Type							
Minor Equipment							
Cost Offsets							
Total Expenses							
Net Revenue/Expense	78,373,590–	78,625,738–	7,537,291–	74,557,824–	74,557,824–	4,067,921–	94
**Total	$78,373,590–	$78,625,738–	$7,537,291–	$74,557,824–	$74,557,824–	$4,067,921–	94

Source: Courtesy of the University of South Alabama Medical Center, Mobile, Alabama.

EXHIBIT 5.13   CareMaps®: The Core of Cost/Quality Care

CareMaps® are the newest breakthrough in cost/quality outcomes management. They have evolved from their longer version, Case Management Plans, and their condensed version, Critical Paths, into "user friendly" documents which

- *replace nursing care plans* as patient care plans.[1]
- describe the contributions of every department.
- show standards of care and standards of practice, and the timed, sequenced relationship between the two for a given case type, DRG, ICD9, or *constellation of problems*.
- individualize care through analyzing and acting upon variances.
- provide a database for Continuous Quality Improvement (CQI).
- integrate with *acuity* systems, *costing* systems, and *research*.

CareMaps® are cause-and-effect grids, that is, staff actions should result in patient/family reactions or responses, which over time are "transformed" into desired outcomes. Staff actions are equivalent to Standards of Practice; patient reactions are equivalent to Standards of Care. CareMaps® are built on a basic formula:

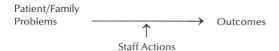

Patient/Family
Problems ——————————→ Outcomes
                 Staff Actions

This basic formula describes very complex practice patterns, which themselves have many sources. *To build a CareMap® requires deep respect for the knowledge, concern, and tradition that the clinicians of each discipline use in the care of their patients.* They reflect good practice, and can never replace good judgement.

Format
CareMaps®, like their Critical Path predecessors, are simplistic charts which graph phenomena associated with a homogeneous patient population on two axes: action vs. time. Critical Paths graph multidisciplinary staffs' actions in terms of interventions against the timeline most appropriate for the phase of treatment of a specific population. CareMaps® go an additional step by including patient/family actions in terms of responses to staffs' interventions.

Classic Critical Path		Time
Patient/Family Actions	problems	
Multidisciplinary Staff Actions	categories	

Patient/Family actions are categorized by problem statements which transform into intermediate goals and, by the last time frame, outcomes. Patient/Family actions are measurable and behavioral, and may include responses in

the realms of physiological, self-care, activities of daily living, follow-up plans, psychological, and absence of complications often related to their medical diagnoses. In 1987, Stetler and DeZell suggested four generic categories that should always be considered for inclusion in problem outcome statements:[2]

1. Potential for complications to self-care. Presence of risk factors that may limit a patient's ability to manage his or her own disease and/or engage in health-promoting activities in the home environment.

2. Potential for injury unrelated to treatment. Presence of risk factors related primarily to the person's general state of health and/or to the specific disease symptom that could lead to physical injury within the institutional setting.

3. Potential for complications related to treatment. Presence of risk factors, at times inherent in the inhospital treatment, that endanger the health and safety of the patient if (a) appropriate preventive measures are not instituted and maintained, and/or (b) on-going observations and monitoring are not instituted.

4. Potential for extension of the disease process. Presence of a specific condition or pathological process that carries with it a risk that endangers the recovery of the patient; that is, presence of a risk that will be increased if a treatable extension or sequela are undetected.

Multidisciplinary staff actions can be categorized in a variety of ways. Over the last 5 years, eight classic categories have emerged:

1. Consults/assessments
2. Treatments
3. Nutrition
4. Meds (IV, other)
5. Activity/safety
6. Teaching (patient, significant other)
7. Discharge planning/coordination
8. Specimens/tests

Additional categories such as "Chest-Tube Management" or "Psychosocial" may be desired depending on the case type. Some institutions have incorporated their intermediate patient/family goals and outcomes into the traditional (staff action) Critical Path. Others have written the staff's actions into the patient/family outcomes section. Yet others have integrated actions and outcomes into their current data flow sheets. *Anytime both the staff's and patient/families' behaviors are graphed against a timeline, the concept of a CareMap®—by whatever name— is being used.*

A CareMap® System
A CareMap® System includes the use of CareMaps® 24 hours a day. The heart of the system is the written CareMap® and the variances that arise from the standard interventions

EXHIBIT 5.13   CareMaps®: The Core of Cost/Quality Care *(Continued)*

and outcomes. In a CareMap® System, variances are not bad; they are real and reflect the way staff are responding to individual patient's needs. Variances can be categorized per patient using standard codes, and when aggregated retrospectively for groups of similar patient populations, form a database for continuous quality improvement.

The ultimate result of a CareMap® system is that unnecessary variance is reduced to a minimum because of an increasingly accurate learning curve that helps clinicians predict, prevent, and manage. It is not unusual for collaborative groups to begin developing CareMaps® for the more straightforward diagnoses, proceed to several varieties of that map, then combine constellations of problems, and finally map care for the patient populations that were initially felt to be totally unpredictable.

Currently, CareMaps® are used either on paper as references only, on paper as permanent documentation, on personal computers, or on mainframes. As institutions and clinicians become increasingly comfortable with CareMap® development, and as computer systems convert to CareMap® systems, higher percentages of patients will be managed by them (with daily or per visit screens). Similarly, variances are presently being handled differently depending on each agency's goals for implementing the system in the first place. Minimally, patient/family and community variances are recorded in the medical record. A few institutions have decided to also include clinician and hospital-generated variances in the chart as well.

Summary

A complete CareMap® System includes variance analysis, use of CareMaps® in change-of-shift report, case con-

sultation, and health-care team meetings for patients at more-than-acceptable variance, and continuous quality improvement. The challenge, of course, is creating a dynamic system of complex care management from a static piece of paper. This can be accomplished with a series of CareMaps® for different phases of treatment (i.e., Acute Myelogenous Leukemia: AML—induction, AML—consolidation, AML—fever and neutropenia, etc.) and the use of blank CareMaps® for anecdotal documentation or for those patients who require a totally individualized map. Any individualized outcomes and interventions written on a CareMap® are generally outside the variance field. When a patient's reason for remaining in the hospital changes in a major way (such as a patient having a craniotomy who remains on a vent), the CareMap® changes as well.

All professional disciplines should be involved in the formation of CareMaps® and education as to their use. Secretaries, computer and medical records department members, and the "forms" department are all integral to the implementation of a CareMap® System. Our future issues will address physician involvement in CareMap® Systems and Case Management, as well as other key development and maintenance factors.

Notes:

1. Brider, P. "Who Killed the Nursing Care Plan?" *American Journal of Nursing* (May, 1991): 35–39.
2. Stetler, C. and DeZell, A. *Case Management Plans: Designs for Transformation* (Boston: New England Medical Center Hospitals. 1987): 26–32.

Source: K. Zander, Ed. "CareMaps®: The Core of Cost/Quality Care." *The New Definition* (South Natick, Mass.: The Center for Case Management) 6(3)1991:1-3.

---

managers to produce the integration of processes, aided by critical paths."[38] Critical paths have been integrated into CareMaps®; see Exhibit 5.13. It should be noted that *the CareMap® is used as the nursing-care plan and for documentation.*

A collaborative team approach is used when integration of care occurs across geographic care units such as ER, CCU, step-down, and ambulatory clinic. Formally oriented primary-care nurses from these units join the team.[39]

The Center for Case Management believes that 100 percent of patients need their care managed by a CareMap®. Approximately 20 percent of patients need a case manager in addition to or instead of a CareMap® System.[40]

In the restructuring of nursing care, Zander places increased emphasis on accountability. This is demonstrated in Exhibit 5.15. It should be noted that case management is not a care delivery system.

Quality assurance is an integral part of the case management system. Total quality management is operationalized by the use of critical paths, CareMaps®, and case management. They provide the tools for accomplishing the nursing process.[41] When interventions and goals are recorded that are different than planned, they

EXHIBIT 5.14 CareMaps®: The Core of Cost/Quality Care

CareMap®: Congestive Heart Failure

	Day 1		Day 2	Day 3	Day 4	Day 5	Day 6
Location	ER 1–4 hours	Floor Telemetry or CCU 6–24 hours	Floor	Floor	Floor	Floor	Floor
			Benchmark Quality Criteria				
Problems							
1. Alteration in gas exchange/profusion and fluid balance due to decreased cardiac output, excess fluid volume	Reduced pain from admission or pain free Uses pain scale O₂ sat. improved over admission baseline on O₂ therapy	Respirations equal to or less than on admission	O₂ sat. = 90 Resp 20–22 Vital signs stable Crackles at lung bases Mild shortness of breath with activity	Does not require O₂ Vital signs stable Crackles at base Respirations 20–22 Mild shortness of breath with activity	Does not require O₂ (O₂ sat. on room air 90%) Vital signs stable Crackles at base Respirations 20–22 Completes activities with no increase in respirations No edema	Can lie in bed at baseline position Chest X ray clear or at baseline	No dyspnea
2. Potential for shock	No signs/symptoms of shock	No signs/symptoms of shock	No signs/ symptoms of shock	No signs/ symptoms of shock Normal lab values	No signs/ symptoms of shock	No signs/ symptoms of shock	No signs/ symptoms of shock
3. Potential for consequences of immobility and decreased activity: skin breakdown, DVT	No redness at pressure points No falls	No redness at pressure points No falls	Tolerates chair, washing, eating, and toileting	Has bowel movement Up in room and bathroom with assist	Up ad lib for short periods	Activity increased to level used at home without shortness of breath	Activity increased to level used at home without shortness of breath
4. Alteration in nutritional intake due to nausea and vomiting, labored		No c/o nausea No vomiting Taking liquids as offered	Eating solids Takes in 50% each meal	Taking 50% each meal	Taking 50% each meal Weight 2 lbs from patient's normal baseline	Taking 75% each meal	Taking 75% each meal

5. Potential for arrhythmias due to decreased cardiac output: decreased irritable foci, valve problems, decreased gas exchange	No evidence of life-threatening dysrhythmias	Normal sinus rhythm with benign ectopy	K(WNL) Benign or no arrhythmias	Digoxin level DNL Benign or no arrhythmias	Digoxin level WNL Benign or no arrhythmias	Digoxin level WNL Benign or no arrhythmias	Digoxin level WNL Benign or no arrhythmias
6. Patient/family response to future treatment & hospitalization	Patient/family expressing concerns Following directions of staff	Patient/family expressing concerns Following directions of staff	Patient/family expressing concerns Following directions of staff	States reasons for and cooperates with rest periods Patient begins to assess own knowledge and ability to care for CHF at home	Patient decides whether he/she wants discussion with physician about advanced directives	States plan for 1–2 days postdischarge as to meds., diet, activity Follow-up appointments Expresses reaction to having CHF	Repeats plans States signs and symptoms to notify physician/ER Signs discharge consent

7. Individual problem

Staff Tasks

Assessments/Consults	Vital signs q 15 min Nursing assessments focus on lung sounds, edema, color, skin integrity, jugular vein distention Cardiac monitor Arterial line if needed Swan Ganz Intake & output	Vital signs q 15 min–1 hr Repeat nursing assessments Cardiac monitor Arterial line Swan Ganz Daily weight Intake & output	Vital signs q 4 hrs Repeat nursing assessments D/C cardiac monitor 24 hr D/C arterial and Swan Ganz Daily weight Intake & output	Vital signs q 6 hrs Repeat nursing assessments Daily weight Intake & output	Vital signs q 6 hrs Repeat nursing assessments Daily weight Intake & output Nutrition consult	Vital signs q 6 hrs Repeat nursing assessments Daily weight Intake & output	Vital signs q 6 hrs Repeat nursing assessments Daily weight Intake & output
Specimens/Tests	Consider TSH studies Chest X ray EKG CPK q 8 hr × 3 ABG if pulse Ox: (range) Lytes, Na, K, Cl, CO_2 Glucose, BUN, Creatinine Digoxin: (range)	B/G	Evaluate for ECHO Lytes, BUN, Creatinine			Chest X ray Lytes, BUN, Creatinine	

(Continued)

EXHIBIT 5.14 CareMaps®: The Core of Cost/Quality Care (*Continued*)

	Day 1	Day 1	Day 2	Day 3	Day 4	Day 5	Day 6
		CareMap®: Congestive Heart Failure					
		Benchmark Quality Criteria					
Location	ER 1–4 hours	Floor Telemetry or CCU 6–24 hours	Floor	Floor	Floor	Floor	Floor
Problems							
Treatments	O₂ or intubate; IV or Heparin lock	O₂; IV or Heparin lock	IV or Heparin lock	DC pulse Ox if stable; D/C IV or Heparin lock			
Medications	Evaluate for Digoxin; Nitrodrip or paste; Diuretics IV; Evaluate for antiemetics; Evaluate for antiarrhythmics	Evaluate for Digoxin; Nitrodrip or paste; Diuretics IV; Evaluate for pre-load after-load reducers; K supplements; Stool softeners	D/C Nitrodrip or paste; Diuretics IV or PO; K supplements; Stool softeners; Evaluate for nicotine patch	Change to PO Digoxin; PO diuretics; K supplements; Stool softeners; Nicotine patch if consent	PO diuretics; K supplement; Stool softeners; Nicotine patch if consent	PO diuretics; K supplement; Stool softeners; Nicotine patch if consent	PO diuretics; K supplement; Stool softeners; Nicotine patch if consent
Nutrition	None	Clear liquids	Cardiac, low-salt diet	Cardiac, low-salt diet	Cardiac, low-salt diet	Cardiac, low-salt diet	
Safety/Activity	Commode; Bedrest with head elevated; Reposition patient q 2 hrs; Bedrails up; Call light available	Commode; Bedrest with head elevated; Dangle; Reposition patient q 2 hrs; Enforce rest periods; Bedrails up; Call light available	Commode; Enforce rest periods; Chair with assist ½ hr with feet elevated; Bedrails up; Call light available	Bathroom privileges; Chair × 3; Bedrails up; Call light available	Ambulate in hall × 2; Up ad lib between rest periods; Bedrails up; Call light available	Encourage ADLs that approximate activities at home; Bedrails up; Call light available	Encourage ADLs that approximate activities at home; Bedrails up; Call light available

Teaching	Explain procedures Teach chest pain scale and importance of reporting	Explain course, need for energy conservation Orient to unit and routine	Clarify CHF Dx and future teaching needs Orient to unit and routine Schedule rest periods Begin medication, teaching	Importance of weighing self every day Provide smoking cessation information Review energy conservation schedule	Cardiac rehab level as indicated by consult Provide smoking cessation support Begin medication teaching Dietary teaching	Review CHF education material with patient	Reinforce CHF teaching
Transfer/Discharge Coordination	Assess home situation notify significant other If no arrhythmias or chest pain transfer to floor Otherwise transfer to ICU	Screen for discharge needs Transfer to floor	Consider Home Health Care referral		Evaluate needs for diet and anti-smoking classes Physician offers discussion opportunities for advanced directives	Appointment and arrangement for follow-up care with Home Health Care nurses Contact VNA	Reinforce follow-up appointments

Note: CareMap® is a registered trademark of the Center for Case Management, South Natick, Mass. Used with permission.

Source: K. Zander, Ed. "CareMaps®. The Core of Cost/Quality Care." The New Definition (South Natick, Mass.: The Center for Case Management) 6(3)1991:1-3.

EXHIBIT 5.15   Expanding Scope of Accountability

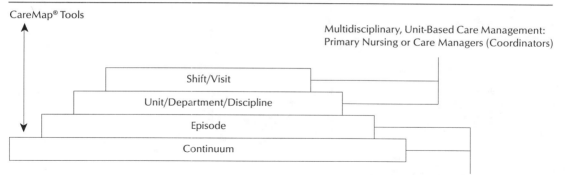

CareMap® Tools

Multidisciplinary, Unit-Based Care Management:
Primary Nursing or Care Managers (Coordinators)

Shift/Visit

Unit/Department/Discipline

Episode

Continuum

Case Management by Clinical
Nursing or Utilization Management

GLOSSARY

Shift or visit: A typical 8-, 10-, 12-hour nursing shift, consult, outpatient, or home health visit by any discipline, etc. A "billable" amount of service.

Unit, department, discipline: The classic ways in which services are organized, i.e., nursing units, satellite pharmacies, dietary departments, GYN services.

Episode: All services given to a patient and family from the first contact to the last contact for that specific set of symptoms or procedures; i.e., chest pain to cardiac rehab, diagnosis through hospice, MD office through surgery and recuperation.

Continuum: An infinite time frame which includes a person's health and life-style. May include chronic but stable states, such as well-maintained diabetes or handicaps.

Primary nursing: A unit-based model for the decentralization of accountability for the outcomes of nursing care from the head nurse to designated staff nurses. Usually all staff nurses who work 4–5 shift equivalents per week are included as primary nurses, making a caseload (not shift assignment) number of 2 to 6.

Accountability: The answerability for outcomes and results. Accountability assumes that the necessary underlying authority to act has been acquired.

Care management: A unit-based model for the decentralization of accountability for the outcomes of nursing care and an acknowledgment of the authority to coordinate all outcomes important to the treatment team. Nurses serve as care coordinators, sometimes in tandem with other professional disciplines. Only several nurses (avg. 1 to 4) are care managers.

Case management: A clinical system that focuses on the accountability of an identified individual or group for coordinating a patient's care across a continuum of care; insuring and facilitating the achievement of quality, clinical, and cost outcomes; negotiating, procuring, and coordinating services and resources needed by the patient/family; intervening at key points for individual patients; addressing and resolving patterns in aggregate variances that have a negative quality-cost impact; and creating opportunities and systems to enhance outcomes.

Responsibility: The fulfillment of distinct behaviors and expectations.

Source: © 1993, The Center for Case Management, South Natick, Mass. Developed by K. Bower; Adapted by K. Zander, 1994. *The New Definition* 9(2)1994:3. Reprinted with permission.

are termed *variances*. Variances show how the CareMap® and reality differ, both positively and negatively. CareMaps® present problems by defining quality as a product.[42] A variance indicates deviations from a norm or standard. Variance indicates intervention that works or does not work. Variances alter discharge dates, expected costs, and expected outcomes[43] (see Exhibits 5.16 and 5.17).

Variance that shows negative outcomes requires action to improve quality. Variance data is collected, totaled, analyzed, and reported. It results in decisions that revise CareMaps®, critical paths, procedures, and other elements of the PDCA cycle (see Exhibit 5.18).

Since CareMaps® can be used to document nursing care, are outcome-based, and have been found to be effective and efficient, nurse managers may want to use a computerized version for documentation.

EXHIBIT 5.16   Sample Variance Sheet

Date	Description	Prob	Path	Source	Action	Initials
1-Feb	Son unavailable: out of town on business		8	A3	Ask ICU to call 2/2	AB
1-Feb	Afib	5	•	A1	Transfer to ICU	CD
	O$_2$ sat + 85%	1	•	A1	Lasix, O$_2$ 6L	
	glucose 250		•	A1	Diabetic regime	
	no Swan Ganz		1	B6		
2-Feb	Unable to transfer to floor	•		C9	Order to drop pt. to general care rate	EF
	•	5		•		
	Afib—benign			A1	No action needed	
2-Feb	Echo not done		2	C9	Schedule for Monday	EF
	Hct 34, Hgb 13				Begin FeSO$_4$	

Source: K. Zander, Ed. "Quantifying, Managing, and Improving Quality. Part III: Using Variance Concurrently." *The New Definition* (South Natick, Mass.: The Center for Case Management) Fall 1992:3. Reprinted with permission.

EXHIBIT 5.17   Variance Source Codes

A	Patient/Family	C	Hospital
	1 Condition		9 Bed/Appt. Availability
	2 Decision		10 Info/Data Availability
	3 Availability		11 Other
	4 Other		
B	Clinician	D	Community
	5 Order		12 Placement/Home Care
	6 Decision		13 Transportation
	7 Response Time		14 Other
	8 Other		

Source: K. Zander, Ed. "Quantifying, Managing, and Improving Quality. Part III: Using Variance Concurrently." *The New Definition* (South Natick, Mass.: The Center for Case Management) Fall 1992:3. Reprinted with permission.

Applied to management and budgeting, the nurse manager sets goals or outcomes that have standards of cost as well as quality. These standards can be used to track costs of personnel programs such as overtime and skill levels, material, supplies, equipment, products, services, DRGs, and many other direct and indirect expenditures as well as revenues.

Controlling techniques may also be stated in terms of standards or norms.

Controlling Techniques

Although operational plans for evaluation are controlling techniques, other specific controlling techniques can be developed including planned nursing rounds by nurse managers from all levels, checklists from ANA *Standards of Nursing Administration Practice,* ANA *Standards of Clinical Nursing Practice,* JCAHO *Accreditation Manual for Hospitals,* and other published standards of third-party payers such as Medicare and Medicaid.

EXHIBIT 5.18   Comparison of Generic Steps in Clinical Decision Making

Scientific Method	CareMap® System Concurrent Use	CareMap® System Retrospective Use	CQI Technique (PDCA)*
1. Assess	Assess		
2. Plan; using problem/ approach statements	Plan; using a CareMap® tool with collaboratively determined outcome measures	CareMap® tool	Plan
3. Intervene	Intervene		Do
4. Evaluate	Evaluate; using variance Compare Consult Analyze Document	Aggregate Variance	Check
5.		Inform Discuss Revise CareMap® if needed Make other changes	Act

*PDCA Control circle: Ishikawa, K. *What Is Total Quality Control? The Japanese Way* (Englewood Cliffs, NJ: Prentice-Hall, 1985):59.

Source: K. Zander, Ed. "Quantifying, Managing, and Improving Quality. Part III: Using Variance Concurrently." *The New Definition* (South Natick, Mass.: The Center for Case Management, Fall 1992). Reprinted with permission.

Nursing Rounds

An effective controlling technique for nurse managers is planned nursing rounds. They can be done on a regular schedule and can include all nursing personnel. Rounds cover such issues as patient care, nursing practice, and unit management. To be effective the results should be discussed with appropriate nursing personnel in a follow-up conference. Part of the evaluation process takes place as a result of the communication occurring during the rounds. Exhibit 5.19 shows a protocol for planned monthly nursing rounds. The rounds may include discussion of pertinent budgeting variances.

Nursing Operating Instructions

Nursing operating instructions or policies become standards for evaluation as well as controlling techniques (see Exhibit 5.20).

The ANA *Standards of Nursing Administration Practice* can be developed into a checklist for evaluating the management processes of nursing services. See Exhibit 5.21 for a format to convert these standards into a usable control tool.

The ANA *Standards of Clinical Nursing Practice* can be implemented in several ways. One way is to convert them into a checklist as in Exhibit 5.21. The entire set of standards can be developed into a checklist along these lines.

Written protocols should be developed to implement a program for the evaluation process. Another way these protocols can be implemented is by using them to develop the evaluation standards, as in Exhibit 5.22.

EXHIBIT 5.19 Protocol for Planned Monthly Nursing Rounds

1. The chair, assistant chair, and other appropriate nursing personnel will make nursing rounds monthly.
2. Time is 10:00 to 11:00 A.M. unless otherwise indicated.
3. Schedule:

Unit	Day
1F	1st Tuesday
2A	1st Wednesday
2B	1st Thursday
2F	2nd Tuesday
ICU	2nd Wednesday
4A	2nd Thursday
3A	2nd Friday
3-OB	3rd Tuesday 10:30 to 11:30 A.M.
3F	3rd Wednesday
4B	3rd Thursday 11:00 A.M. to 12:00 noon
5A, CCU	4th Tuesday
5B	4th Wednesday

4. All unit nursing personnel are welcome to attend these rounds with their head nurse. Patient-care needs come first. The following areas will be covered as rounds are made to each patient's bedside:
   a. nursing histories
   b. nursing care plans
   c. nursing notes
   d. nurses' signatures on necessary documents
5. Other management areas of note will be discussed after bedside rounds:
   a. equipment and supplies
   b. staffing and assignments
   c. narcotic registers

EXHIBIT 5.20 Operating Instructions

1. Special care units will maintain policies and procedures relative to their mission. These procedures will be reviewed, updated, and signed at least annually.
   a. intensive care unit
   b. critical care unit
   c. newborn/intensive care unit nursery
   d. renal dialysis
2. Special care units will maintain a list of equipment needed to achieve their mission.
3. Supplies and equipment
   a. Blount resuscitator will have percent adaptor to increase oxygen concentration.
   b. Ambu resuscitator will have tail on to increase oxygen concentration.
   c. Humidification will not be used with oxygen with Ambu resuscitator.
   d. Trays from Central Sterile Supply will be returned as soon as used so that instruments will not be lost or misplaced.

EXHIBIT 5.21 Format for Converting the ANA *Standards of Nursing Administration Practice* into a Usable Control Tool

Standard No. _____

Measurement Criteria	Yes	No
(List)		

Gantt Charts

Early in this century, Henry L. Gantt developed the Gantt chart as a means of controlling production. It depicted a series of events essential to the completion of a project or program. It is usually used for production activities that include budgeting.

Exhibit 5.23 shows a modified Gantt chart that could be applied to a major nursing administration program or project. The five major activities that the nurse administrator has identified are segments of a total program or project. It could be applied to a project such as implementing a modality of primary nursing or implementing case management. The following are possible nursing actions for a project:

1. Gather data.
2. Analyze data.
3. Develop a plan.
4. Implement the plan.
5. Evaluate, give feedback, and modify.

Exhibit 5.23 is only an example. Application of this controlling process by nurse managers would be specific to the project or program, and the time

EXHIBIT 5.22   Standards for Evaluating the Controlling (Evaluating) Function
of Nursing Administration of a Division, Service, or Unit

1. An evaluation plan exists and is used for each nursing department, service, or unit.
2. Each evaluation plan is specific to the needs and activities of the individual department, service, or unit.
3. Evaluation findings are given in immediate feedback to subordinate nursing personnel.
4. Standards are accurate, suitable, and objective.
5. Standards are flexible and work when changes are made in plans and when unforeseen events and failures occur.
6. Standards mirror the organizational pattern of the nursing division, service, or unit.
7. Standards are economical to apply and do not produce unexpected results or effects.
8. Nursing personnel know and understand the standards.
9. Application of the standards results in correction of deficiencies or variances.

EXHIBIT 5.23   Modified Gantt Chart

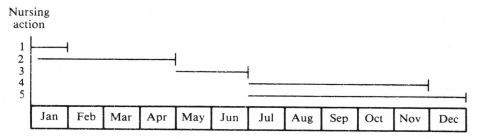

Note: Five nursing actions are needed to complete a program planned to start in January and end in December. In Exhibit 5.24, these five actions are translated into milestones and critical control points.

elements for the various activities would vary accordingly. Also, these five major activities could be modified by using subcategories of activities with estimated completion times. The nurse manager's goal is to complete each activity or phase *on or before* the projected date and at the cost budgeted for it.

Milestones and Critical Control Points

Master evaluation plans should have critical control points. *Critical control points* are specific points in production of goods or services at which the nurse administrator judges whether the objectives are being met, qualitatively and quantitatively. They tell whether the plan is progressing satisfactorily. They pinpoint successes and failures and the causes. Critical control points tell managers whether they are on target with regard to time, budget, and other resources. Milestones are segments or phases of specific activities of a project or program that are projected to occur within a time frame.

Exhibit 5.24 represents a modified Gantt chart with networks of milestones and critical control points. The critical path is 1 → 2 → 3 → 4 → 5 → 6 → 7 → 8 → 9 → 17 → 18. Line 5 represents evaluation of all other nursing actions. This is a simplified illustration of control techniques.

Case management also uses critical paths with milestones and control points. Any major nursing program could have dozens or even hundreds of milestones

EXHIBIT 5.24   Milestones and Critical Control Points

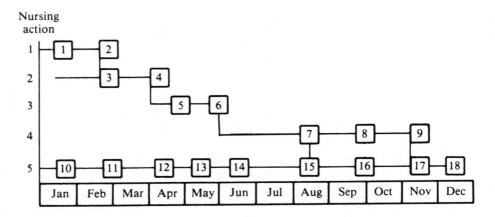

Modified Gantt chart with milestones and critical control points and network of milestones

and critical control points. This system may also be known by the name PERT (Program Evaluation and Review Technique).

Application of the milestone technique involves establishing a network of controllable pieces when planning a project or program. Each piece of the project or program is allocated a prorated portion of the total budget. A nurse manager could use this technique to evaluate the actual expenditure versus estimated budget at the end of each step of activity (or monthly) of the project or program. These evaluations would be the critical control points because each would culminate in the achievement of a milestone. Each event could represent a budgeting allocation, a period of time or time span, or a continuum of several or all of these elements. Bar graphs are frequently used to depict milestone budgeting. Budgeting in any of its forms is a major controlling technique.[44]

Program Evaluation and Review Technique

The Program Evaluation and Review Technique (PERT) was developed by the Special Projects Office of the U.S. Navy and applied to the planning and control of the Polaris weapon system in 1958. It worked then; it still works; and it has been widely applied as a controlling process in business and industry.

PERT uses a network of activities. Each activity is represented as a step on a chart. A time measurement and an estimated budget should be worked out to include:

1. The finished product or service desired.
2. The total time and budget needed to complete the project or program.
3. The starting date and completion date.
4. The sequence of steps or activities that will be required to accomplish the project or program.
5. The estimated time and cost of each step or activity.

6. Three paths for steps 4 and 5:
   A. the optimistic time,
   B. the most likely time, and
   C. the pessimistic time.
7. Calculation of the "critical path," the sequence of events that would take the greatest amount of time to complete the project or program by the planned completion date. The reason this is the critical path is because it will leave the least slack time.[45]

Why should nurse managers use the PERT system for controlling? It forces planning and shows how pieces fit together. It does this for all nursing line managers involved. It establishes a system for periodic evaluation and control at critical points in the program. It reveals problems and is forward-looking. PERT is generally used for complicated and extensive projects or programs.

Many records are used to control expenses and otherwise conserve the budget. These include personnel staffing reports, overtime reports, monthly financial reports, expense and revenue reports, and others. All these reports should be available to nurse managers to help them monitor, evaluate, and adjust the use of people and money as part of the controlling process.[46]

Benchmarking

Benchmarking is an offshoot of total quality management, and is a technique whereby an organization seeks out the best practices in its industry so as to improve its performance. It is a standard, or point of reference, for measuring or judging quality, values, costs, and other factors. Examples of benchmarks that could apply to nursing are:

- Establishing a skill mix of nursing employees to obtain the highest quality of patient care at the lowest cost. This is called *vertical leveraging*. *Horizontal leveraging* uses cross-training to boost productivity. If the average for the industry is a ratio of 60 percent R.N. to 40 percent other nursing personnel, the institution would make a decision to meet or exceed this ratio.
- An OR utilization rate of 80 percent or higher if the industry rate is 75 percent.
- An average turnover time between cases of 15 minutes if the industry rate is 20 minutes.
- A reduction of 10 percent from the average for industry cost of supplies per patient day.
- A reduction of 30 percent from the average for industry rate of hospital-acquired infections.[47]

Standards of practice and standards of care are the benchmarks for nursing practice in all domains. Standards of care define the levels of care that a patient can expect to receive in a given situation or on a given nursing unit. They are clinical benchmarks and are the foundation for quality improvement programs. Quality occurs when personnel meet the established standards.

Structure standards describe the environment in which care is delivered.

Process standards describe a series of activities, changes, or functions that bring about an end or result.

Clinical standards, a subgroup of process standards, are developed to include clinical issues specific to areas of practice—both standards of care and standards of professional performance. According to the American Nurses' Association, standards of care are authoritative standards describing a competent

EXHIBIT 5.25 Generic Nursing Care Plan

ST. JOHN MEDICAL CENTER
Medical Excellence • Compassionate Care

GENERAL SURGERY

Date	Nursing Diagnosis/Problems	Init	Interventions/ Discharge Plans	Goals	Date Reslv'd
	☐ Anxiety related to fear of surgical procedure as evidenced by ☐ call light on frequently ☐ multiple questions ☐ inability to sleep ☐ _____ _____ _____		☐ Preoperative teaching method _____ _____ _____ ☐ Provide reassurance and comfort _____ _____ _____	☐ Patient will express feelings of comfort and decreased anxiety	
	☐ Alteration in comfort related to surgical procedure as evidenced by: ☐ protecting the surgical site ☐ inability to stand upright ☐ shallow respirations ☐ _____ ☐ _____ _____		☐ Position for comfort _____ _____ _____ ☐ Instruct patient on splinting of incision ☐ Anticipate patient's needs for analgesics _____	☐ Pain is minimized or controlled with good muscle relaxation and ventilation	

Source: M. McAllister. "A Nursing Integration Framework Based on Standards of Practice," *Nursing Management* (April 1990):31. Reprinted with permission of Springhouse Corporation.

level of nursing practice. Standards of professional practice are authoritative statements describing a competent level of behavior in the professional role.[48] Outcome standards are the results to be achieved.

Standards of practice to be achieved are used to structure the quality assessment (QA) program. They are linked to development of policy and procedure, and to job descriptions and performance appraisal. Implementation of standards is done through use of generic nursing care plans and the computer. The latter provides generic nursing care plans and nursing diagnoses. See Exhibit 5.25 as an example of a generic nursing care plan.[49]

Benchmarking is enhanced when quality teams perform at the highest level of service by sharing their best practices and processes with similar committees or teams in other institutions and organizations. Total quality management is a necessary element of benchmarking. Benefits of benchmarking include:

• setting goals and objectives and obtaining full team support to meet them,
• continual improvement of practices, processes, and outcomes,
• commitment and accountability for excellence, and
• seeking out, learning about, and adapting new approaches.

The benchmarking program includes planning during team meetings, collection of specific data, analysis of data to determine gaps, integration through keeping all team members informed, action, and follow-up and monitoring.[50]

Variance Statistics

Variance as a statistic represents the sum of squares of deviation about the mean. Graphically, the statistical mean is a point on the horizontal axis which corresponds to the centroid, or center of gravity, of the distribution. The point on the horizontal axis where the ordinate divides the total area under the curve into two equal parts is the median.[51] The arithmetic mean is the average of a distribution and is more generally preferred to the median.

Variance statistics including mean, median, and standard deviation are used in applications of quality management. A manager should plan a statistics course tailored to the organizational objectives to be achieved by employees. Deming used variance statistics extensively in his theory of management. As an example:

Deming used the formula $\overline{X} \pm 3\sqrt{X}$ to describe the limits of variation attributable to the system. Applying this formula to performance evaluation for eight employees:

Name	No. of errors
Janet	10
Andrew	15
Bill	11
Frank	4
Dick	17
Charlie	23
Alicia	11
Tom	12
Joanne	10
Total	113

Therefore,

$$\overline{X} = \frac{113}{9} = 12.55$$

Limits of variation attributable to the system are

$$\text{upper limit} = 12.55 + 3\sqrt{12.55} = 23.2$$
$$\text{lower limit} = 12.55 - 3\sqrt{12.55} = 1.9$$

Who falls outside limits? It seems apparent that there are no statistical differences among the nine employees. Thus we see that variance has visual effects as well as objective effects depending upon whether we apply the concepts to quantitative or qualitative outcomes.[52]

Personnel Budgets

The cost of personnel is usually the greatest single expenditure for the nursing cost center and is generally the part of the budget over which the nurse manager exercises most control. Consideration must be given to full-time equivalents, productive and nonproductive hours, staffing requirements, target hours per workload unit, and distribution by mix and shift. Chapter 2 describes in

detail such concepts incorporated into personnel budgets. Francisco describes the flexible budgeting method that allows the nurse manager to take any budget variances and subdivide them into three distinct variance elements: an acuity-volume variance, a price variance, and a quantity or use variance.[53]

Variability in patient acuity and volume is the amount of variance attributed to the acuity-volume variance. The nurse manager is held accountable for the expense variance, however is generally not credited for increased revenues. Budgets that are flexed can move in both directions, up as well as down. Price or rate variance as well as quantity or use variance also factor into the equation.

As previously described, supplies, nursing hours, number of visits, and acuity-volume are driven by price/rate and/or quantity. The nurse manager is accountable for any variances incurred by such. In addition, Exhibit 5.26 illustrates an example of a personnel budget that factors in quality improvement. This in turn gives a budgeted cost for such improvement. It incorporates Deming's quality management approach to variance analysis in the personnel budgeting process.

Supplies and Equipment Budgets

Workload, supplies, and equipment costs make up the operating budget. The operating budget outlines and projects the organization's anticipated activity, necessary resources, and associated revenue and expenses for a specified period of time. Such time frames are generally one year. The functional unit is based on a cost center that generates costs within the organization. The term *responsibility center* is often used interchangeably with *cost center*; cost centers may be revenue-producing (pharmacy, diagnostics) or non-revenue producing (administration, maintenance). Supplies and equipment costs are resources needed to operate the business. Reducing variation in incoming supplies reduces scrap, rework, and the need to adjust to accommodate variation. Although the goal is not necessarily to have single suppliers, single sourcing may contribute to reduction of variation. In addition, single sourcing facilitates reduction of the supplier base and promotes a longer-term relationship between customer and supplier. Such may allow the supplier greater volume and therefore greater opportunity to fine-tune and improve its process. The goals are to reduce administrative cost and allow more time to be spent on improving product and process rather than on crisis intervention.

Franciso describes a supply budget using flexible budgeting and variance analysis.[54] See Exhibit 5.27. Supply and equipment costs can also be plotted on a control chart that identifies variances as common (predictable) or special (sporadic) causes. Quantifiable data provide objective information for understanding variance in use of supplies. Variance analysis would further guide the nurse manager in intervening when necessary.

Capital Budgets

Capital budgeting refers to planning for the acquisition of long-term investments. A capital item is one that when purchased has a lifetime beyond the year of

EXHIBIT 5.26 Allocation of Expenditures to Performance Areas

Cost Item	Total	Quality	Staffing	Cost Control	Productivity	Patient Satis.	Staff Satis.	Innov.	Direct Care	Indirect Care	Other
Performance Areas											
Nurse Manager	$ 50,000	$ 7,500	$7,500	$10,000	$10,000	$ 5,000	$2,500	$ 7,500	$ 0	$ 0	$ 0
Staff Salary	800,000	40,000	0	40,000	16,000	40,000	0	0	240,000	240,000	184,000
Education	20,000	4,000	0	4,000	4,000	2,000	2,000	4,000	0	0	0
Supplies	40,000	0	800	800	0	0	0	0	36,000	2,000	400
Overhead	90,000	0	0	0	0	0	0	0	90,000	0	0
Totals	$1,000,000	$51,500	$8,300	$54,800	$30,000	$47,000	$4,500	$11,500	$366,000	$242,000	$184,400

Source: S. A. Finkler. "Performance Budgeting." *Nursing Economics* (Nov.-Dec. 1991):405. Reprinted with permission of Jannetti Publications, Pittman, New Jersey.

EXHIBIT 5.27 Flexed Variances

A. Flexed Supply Price Variance

Actual Price:	7843 × Y	=	$7843	
				$0.00
Budgeted Price:	7843 × $1.00	=	$7843	

B. Flexed Supply Quantity Variance

Actual Quantity:	7843 × $1.00	=	$7843	
				$400 F
Flexed Quantity:	8243 × $1.00	=	$8243	

C. Flexed Supply Quantity Variance

Budgeted Supply Cost:		=	$7343	
				$900 U
Flexed Supply Cost:		=	$8243	

Note: F = favorable; U = unfavorable

Source: P. D. Francisco. "Flexible Budgeting and Variance Analysis." *Nursing Management* (Dec. 1989):43. Reprinted with permission of Springhouse Corporation.

purchase. A capital item must be considered useful in future years in order to be identified as such. The capital budget is treated separately from the regular operating budget. Expenses on capital items are accounted for separately from ongoing operating budget expenses. Chapter 4 further describes the capital budgeting process.

Exhibit 5.28 illustrates an example of a capital item expense, projected revenue, and value of the item. Variances would be accounted for per use with actual costs of use subtracted from projected use. An example of this would be more or fewer than 10 transactions per day or 2600 per year. Common cause variances would be differentiated from special or abnormal causes, thereby further guiding the nurse manager in the need to intervene with regards to capital expenditures. A common cause variance would be fewer or more patients; a special cause an increase or decrease in personnel productivity.

Summary

This chapter defines and describes variance analysis as an integral component of the budgeting process. Variation is a part of everything—of the supplies used by nurses, of employee performance, and of many other activities. Variance analysis is the aspect of the budgeting process by which actual monetary results are compared to anticipated budgetary outcomes. A variance describes the difference between the experienced result and the planned result. Variance analysis in the budgetary process identifies the quantified results (dollars and cents) that vary from the expected outcomes. As a critical factor in the quality management equation, variance analysis provides hard data in the measurement of outcomes. Using Deming's quality management model, variance analysis in the budgeting process identifies methods and strategies to better understand and reinforce organizational standards of practice.

EXHIBIT 5.28   Figuring Charges per Procedure

Item: PC with accessories
1. Cost of item: $8,000
2. Useful life (years): 3
3. Depreciation cost per year (1 divided by 2): $8,000 ÷ 3 = $2,666
4. Number of transactions per year: 260 days × 10 = 2,600
5. Average time per transaction (minutes): 15
6. Average personnel cost per transaction: $22
7. Average supply and service cost per transaction: $0.50
8. Average cost per transaction (3 divided by 4 plus 6 plus 7): $1 + $22 + $0.50 = $23.50
9. Charge = $23.50 + $10 profit + $12 losses for unpaid bills = $45.50 per transaction

Experiential Exercises

1. Identify the norms or standards used to measure variance in a nursing department's or unit's budget. List them. How are the causes of variance identified? How are identified causes of variance corrected?
2. Identify an element of the budget you wish to study related to personnel, supplies, equipment, or capital items. What norms or standards identify variances? If none exist, develop a set of norms or standards. Use them to measure variances, identify causes of the variances, and establish plans for correcting negative causes of variances.

Notes

1. J. Oberle. "Quality Gurus: The Men and Their Message." *Training* (Jan. 1990):47-52.
2. S. A. Finkler. *Budgeting Concepts for Nurse Managers*, 2d. ed. (Philadelphia: W. B. Saunders, 1992):1-370.
3. B. L. Joiner and M. A. Gaudard. "Variation, Management, and W. Edwards Deming." *Quality Progress* (Dec. 1990):29-37.
4. M. Tritus. "Deming's Way." *Mechanical Engineering* (Jan. 1988):28.
5. W. J. Duncan and J. G. Van Matre. "The Gospel According to Deming: Is It Really New?" *Business Horizons* (Jul.-Aug. 1990):3-9.
6. A. E. Francis and J. M. Gerwels. "Building a Better Budget." *Quality Progress* (Oct. 1989):70-75.
7. T. A. Smith. "Why You Should Put Your Safety System under Statistical Control." *Professional Safety* (Apr. 1989):31-36.
8. B. L. Joiner and M. A. Gaudard, op. cit.
9. S. A. Finkler and C. T. Kovner. *Financial Management for Nurse Managers and Executives* (Philadelphia: W. B. Saunders, 1993):348-378.
10. R. Kirk. "The Big Picture Total Quality Management and Continuous Quality Management." *Journal of Nursing Administration* 9(4)1992:24-31.
11. S. A. Finkler and C. T. Kovner, op. cit.
12. Ibid.
13. Ohio Quality and Productivity Forum. "Deming's Point Four: A Study." *Quality Progress* (Dec. 1988):31-35.
14. W. E. Deming. *Out of the Crisis* (Cambridge: Massachusetts Institute of Technology, Center for Advanced Engineering Study, 1986):1-82. Dr. Deming was an early advocate of the principles of management for quality. According to personnel of the MIT Center for Advanced Engineering Study, he rejected the concept of Total Quality Management (TQM), saying it was undefined.

15. L. E. Mainstone and A. S. Levi, op. cit.

16. Ibid.

17. Ibid.

18. Ibid.

19. H. S. Gitlow and S. H. Gitlow. *The Deming Guide to Quality and Competitive Position* (Englewood Cliffs, NJ: Prentice-Hall, 1987):1-92.

20. W. W. Notz, I. Boschman, I and S. S. Tax. "Reinforcing Punishment as Extinguishing Reward: On the Folly of OBM without SPC." *Journal of Organizational Behavior Management* 9(1)1987:28-34; L. E. Mainstone and A. S. Levi, op. cit.

21. H. S. Gitlow and S. H. Gitlow, op. cit.

22. L. A. Heinzlmeir. "Under the Spell of the Quality Gurus." *Canadian Manager* (Spring 1991):22-23.

23. Ibid.

24. J. T. Burr. "The Tools of Quality Part VI: Pareto Charts." *Quality Progress* (Nov. 1990):59-61.

25. Ibid.

26. B. L. Joiner and M. A. Gaudard, op. cit.

27. L. Cohen. "Quality Function Deployment: An Application Perspective from Digital Equipment Corporation." *National Productivity Review* (Summer 1988):197-208.

28. B. Rudin. "Simple Tools Solve Complex Problems." *Quality* (Apr. 1990):50-51.

29. S. A. Finkler. *Budgeting Concepts for Nurse Managers* 2nd. ed. (Philadelphia: W. B. Saunders, 1992):258-281.

30. S. A. Finkler and C. T. Kovner, op. cit.

31. Ibid.

32. A. E. Francis and J. M. Gerwels, op. cit.

33. Ibid.

34. Ibid.

35. Ibid.

36. K. Zander. "Toward a Fully Integrated CareMap® and Case Management System." *The New Definition* (Spring 1993):1.

37. K. Zander. "Part 1: Rationale for Care-Provider Organizations." *The New Definition* (Summer 1994):1.

38. Ibid.

39. Ibid.

40. Ibid.

41. "Quantifying, Managing, and Improving Quality Part I: How CareMaps® Link CQI to the Patient." *The New Definition* (Spring 1992):1.

42. Ibid.

43. "Quantifying, Managing and Improving Quality Part III: Using Variance Concurrently." *The New Definition* (Fall 1992):1-2.

44. H. Koontz and H. Weihrich, *Management*, 5th ed. (New York: McGraw-Hill, 1990):424; R. M. Hodgetts, *Management: Theory, Process, and Practice*, 5th ed. (Orlando, Fla: Harcourt Brace Jovanovich, 1990):243; H. S. Rowland and B. L. Rowland, *Nursing Administration Handbook*, 3rd ed. (Gaithersburg, Md: Aspen, 1992):36; R. M. Fulmer and S. G. Franklin, *Supervision: Principles of Professional Management*, 2d ed. (New York: Macmillan, 1982):221-227.

45. H. Koontz and H. Weihrich, op. cit., 424-428, R. M. Hodgetts, op. cit., 240-242.

46. J. M. Ganong and W. L. Ganong, *Nursing Management*, 2d ed. (Gaithersburg, Md: Aspen, 1980):257.

47. P. Patterson. "Benchmarking Study Identifies Hospitals Best Practices." *OR Manager* (Apr. 1993):11, 14-15.

48. American Nurses' Association. *Standards of Clinical Nursing Practice* (Washington, DC: 1991):21.

49. M. McAllister. "A Nursing Integration Framework Based on Standards of Practice." *Nursing Management* (Apr. 1990):28-31.
50. J. A. Murray and M. H. Murray. "Benchmarking: A Tool for Excellence in Palliative Care." *Journal of Palliative Care 8*, 4(1992):41-45.
51. G. A. Ferguson. *Statistical Analysis in Psychology and Education*, 4th ed. (New York: McGraw-Hill, 1976):55, 61.
52. W. E. Deming, op. cit., 112-113.
53. P. D. Francisco. "Flexible Budgeting and Variance Analysis." *Nursing Management* (Nov. 1989):40-43.
54. Ibid.

References

American Nurses' Association. *Standards of Nursing Administration Practice and a Statement on the Scope and Levels of Nursing Administration Practice and Qualifications of Nurse Administrators Across All Settings* (Washington, DC: 1988). In revision.

American Nurses' Association. *Standards of Clinical Nursing Practice* (Washington, DC: American Nurses' Association, 1991).

Bryce, G. R. "Quality Management Theories and Their Application." *Quality* (Jan. 1991):15-18.

Crosby, P. B. *Quality without Tears: The Art of Hassle-Free Management* (New York: McGraw-Hill, 1984).

Deutsch, B. J. "A Conversation with Philip Crosby." *Bank Marketing* (Apr. 1991):22-27.

Ferguson, G. A. *Statistical Analysis in Psychology and Education*, 4th ed. (New York: McGraw-Hill, 1976).

Finkler, S. A. "Performance Budgeting." *Nursing Economic$* (Nov.-Dec. 1991):401-408.

Finkler, S. A. *Budgeting Concepts for Nurse Managers*, 2d. ed. (Philadelphia: W. B. Saunders, 1992).

Joint Commission on Accreditation of Healthcare Organizations (JCAHO). *Accreditation Manual for Hospitals 1995* (Chicago: American Hospital Association, 1994).

Juran, J. M. "Universal Approach to Managing for Quality." *Executive Excellence* (May 1989):15-17.

Kiehl, E. M. "A Strategy for Budgeting Obstetrical Costs." *Nursing Management* (Oct. 1991):50-52.

Manthey, M. "Budgeting: Controlling the Ominous Art." *Nursing Management* (Mar. 1992):14.

McGrail, G. R. "Budgets: An Underused Resource." *Journal of Nursing Administration* (Nov. 1988):25-31.

Moss, M. T., and S. Shelver. "Practical Budgeting for the Operating Room Administrator." *Nursing Economic$* (Jan.-Feb. 1993):7-13.

O'Neal, C. R. "Its What's Up Front That Counts." *Marketing News* (Mar. 4, 1991):9, 28.

Piczak, M. W. "Quality Circles Come Home." *Quality Progress* (Dec. 1988):37-39.

Port, O. "How to Make It Right the First Time." *Business Week* (June 8, 1987):142-143.

Reilly, D. E. "Issues in Budgeting an Outreach Program." In *Graduate Professional Education Through Outreach: A Nursing Case Study* (NLN Publication 15-2340 1990):109-132.

Reimer, M. S. "Computerized Cost Analysis for the Nursing Skills Laboratory." *Nurse Educator* (Jul.-Aug. 1992):8-11.

Schaaf, D. "Beating the Drum for Quality." *Quality* (Mar. 1991):5-6, 8, 11-12.

Schrage, M. "Fire Your Customers." *The Wall Street Journal* (March 16, 1992):A12.

SV. "Quality Can't Be Delegated." *Supervision* (May 1988):6-7.

Taguchi, G., and D. Clausing. "Robust Quality." *Harvard Business Review* (Jan.-Feb. 1990):65-75.

Vasilash, G. S. "Crosby Says Get Fit For Quality." *Production* (Jan. 1981):51-52, 54.

"What's Next On the Quality Agenda?" *Quality* (Mar. 1991):42.

6

A Model for Costing and Pricing Nursing Service

Russell C. Swansburg, Ph.D., R.N.
Richard L. Sowell, Ph.D., R.N., F.A.A.N.

Confronted with new realities posing unknown consequences, people try to guess what those consequences might be. Thoughtful and ambitious professionals translate these guesses into hypotheses and test them. Their results support or disprove the hypotheses and only then can facts replace the guesses. Since the advent of diagnosis related groups (DRGs) in 1983, nurse administrators, educators, and researchers have been investigating hypotheses related to the effects of DRG reimbursement on nursing care. Their subsequent study on the effects of the Prospective Payment System (PPS) has added to the theory base of nursing administration.[1]

Health-care planners, hospital administrators, and third-party payors have expounded on the merits of early discharge of patients to make DRGs profitable. However, public outcry and congressional inquiry have followed. The PPS has saved billions of health-care dollars, even with the adjustments needed to accommodate the shift in geographic site of care from hospital to outpatient settings.

A second assumption of the DRG reimbursement system was that the age of patients increased complication or co-morbidity (CC) and subsequent cost. Price and Kominski "analyzed inpatient charges for 1984 and found that the use of age in combination with CC is inappropriate for grouping Medicare patients. The original DRGs resulted in underpayment for CC patients and overpayment for patients 70 years or older without a CC." As a consequence, "as of October 1987 patient age was no longer used in combination with the presence of a

complication or co-morbidity to define DRGs."[2] Munoz and colleagues report a study of 6331 patients to show that "older patients (65 years of age and older) who were treated in the ICU had longer hospital lengths of stay, higher mortality rates, and a greater percentage of outlier patients, as compared with younger patients (under 65 years of age)."[3] Their pitch is for higher reimbursement rates for patients with greater acuity who use more hospital resources. However, their study raises more questions than it answers.

1. The cost-to-charge ratio for blood, surgical pathology, operating room, recovery room, and electrocardiology were greater than 1.00 indicating a financial management problem. They are not charging to cover costs.

2. The mean total cost per patient for all patients was $18,332. Since at least 50 percent of all patients in every age category required emergency admission and patients 85 years of age and older had the highest emergency admissions, one might suggest studies to assess overtreatment, appropriate treatment, and consideration of quality-of-life factors. Since diagnoses are not listed, one wonders if these patients were not overtreated for emergency conditions. Intensive care does not equate necessarily to high quality of care! Further studies could be done on cost management to determine appropriateness of procedures, coordination to prevent different specialists from writing multiple sets of orders on the same patients, and whether patients come to the hospital to die peacefully but get intensive treatment instead.

Issues related specifically to intensity of nursing care were addressed in research reported by Trofino.[4] These studies indicated that (1) 73 percent of DRGs studied showed no statistically significant differences between the mean patient length of stay (LOS) at $p < .01$ and (2) 83 percent showed no difference at $p < .001$. There was a statistically significant positive correlation ($p < .01$) between nursing care hours (NCHs) and patient LOS found in 166 tests performed. NCHs were determined by patient LOS. This suggests that nurses have adopted a businesslike approach and are adjusting care to meet the adjusted LOS. Trofino indicates that correlation of NCH and LOS now can be used to put a price on NCHs. Further data on linkage can lead to standard NCHs per DRG category and allow NCHs to be the basis for nursing reimbursement per DRG category.

For years, a resource has been available that can be used to cost out nursing services in hospitals: the *Hospital and Hospital Health Care Complex Cost Report Certification and Settlement Summary* or Medicare Cost Report (MCR). Every hospital being reimbursed by Medicare submits data annually based on its cost/charge ratios from the previous year; this information collectively comprises the MCR. This serves as a standard data source on which the hospital industry determines reimbursement under PPS. Generally, nurse administrators can obtain the report from the hospital finance administrator; it is available to the public on request under the Freedom of Information Act.

Thus the Health Care Financing Administration (HCFA) has gathered a huge database of financial information about U.S. hospitals since Medicare and Medicaid were established in 1965. These data, collected annually by HCFA through the Medicare Cost Report, are used to (1) support PPS analyses and initiate

special congressional studies and legislation and (2) provide data support to the General Accounting Office, the Office of the Inspector General, and the Congressional Budget Office.

To determine nursing costs accurately, it is essential to define the nursing product in terms of output, or process, or a combination of both. Currently, the patient classification system (PCS) is being used for staffing and for personnel budgeting and some nurse administrators use it for productivity management.[5] By charging patient care hours on a daily basis, a database can be developed. The daily charges enter into the total charges as an outcome measurement, thus becoming the charges on the patient's bill per discharge and DRG category. Together with the MCR, the patient's bill becomes part of the databank of Medicare and a source of information for financial research in nursing administration.

Designing a Model for Costing and Pricing Nursing Services

The authors propose a model for unbundling the hospital bill, for establishing both a cost and a price for nursing services and for budgeting (Exhibit 6.1). Generally, nursing service costs are grouped with those of nutrition and dietary services and intern and resident services. Also, several cost centers include both adult and pediatric unit groups. Nursing research could be done to determine if there is a higher use of resources in pediatric cases. If a difference were found, HCFA might change the cost accounting procedures of the MCR to separate these two entities. Units separated for cost analysis and definition include intensive care, surgical intensive care, coronary care, burn intensive care, adults and pediatric (general routine care), and the nursery.

The first decision to be made by the nurse administrator is which services to cost to nursing as direct and indirect expenses (Exhibit 6.2). Costs shown are extracted from the MCR for a University Medical Center, using the authors' groupings. Similar costing techniques could be used to establish these costs for individual units within these combined adult and pediatric areas.

To establish a productivity unit or relative value unit (RVU), necessary information can be gained from any patient classification system. In Exhibit 6.3A, data for 120 continuous days are taken directly from the Medicus PCS. The costs for 365 days are used to determine nursing costs per day (Exhibit 6.3B). The base unit or RVU represents direct nursing care of a type 1 patient for 1 hour in a 24-hour period, plus related overhead costs as variances. The cost of 1 unit of care (RVU) is determined by dividing the cost of nursing services (Exhibit 6.2) by the total RVUs (Exhibit 6.3B). Multiplied by the nursing hours per patient, it is possible to determine accurately the cost of nursing care for patients of all acuity types (Exhibit 6.3B).

Now it is possible to proceed by first applying the inflation rate for the period, obtained from the American Hospital Association. In this study, it was 8.0%, which is figured in to each item's cost per day using this formula:

$$(\text{total cost} \times \text{no. of days}) + (\text{cost of total stay} \times \text{inflation rate})$$
$$= \text{cost per day}$$

EXHIBIT 6.1   Steps in Unbundling the Costs of Nursing Services

1. Separate nursing from other services using the Medicare Cost Report.
2. Identify direct expenses and indirect expenses attributable to nursing services using the Medicare Cost Report.
3. Identify a productivity unit or relative value unit (RVU) for nursing services using the patient classification system.
4. Translate RVUs into costs per day.
5. Identify costs per day of hotel services.
6. Identify costs per day for nutrition and dietary services.
7. Identify costs per day for interns and residents.
8. Summarize costs per day.
9. Apply inflation rate to total costs per day.
10. Apply cost-to-charge ratios.
11. Bill charges.

EXHIBIT 6.2   Costs of Nursing Services

Direct Expenses (Directly Assigned)	
Salaries	$5,396,503
Employee benefits	1,321,111
Supplies (Central Supply)	86,542
Total Direct Costs	$6,804,156
Indirect Expenses	
General Administration	275,367
Nursing Administration	378,689
Pharmacy (floor stock)	3,931
College of Nursing	315,840
Total Indirect Costs	973,827
Total Costs	$7,777,983

As an example, we can refer to Exhibit 6.5 for a type 1 patient hospitalized for 4 days:

$$(\$145.26 \times 4) + (\$581.04 \times .08) = \$627.52$$

The cost-to-charge ratio is the amount that has to be charged to meet costs. If $1.32 has to be charged for every $1.00 of cost, the amount to be charged can be calculated:

$$\text{Final charge} = 1.32 \times \text{calculated charge (corrected for inflation)}$$

Exhibit 6.5C thus provides all the information needed to bill the patient accurately for nursing care. For example, the cost of nursing care of a type 1 patient for 4 days would be:

$$\$37.24 \times 4 = \$148.96$$

EXHIBIT 6.3   Calculating Cost per Unit of Care

A. Nursing Hours Required

PCS Type	Patients Classified(%)	Acuity	Nursing Hr/ Patient/24 Hr	Average NHPP
1	21%	0.5	0–2	1
2	36	1.0	2–4	3
3	42	2.5	4–10	7
4	1	5.0	10–24	17

B. Nursing Costs per Day

PCS Type	Patients Classified(%)	Patient Days	RVUs	NHPP	Cost/Unit of care
1	21%	14,223	14,223	1	$ 26.12
2	36	24,382	73,146	3	78.36
3	42	28,445	199,115	7	182.84
4	1	677	11,339	17	444.04
Totals		67,727	297,823		

EXHIBIT 6.4 Cost per Day for Hotel Services

Capital Related Costs—buildings and fixtures	$ 201,691
Capital Related Costs—moveable equipment	37,273
Communications	25,059
Data Processing	127,459
Purchasing	10,839
Admitting	87,630
Patient Accounts	191,073
Plant Operations	1,112,362
Biomedical	19,483
Laundry	365,753
Housekeeping	548,909
Patient Transport	120,682
Medical Records	735,716
Social Services	260,881
Total Indirect Costs	$ 3,844,810

$$\text{Cost per day} = \frac{\text{total cost}}{\text{patient days}} = \frac{\$3,844,810}{67,727} = \$56.77$$

EXHIBIT 6.5 Summary of Costs to Nursing

A. Total Costs

	Total	Cost per Day
Nursing Services	$ 7,777,983	Varies by pt. type
Hotel Services	3,844,810	$56.77
Nutrition & Dietary	1,710,619	25.26
Interns & Residents	2,513,085	37.11
Total Costs	$15,846,497	

B. Costs per Day

Patient Type	Nursing	Hotel	Nutrition	Interns	Total
1	$ 26.12	$56.77	$25.26	$37.11	$145.26
2	78.36	56.77	25.26	37.11	197.50
3	182.84	56.77	25.26	37.11	301.98
4	444.04	56.77	25.26	37.11	563.18

C. Charge per Day
(Cost per day corrected for inflation and cost-to-charge ratio)

Patient Type	Nursing	Hotel	Nutrition	Interns	Total
1	$ 37.24	$80.93	$36.01	$52.91	$207.09
2	111.71	80.93	36.01	52.91	281.56
3	260.66	80.93	36.01	52.91	430.51
4	633.02	80.93	36.01	52.91	802.87

For another example, the cost of nursing care of a patient who is classified as type 4 for 4 days and type 3 for 6 days would be:

$$\$633 \times 4 = \$2532.00$$
$$261 \times 6 = \underline{1566.00}$$
$$\text{Total} \quad \$4098.00$$

Use of the MCR for Costing Nursing Services

Among the reasons for using the MCR for costing and pricing nursing services are the following.

1. In developing annual budgets, nurse administrators can compare actual direct and indirect costs of the past year with costs predicted for the current year. Over a period of years, a nursing care price index can be developed.[6] Exhibit 6.4 details the breakdown of hotel costs and the calculation of cost per day, and Exhibit 6.5 shows a summary of nursing service costs.

2. Research questions on budgeting, costing, and pricing can be formulated using hospital-specific data.

3. Research can be done on costing nursing services using regional data, hospital size, or specific mission.

4. Combined with the PCS:
- Staffing and other needs are documented on the basis of patient classification.
- Nurses account for care given as it is quantified and priced.
- Costs are controlled as resources match demands.
- Fair and accurate billing for actual care received is possible.
- Nurses see themselves as providing valued services.

5. The PPS is a cost-driven reimbursement system based on individual and collective MCRs. Nurse administrators have this accurate information even before it is available to the HCFA.[7]

A goal of professional nurses is third-party payor reimbursement specifically for nursing services. Achievement of this goal depends on quantification of price per unit of nursing service to patients. Such outcome measures of nursing services are available to hospital and nursing administrators in increasing revenues. Perhaps most important of all, it serves to enhance the self-esteem of nurses and to build a positive organizational culture.

Experiential Exercise

1. Using this form, prepare a budget for an adult and pediatric unit. Use Exhibits 6.1 through 6.5 to unbundle the hospital bill for this nursing cost center. Refer to the PCS, payroll records, Medicare Cost Report, and consult with the person who prepares the Medicare Cost Report. All the information may be available from the nursing administration office.

Units: Adult and Pediatrics	Revenue Center
General	Number(s)_____
Routine care	
1. Nursing Services	
Direct Expenses (directly assigned)	
Salaries (attach position questionnaire for new ones)	$_____ . _____
Employee Benefits	$_____ . _____
Personnel Services	$_____ . _____
Supplies	$_____ . _____
Other	$_____ . _____
TOTAL DIRECT	$_____ . _____

Indirect Expenses
  Worker's Compensation $_____ . _____
  Life Insurance $_____ . _____
  General Administration $_____ . _____
  Nursing Administration $_____ . _____
  Pharmacy (floor stock) $_____ . _____
  College of Nursing $_____ . _____
  TOTAL INDIRECT $_____ . _____

  TOTAL COSTS (direct + indirect) $_____ . _____

When unbundling the bill, a decision is made to exclude specific costs from nursing and include them in nutrition or hotel cost categories. This reduces the Total Indirect, Total Costs categories.

Collect PCS data for 120 days and multiply by 3.0416 = 365 days (120 days as sample)

  Type 1 patients = _____ patient days × 3.0416 = _____
  Type 2 patients = _____ patient days × 3.0416 = _____
  Type 3 patients = _____ patient days × 3.0416 = _____
  Type 4 patients = _____ patient days × 3.0416 = _____

Base Unit or Relative Value Unit (RVU) = Type 1 patient. A Base Unit or RVU = a patient requiring 1 hour of direct nursing care within a 24-hour period plus related overhead costs as variances.

Total units (RVUs) for adult and pediatric units

  Type 1 patients   1 × _____ (patient days)   = _____
  Type 2 patients   3 × _____ (patient days)   = _____
  Type 3 patients   7 × _____ (patient days)   = _____
  Type 4 patients   17 × _____ (patient days)   = _____
     Total units (RVUs) of care   = _____
  Cost of 1 unit (RVU) of care = (TOTAL COSTS) $_____ . _____
     divided by TOTAL UNITS (RVUs) OF CARE $_____ . _____
                                                       = $_____ . _____

Charges per day (24-hours)

  Type 1 patient   1 × $_____ . _____ (cost per RVU) = $_____ . _____
  Type 2 patient   3 × $_____ . _____ (cost per RVU) = $_____ . _____
  Type 3 patient   7 × $_____ . _____ (cost per RVU) = $_____ . _____
  Type 4 patient 17 × $_____ . _____ (cost per RVU) = $_____ . _____

2. Hotel Services
   Indirect Costs (to nursing)
     Depreciation of Capital Buildings and Fixtures $_____ . _____
     Capital Equipment (moveable) $_____ . _____
       (attach requests for new items)
     Communications $_____ . _____
     Data Processing $_____ . _____
     Purchasing $_____ . _____
     Admitting $_____ . _____
     Patient Accounts $_____ . _____
     Plant Operations $_____ . _____
     Biomedical $_____ . _____
     Laundry $_____ . _____
     Housekeeping $_____ . _____
     Patient Transport $_____ . _____
     Central Supply $_____ . _____
     Medical Records $_____ . _____
     Social Service $_____ . _____
   TOTAL INDIRECT $_____ . _____

The cost per day for hotel services is total indirect cost divided by patient days:
  $_____ . _____ ÷ _____ = $_____ . _____ per day.

3. Nutrition and Dietary
   Indirect costs (to nursing) $ _____ . _____

   The cost per day for nutrition and dietary services is
   $ _____ . _____ ÷ _____ patient days = $ _____ . _____ per day.

4. Interns and Residents
   Indirect costs (to nursing) $ _____ . _____

   The cost per day for interns and residents is
   $ _____ . _____ ÷ _____ patient days = $ _____ . _____ per day.

5. Summary
   Charges (projected)
       Nursing Services $ _____ . _____
       Hotel Services $ _____ . _____
       Nutrition and Dietary $ _____ . _____
       Interns and Residents $ _____ . _____
       TOTAL $ _____ . _____

6. Daily Charges

	Nursing	Hotel	Nutrition	Interns	Total
Type 1	$ ____ . ___	+ $ ____ . ___	+ $ ____ . ___	+ $ ____ . ___	= $ ____ . ___
Type 2	$ ____ . ___	+ $ ____ . ___	+ $ ____ . ___	+ $ ____ . ___	= $ ____ . ___
Type 3	$ ____ . ___	+ $ ____ . ___	+ $ ____ . ___	+ $ ____ . ___	= $ ____ . ___
Type 4	$ ____ . ___	+ $ ____ . ___	+ $ ____ . ___	+ $ ____ . ___	= $ ____ . ___

Once the patient room bill is unbundled, the charges will equal the costs of providing these services and the cost-to-charge ratio will be 1:1. The so-called revenue departments will have balanced budgets developed to reflect the true costs of operations. There will be no further need to have cost-to-charge ratios.

The following list specifies cost centers that would be revenue centers along with nursing, hotel, nutrition, and interns:

Operating Room	Recovery Room
Delivery Room and Labor Room	Anesthesiology
Radiology	Laboratory
Respiratory Therapy	Physical Therapy
Electrocardiology	Fiberoptic
Medical Supplies Charged	Drugs Charged to Patients
to Patients	Renal Dialysis
Cast Room	Emergency

Notes: Other services are included in the foregoing cost centers.

Only for-profit hospitals are allowed a return on equity by Medicare. Bad debts are not allowed hospitals as a legitimate cost of doing business by third-party payers. Because most hospitals are not allowed a return on equity or bad-debt adjustment, they charge disproportionate prices for other services such as drugs.

Source: Courtesy of the University of South Alabama Medical Center, Mobile, Alabama.

Notes

1. S. Thomas and R. G. Vaughn. "Costing Nursing Services Using RVUs." *Journal of Nursing Administration,* 16(12)1986:10-15; L. Strasen. "Standard Costing/Productivity Model, for Nursing." *Nursing Economics,* 5(4)1987:158-161; M. D. Sovie, M. A. Tarcinale, A. W. Vanputee, and A. E. Sturden. "Amalgam of Nursing Acuity, DRGs and Costs." *Nursing Management,* 16(3)1985:22-42; and R. C. Swansburg and P. W. Swansburg. *The Nurse Manager's Guide to Financial Management* (Rockville, Md: Aspen, 1988):268-286.

2. K. F. Price and G. F. Kominski. "Using Patient Age in Defining DRGs for Medicare Payment." *Inquiry,* 25(4)1988:494-503.

3. E. Munoz, J. Josephson, N. Tenenbaum, J. Goldstein, A. M. Shears, and L. Wise. "Diagnosis-Related Groups, Costs and Outcome for Patients in the Intensive Care Unit." *Heart and Lung*, 18(6)1989:627-633.

4. J. Trofino. "JCAHO Nursing Standards, Nursing Care Hours and LOS per DRG— Parts I and II. *Nursing Management*, 20(1)1989:29-35.

5. R. C. Swansburg. *Management and Leadership for Nurse Managers* (Boston: Jones and Bartlett, 1990):88-93.

6. J. Bauer. "A Nursing Care Price Index." *American Journal of Nursing*, 72(7)1977:1150-1154.

7. Because the HCFA by law (OBRA) is changing costing formulas, some changes in the MCR may occur on an annual basis. Nurse managers should become familiar with the MCR on an annual basis.

References

Burik, D., and T. J. Duvall. "Hospital Cost Accounting: Implementing the System Successfully." *Healthcare Financial Management* 39(5)1985:76-88.

Lee, V. "What's the Cost of Nursing Care?" *Hospitals* 60(21)1986:48-52.

McClosky, J. C. "Implications of Costing Out Nursing Services for Reimbursement." *Nursing Management* 20(1)1989:44-46, 48-49.

Merrill, T. "Medicare Cost Report Needs Major Overhaul." *Hospitals* 61(4)1987:22.

Newhouse, J. P., S. Cretin, and C. J. Witsberger. "Predicting Hospital Accounting Costs." *Health Care Financing Review* 11(1)1989:25-33.

Ryan, J. "The Basic Need for Hospital Cost Accounting Expands." *Healthcare Informatics* 7(4)1990:22-24.

Wagner, L. "Hospital Cost Report Predicts Future Shock." *Modern Healthcare* 20(18)1990:14.

7

Cost Management and Trends

Russell C. Swansburg, Ph.D., R.N.
Philip W. Swansburg, M.S.N., R.N.
Richard J. Swansburg, M.S.C.I.S., R.N.

Events of the 1990s have slowed the annual rate of increase in health-care costs but have not held them to the level of diminished increases in other goods and services related to the consumer price index.

Hospitals are at risk in today's health-care environment. Most third-party payers reimburse hospitals at rates less than charges. Adding new supplies and equipment will no longer add to reimbursement, except from a very few commercial insurance payers. The bill has become too expensive for business and industry. Therefore, "less is best" is a difficult concept to get across to physicians and to employees of hospitals.

If the hospital admission is not justified to the Peer Review Organization (PRO), the bill will not be paid. Exhibit 7.1 illustrates rejection of a bill for an unjustified admission, rejection of certain charges for payment, and reversal of a rejection. Many procedures will be paid for only on an outpatient basis. Each mail brings new rules for reimbursements from Medicaid, Medicare, and other insurers.

Beginning in 1981, the medical care price index (10.7 percent) exceeded the consumer price index (10.3 percent). See Exhibit 7.2. Some of the significant factors related to the burgeoning costs of health care include billions of dollars spent on paperwork, unnecessary procedures, tests, caesarean operations, breast surgeries, hysterectomies, and spine operations.[1]

The U.S. health-care system is dominated by unrestricted and advanced technological growth, high costs, and limited access to services. Low insurance

EXHIBIT 7.1   Letter Denying Admission and Charges, and Reversal of Rejection

To: USA MEDICAL CENTER
    S. S.
    2451 FILLINGIM STREET
    MOBILE AL 36617
    Date: 4/12/19xx

Patient:
HICN:
Admitted:
Provider: USA MEDICAL CENTER
Doctor:
EXP. DATE: Control#

Re: ADMISSION DENIAL PROPOSED INITIAL NOTIFICATION

Selected for: HCFA UCDS Sample   Beneficiary Sample

_____ is the Peer Review Organization (PRO) authorized by the Health Care Financing Administration to review inpatient hospital services provided to Medicare beneficiaries in the State of _____. By law, we review Medicare cases to determine if the services meet medically acceptable standards of care, are medically necessary, and delivered in the most appropriate setting. Our Physician Reviewers have reviewed information concerning this hospital admission.

AFTER REVIEW OF THE MEDICAL RECORD, AN _____ PHYSICIAN REVIEWER HAS DENIED THIS ADMISSION. THE PATIENT HAD CHRONIC INTERMITTENT HEMOPTYSIS, BUT NO OTHER ACUTE MEDICAL PROBLEMS. IT WAS FELT THAT HIS EVALUATION COULD HAVE BEEN PERFORMED ON AN OUTPATIENT BASIS.

If you feel these findings are in error and you would like to discuss this case, a Physician Reviewer will be available Monday through Friday 8 A.M. to 4 P.M. If you do not wish to discuss the case, please state your rebuttal on this form in the space provided below and return to our office by the expiration date noted above. The Physician Reviewer will approve or deny the case from your rebuttal information. If you are unable to meet this time frame, you may request a reconsideration within sixty (60) days of the denial notice.

_____ as the Medical Review Agent for the State of _____ , is taking this action pursuant to Public Law 97-248 amended Part B of Title XI of the Social Security Act. If you have any questions, you may call our office.

Sincerely,
_____ , M.D.
Medical Director

This letter is in addition to any other correspondence you may have received from the Foundation and requires a separate response.

REBUTTAL: _____

_____

_____

_____

_____

_____

*(If you need more space, please use back of form.)

Signature: _____ , M.D.   Phone # _____

Provider: _____

cc: Administrator
    Attending Physician
    Surgeon

(Continued)

EXHIBIT 7.1 Letter Denying Admission and Charges, and Reversal of Rejection *(Continued)*

Example: THE FOLLOWING ITEMS PROVIDED TO THIS PATIENT ARE NOT BILLABLE UNDER PART A MEDICARE. PLEASE SEE THE ATTACHED LIST FOR DETAILS.

COST OUTLIER WORKSHEET

DATE	Items/Services with disallowed Medicare charges	No Med. Nec.	Frag. Chg.	Part A Non-Billable	Duplic.	No Order	# Not Rec.	# Rec.	# Billed	Physician Ref.	Unit Price		$ Amount Dis-Allowed		Rev. Code
3/17	Cepacol Mouthwash			X					1		6	25	6	25	250
3/17	Vaseline			X					1		8	00	8	00	250
3/17	Diaper Adult			X					2		15	75	31	50	270
3/17	Pad incontinent, flexicare			X					26		12	50	325	00	270
3/17	Enteros therapy initial			X					1		62	75	62	75	940
3/18	Bld Processing Cost	X												⟶	390
3/19	Handling charge	X												⟶	300
3/22	Towel Hand			X					5		5	75	28	75	270
3/23	Gown - sterile			X					5		5	75	28	75	270
3/23	Enteros skin care per minute			X					8		16	20	129	60	940
3/29	Thermometer kit			X					2		10	75	21	50	270
4/1	Vent (initial setup durable)			X					1		97	75	97	75	410

RC Comments: _____

_____

_____

_____

_____

_____

_____

 * DO NOT REFER "FRAGMENTED" CHARGES TO P.A.
** See other side for definition of categories of review findings.

(Continued)

EXHIBIT 7.1   Letter Denying Admission and Charges, and Reversal of Rejection *(Continued)*

Re: DENIAL REVERSAL

Our physician reviewers have reviewed information concerning this hospital admission.

A Re-review was requested and performed on the above case. The information submitted from you has been reviewed and the decision to deny payment has been withdrawn. Thank you for providing additional information with which to make a more appropriate decision.

AFTER REVIEW OF THE MEDICAL RECORD AND THE REBUTTAL INFORMATION PROVIDED, AN _____ PHYSICIAN REVIEWER IS REVERSING THE DECISION TO DENY THE PROCEDURE, REMOVAL OF FALLOPIAN TUBE.

---

deductibles and co-payments increase use. A Rand Corporation study showed that increased co-payment resulted in 50 percent reduction in costs with minimal negative impact on health status.[2]

The list seems endless, and it is only the tip of the iceberg. Although some causes of high health-care costs concern bioethical issues that are not easily resolved, many causes result from poor judgment, mismanagement, and fraud. In any case, nurse managers need to be aware of these issues. They are in a position to provide accurate data and contribute to ethical decisions, thereby reducing costs.

Economics of Cost Control

Rational Choice

Rational choice is the cornerstone of economic analysis. Every decision made by a nurse administrator involves rational choice. For example, consider the following scenario. A physician notes that respirator monitoring alarms are turned off in the pediatric intensive care unit (PICU). When confronted, the nurses claim the alarms are too sensitive and sound constantly. Since more are to be purchased by bid, and this model is the lowest bid, the physician tells the nurse administrator to reject the low bid. The nurse administrator involves the biomedical engineer, the circulation technologist, the head nurse of PICU, and a company representative. Changes are made in the software, the models are tested, and it can be shown that the lower bid will meet the specifications. This action demonstrates the economic necessity of arriving at a rational choice, in this case with the same supplier.

It is not necessary to have scarce resources wasted or even used up without using the decision-making skills required by rational choice. In this instance, an alternative course of action saves money to use for other requirements. Cost-benefit analysis and decision making are the tools of economics.

In nursing, the economic system functions as in other divisions of the health-care system. It "(1) transforms available resources into goods and services, (2) determines the types of goods and services produced, and (3) determines the distribution of these goods and services among individuals."[3] This leads to satisfaction of the wants of consumers through the best allocation of scarce resources.

EXHIBIT 7.2 Medical Care Price Index Compared to Consumer Price Index

| Year | Annual Percent Change | |
	Medical Care Price Index	Consumer Price Index
1970	*6.6	5.7
1975	12.0	9.1
1978	8.4	7.6
1979	9.2	11.3
1980	11.0	13.5
1981	10.7	10.3
1982	11.6	6.2
1983	8.8	3.2
1984	6.2	4.3
1985	6.3	3.6
1986	7.5	1.9
1987	6.6	3.6
1988	6.5	4.1
1989	7.7	4.8
1990	9.0	5.4
1991	8.7	4.2
1992	7.4	3.0
1993	5.9	3.0
1994	4.8	2.8
1995		2.6

*Change from 1969

Source: U.S. Bureau of the Census. *Statistical Abstract of the United States 1995.* 115th ed. (Washington, DC: U.S. Government Printing Office, 1995).

Economic Choice

Many activities affect the economic system and can be observed and modified by the nurse manager. For example, with knowledge of what has proved effective in other places, the nurse manager can discuss with clinical nurses the value of providing brief psychological intervention by the nursing staff. Forty-nine studies have indicated such interventions reduced hospital stays by 1¼ days. It will be necessary to determine which nursing diagnoses benefit from psychological interventions.[4]

Technological limitations put constraints on the productive capabilities of nurse administrators. For example, if the supply system is not computerized and the operating room supervisor cannot obtain sutures quickly, the economic impact on the operating room can be great. To reduce it to its marginal limits, the system at the supply source must also be computerized, for "just in time" inventory control. Costs under these conditions will be variable. They will become fixed when the supply system is computerized and costs of production can be standardized.

Hospitals produce health care as output. In this production, personnel decide what diagnostic tests and procedures they will use. They decide treatment modalities to be applied. These decisions determine the kinds of personnel, supplies, and equipment that will be used as input. Hospitals are either profit

or not-for-profit. However, none want to lose money. Nurse administrators make decisions based on fluctuations in census, patient acuity, and other factors that influence profits or losses. They even make product quality decisions based on profits or losses.

Labor Supply

The supply of labor has been an economic factor for nurse administrators for years. It has influenced wage rates and the individual preferences of nurses. Labor supply has increased, and hospitals have reduced use of agency nurses. The economic conditions impacting labor supply will change as more students enter a crowded field and women enter professions and occupations not previously available to them.

Competition versus Regulation

The health-care industry is in a competitive market stage. There are many sellers of identical health services including hospital care, ambulatory care, home care, wellness care, and other types of care. Most people buy the health care they can afford. The enormity of the health-care market makes buyers and sellers seem small. Even mergers of providers does not change the competitive market when the distribution of facilities and services is broad. Entry of providers into the health-care industry is restricted by certificate of need (CON) laws and other state and federal laws. This factor does not restrict the economics of the competitive market and will eventually bankrupt more health-care firms. As it does, the licensed services will be sold to other providers.

In communities where a health-care monopoly exists, services can be curtailed to inflate prices. While third-party payers regulate prices, services can be cut to maximize profits. Provision of emergency medical services can be a source of access for people without adequate insurance or money to pay for these output problems. Compromise has to be reached to improve productivity, the givens being that patients will not be held beyond need and alternative groups of patients will be admitted to empty beds.[5]

Samson states that health-care markets do not respond to price competition as do other industries.[6] There is evidence that this is changing:

- In Cleveland, Ohio, businesses and industries reduced health-care costs by joining together to build purchasing power. They built partnerships with provider leaders forming a nonprofit organization. They agreed on uniform measures of provider performance: mortality, complications, length of stay, and hospital-acquired infections. Systems are tested and methods modified.
- Some employers are implementing new employee incentive benefit plans; choice of preferred providers gives employees additional benefits.[7]
- In Memphis, Tennessee, employers formed a coalition and bid hospital insurance saving tens of millions of dollars. Coalition members saved $4 to $6 for every dollar invested in the group. The lithotripsy procedure was negotiated from $7,100 down to $5,000 per procedure.
- There are more than 90 coalitions in the United States of America. Costs are being brought down and productivity up by competition. Businesses are developing information systems on provider efficiency.[8]

Economics

Economics is "the social science concerned with the production and distribution of goods and services produced by firms employing workers and other scarce factors of production of an economy. An economy is composed of everything in a geographic area that is related to production and distribution. An economic system is the way production and distribution occur."[9]

Economics has become so important to the healthy survival of nurses and of nursing that it may well warrant inclusion as a vital course in the education of both clinical practitioners and nurse managers. It should become continuing education for both.

Accelerating health-care costs threaten scarcer resources, including providers and raw materials. How much of the nation's resources can be spent on health care? It is already at 15 percent of the GNP. Until recently the health-care market demanded treatment and cure of disease and injury. There is now some limited focus on maintaining health through wellness and fitness programs. While this has increased the overall cost of health care, there is no evidence available that the cost of disease and injury have decreased. The opposite is apparent. As an example, gunshot wounds cost $116.4 billion annually in hospital and medical care. In 1992 one thousand people were killed on the job, 80 percent from gunshot wounds. In 1991 more than 8,000 young people were murdered.[10]

Demand for health care and nursing care is increased (or decreased) by the availability of health insurance. Increased availability of providers influences demand. Given the increased availability of wellness care, nurse managers will need to know its impact upon demand. Will people elect wellness care as an alternative to illness care? Evidence points to their doing so, even paying for it from their own pockets.

Exercise appears to be increasing as more people choose to jog, walk, and so on. Business and industry are building exercise facilities. Individuals are buying diet and nutrition services. It only remains for third-party payers to incorporate wellness into their payment mechanisms. This is already being done by a few health maintenance organizations (HMOs). When able to afford it, consumers will buy inefficient health insurance policies and supplemental policies that, when combined, technically will pay more than the charges. However, benefits are coordinated by third-party payers and the insured do not get refunds. In addition, consumers who know the value of health insurance consider it when seeking employment. They include it in their budgets as a priority when given alternatives because health insurance is an investment in future income.

Economies of Scale

Nurse managers have given some attention to economies of scale. They have entered joint ventures for staff development programs. Consortiums produce quality programs for individual nursing departments at a split cost each can afford. They can then send many nurses to such programs for this one split cost.

Other economies of scale could be developed to contain cost for expensive but scarce clinical nursing specialties. They could include enterostomal therapy nurses, chemotherapy nurses, hyperalimentation therapy nurses, and other

advanced practitioners. Nurse managers have barely touched this area of cost management. It could be shared among hospitals, nursing homes, home health care agencies, and other health-care institutions.

Even within one institution nurse managers can increase productivity by cross-training nurses in families of specialties and skills. Nurses can be prepared to function between PICU and NICU and among adult ICUs. The possibilities are endless.

Productivity Research

Nurse managers need to study productivity by establishing research protocols. In a cardiac rehabilitation program paid for by third-party payers, nurses could study the cost-effectiveness with a control group of uninsured (also called self-pay, or nonpaying) patients denied access to the system. Effectiveness would be measured by differences between the two groups in medication compliance, visits to providers, hospitalizations, complications, and deaths.

Nurse managers and researchers would enhance the validity of the nursing process if nursing output could be quantitatively related to patient outcome. This is true of both wellness and illness programs. What is the cost-effectiveness of nursing as measured by comparing efficiency of one nursing treatment with another? What are the outcome criteria?

Another area of research into productivity is a study of the effects of different levels of nurses upon outcomes. The outcomes can all be economics based including costs of salaries, consumption of resources, lengths of stay, among others. Are nurses with bachelor's degrees more productive than nurses with high school diplomas or associate's degrees? The same question can pertain to nurses with master's degrees and doctorates, if they are working at the clinical nurse level.

In-hospital time and medical costs were reduced and patient satisfaction increased when a nurse practitioner was introduced into a cardiology clinic of a Puerto Rican hospital.

Analysis of supplies and equipment expenditures has saved as much as 15 percent of the supplies budget in a hospital. Stocks were reduced, recycling of equipment was improved, ordering of supplies was coordinated, and cost-effective alternative sources of equipment and supplies were identified.

Redesign of forms and flowsheets has saved $500,000 in a large hospital. Unnecessary tests and procedures have been reduced in many instances. Patient LOSs have been decreased. Improved physician and nurse collaboration has saved millions of dollars in several hospitals. Nurse-led research is needed for cost-effectiveness.[11]

Normative Economics

An analysis of what is and what ought to be is termed *normative economics*. In the United States the prevailing theory is that free-market competition is superior to government regulation of most business enterprises. There are three exceptions: public goods such as national defense, externalities such as pollution control, and monopolization of an industry such as communications. The health-care industry is in a transition between being a monopoly of hospitals and physicians and being more open to out-of-hospital and other-than-physician

markets. If physicians' fees do not respond to market demand and physician supply, prices will continue to increase as physicians increase in numbers. In the latter instance, if physicians' waiting-room times decrease and physicians spend more time with patients, then the price in time of physician visits decreases and so does the real price.

Other theories are (1) physicians target income and raise fees if numbers of clients decline, and (2) as numbers of physicians increase they induce people to consume more of their services.[12]

Alabama exceeded the goal of 1 physician per 1,000 people and had 1 for each 787 people in 1985. There is still a maldistribution in geographic location as well as the mix of specialties within the physician workforce. Only future studies will tell how this oversupply will affect the economics of health care in this state.[13]

The mean net income of all physicians increased $6,800, from $170,600 in 1991 to $177,400 in 1992. In addition their professional expenses increased $10,600, from $168,400 in 1991 to $179,000 in 1992.[14]

Increased Interest by Health Providers and Consumers

Rising health-care costs have sparked increased interest in health care as an industry by providers, consumers, and economists. Increased use has limited the availability of health-care resources. Increased costs leading to shortages of revenues have resulted in debate of the question of social policy for the right to health care. Since there is no constitutional right to health care in the United States, who will care for the poor? Will society's compassion be inspired to change the law and mandate health care as a right? Will private sources provide health-care services? They do to some extent, however they are usually targeted to some individual whose condition has aroused public support via the efforts of the news media. A few categories of people have private sponsors, such as children suffering from burns, muscular dystrophy, and other specific conditions. Some private support is limited, such as that for cancer and heart disease. Most efforts in these categories have focused upon research.

Economists study the efficient allocation of scarce resources among competing users. In doing so they identify the product, methods of producing it, the quantities to be produced, and the people who will produce and use the product. From the economist's viewpoint, economic theories are analyzed to produce nonbiased information, which is then used to make biased judgments.

More and more we are faced with the question of rationing health care. Who will do the rationing? Will it be the insurance industry? Today the people who can afford to buy it receive greater amounts while paying more out-of-pocket costs in deductibles and co-payments. No segment of the provider system has decided to provide health care as a basic human right of United States citizens.

An organization survives economically when revenues exceed costs. Revenues to exceed health-care costs must come from consumers via insurance, cash, or government payments. Hospitals have to reduce costs to match reduced revenues. Nurses must be realistic and reduce costs also. Otherwise when the hospital goes bankrupt they will be out of jobs. Alternatives can be two levels of care based on ability to pay and the replacement of registered nurses by licensed

and nonlicensed technicians or extenders. The focus on nursing productivity will be on outcome rather than on process.

Nurses will develop new models of nursing-care delivery to reduce readmission rates of patients, reduce lengths of stay, reduce turnover, and reduce absenteeism. Reduction of numbers of nurses is necessary to increase salaries. Spitzer recommends a professional practice model of nursing with the following characteristics:

1. The professional nurse is responsible for the care of the patient from admission to discharge.
2. The professional nurse is accountable for the quality of care delivered and documented.
3. Continuity of care is provided inasmuch as feasible.
4. The professional nurse maintains communication with the patient, family, physician, and other members of the health-care team in an ongoing, timely, and appropriate manner.
5. Documentation and evaluation of the nursing process and the response to care is maintained in the patient's record.
6. The nurse is responsible and accountable for meeting and expanding his or her scope of knowledge and practice through continuing education.[15]

State and federal government programs that have attempted to control costs have included:

1. An economic stabilization program to freeze wages and prices.
2. Social Security amendments of 1972.
3. The National Health Planning and Resource Development Act of 1972.
4. Budget review to set or approve reimbursement rates based on detailed review of projected budgets of individual hospitals and their departments.
5. Formulas to determine rates of payments or ceilings.
6. Negotiated rates between hospitals and rate setters.
7. The Hospital Cost Containment Act of 1977.
8. The Rostenkowski Voluntary Effort of 1977.
9. The Talmadge Bill.
10. Competition of for-profit hospital chains, which are reputed to reduce nursing hours per patient day, extraneous tests, and professional/technical personnel ratios. Medicare and Medicaid patients went to teaching and community hospitals.[16]

To these efforts can be added:

11. Prospective payment system (PPS) and diagnosis related groups (DRGs). The Tax Equity and Fiscal Responsibility Act (TEFRA) of 1982 went into effect in 1983. It is usually modified with each annual congressional office of the budget reconciliation act (COBRA).
12. In 1993 the Health Care Financing Administration (HCFA) implemented a new reimbursement plan for physicians, the Resource-Based Relative Value Scale (RBRVS).[17]

The Recession-Proof Medical Supply Industry

For the most part the health-care supply industry has been recession proof. It increased supply sales 550 percent in the decade from 1970 to 1980. To the

industry this represents a projected bonanza of $10 billion per year in sales during the 1980s. Although there have been cutbacks and competition has increased, the industry is still healthy. Among the reasons for this strength are that:

- People will pay any amount of money when it comes to their own health.
- There are a large number of third-party payers and the number is increasing.
- The seller dictates to the buyer what shall be bought.[18]

As an example of the seller dictating to the buyer, if an elderly male patient is cared for in the home by his family, his external catheter and urinary drainage bag are washed and reused daily. In the nursing home or hospital they are disposable, used and discarded on a daily basis. The cost is charged to the patient, insurer, or the family, with a markup for profit. (The industry looks forward to increasing numbers of the population older than 65 because they use more health services.)

The over 65 age group, approximately 18 percent of the population, now consumes 35 percent of health care. The number of persons over age 85 is increasing at three times the rate of the population at large.[19] Per capita spending for the elderly was $11,152 in 1990 compared to $4,166 for children. Forty percent of the $110 billion spent on Medicaid in 1992 went to people over 65. Since 1960 the number of seniors below the poverty line has shrunk from 35 percent to about 12.2 percent. This is less than the 13.5 percent of the total population below the poverty level and much less than the 20.6 percent of persons under 18 below the poverty level.[20]

Another example of the seller dictating to the buyer is the case of the surgeon in the OR who specifies the sutures he or she will use and they are manufacturer specific. When new technology is available, the seller sells it to physicians, who then demand it of hospitals.

Now that the public has raised the specter of cost management, the industry has had to look at its methods. Hospitals have joined together to buy supplies at better economies of scale. A majority of hospitals are now doing this. In addition, hospitals are bidding supplies, equipment, and services such as ambulance service. When bid specifications are set by buyers, they can frequently buy the lowest bid item with the same standard of quality and service. Remember Deming's theory that it is best to stay with one supplier.

Standardization of supplies has been achieved by the American Hospital Supply and other companies who have computerized inventories and serve as distributors, manufacturers, and service companies to their clients. Elimination of small suppliers, with manufacturers selling directly to users, could cut costs. There is also a danger in supply companies becoming too big and creating a monopoly leading to higher costs and diminished service. Although durable medical equipment has become a product line within vertically integrated hospital corporations, the medical supply industry will take on another new look with the rampant hospital mergers.

Many of today's markets are aimed at home health care and physical therapy. Home health care uses oxygen supplies and durable medical equipment, items that may shore up the small independent medical supplier. Physical therapy is moving out of hospitals and into clinics and homes. Increasingly, attempts are being made to change state laws to allow physical therapists reimbursement for services without physician orders. All of this means that health care is shifting out of hospitals, but the price is no different. It is just paid to a different provider.

Elasticity of Health-Care Costs

Emergency care is price inelastic because it requires an immediate medical response. Nonemergency care is price elastic because people can choose whether to pay its price. This trend was proven in a California study in which 26 percent of Medicaid beneficiaries were charged a minimum co-payment. They paid $1.00 for each of the first two office visits in a month and $.50 for each of the first two prescriptions in a month. Office visits were reduced by 8 percent. Since nonemergency care represents about 60 percent of the market responsive to price changes, it is an area for cost management. Employers have increasingly taken advantage of this elasticity and have increased deductibles and co-payments, thereby reducing cost and use.[21]

Because of third-party insurance with low deductibles, high-cost procedures with low-value results to the patient have frequently been ordered. This process is termed "moral hazard." According to Chang:

> Economic analysis of demand suggests that the amount of waste resulting from overconsumption of medical care varies directly with elasticity of demand; the more responsive the demand is to changes in price, other things being the same, the larger the waste of resources due to overconsumption of medical care.[22]

Health-care consumers need to be informed about the benefits of a treatment relative to the purchase price. Consumers seldom call providers and obtain comparative information on either product or price. This behavior is another area for nursing research.

Definitions and Principles

What Is Cost Management?

Cost containment, cost control, cost-effectiveness, cost-benefit analysis, and *cost reduction* are all terms frequently heard in illness care facilities. While each can be defined separately, together they make a generic entity called *cost management.* They all mean that we must make maximum use of our resources—people, materials, money—to contain the spiraling costs of illness. People still want increasingly higher wages. Even though the overall cost-of-living index was down to 2.6 percent for 1995, health-care costs were projected to top $1 trillion in 1994, an increase of $118 billion over 1993. The 1999 projected cost is $1.99 trillion. Reasons include 25 percent overhead, which is only 11 percent or lower in other industrialized countries.[23] Inflation is being controlled in the non–health-care sector, oil and gas prices remain constant, and some salaries and wages are being decreased.

The flexible budget is considered by some financial managers to be an important technique for cost control. A fixed budget describes the degree to which actual results have compared with expected results. The flexible budget provides results that describe the degree to which the actual results were appropriate. One pertinent example is to prepare a flexible staffing budget that is based on the results of monthly samples of patients' acuity ratings and a monthly bed occupancy rate for each unit. Staffing is then adjusted according to workload. Budgeting should involve both fixed and flexible techniques.

Insurers and consumers can benefit from cost management. Providers face public and private financial restraints on practice and services provided. True cost management reduces the total cost of health care, or it limits the inflationary rate increases. Some cost-management measures merely shift the cost away from insurer onto the provider or patient.

Nurse Personnel Pool

A nurse personnel pool is an example of creatively managing costs. When the census fluctuates there must be ways of increasing and decreasing staffing without stretching staff beyond the breaking point or firing them. What kinds of educated and experienced nurse personnel are available? Is there a need to recruit more personnel with certain qualifications? How many to hire into the pool as temporary employees must be decided and a paid orientation provided for them. Policies must be set for their hours of work and assignments. Perhaps they will be employed on all shifts as needed. They will work no more than 8 hours per day or 80 hours in one pay period if overtime is to be avoided. They will be employed full time as vacancies occur and on a seniority and competency basis. Other policies will be the same as for temporary workers.

Other sources of nurse personnel for such a pool are RNs and LPNs who want to work only part time. In addition, some persons want to supplement full-time jobs in other institutions.

Cost-effectiveness has been described by Koontz and O'Donnell as a technique for choosing from among alternatives to identify a preferred choice when objectives are far less specific than the quantitative facts of sales, costs, or profits. They state that the major features that distinguish cost-effectiveness from any other planning decision are:

1. Objectives are normally output- or end-result–oriented and usually imprecise.
2. Alternatives ordinarily represent total systems, programs, or strategies for meeting objectives.
3. The measures of effectiveness must be relevant to objectives and set in as precise terms as possible, although some may not be subject to quantification.
4. Cost estimates are usually traditional and normal but may include nonmonetary as well as monetary costs, even though the former may be eliminated by expressing them as negative factors of effectiveness.
5. Decision criteria, while definite but not usually as specific as cost or profit, may include achieving a given objective at the least cost, or attaining it with resources available, or providing for a trade-off of cost for effectiveness particularly in the light of the claims of other objectives.[24]

Cost management in nursing includes conceptual and physical acts to curb unnecessary spending through planned and practical use of personnel, material, and physical resources for maximum productivity.

Views of the American Public

In a survey by Louis Harris and associates for the Equitable Life Assurance Society of the United States, it was found that the American public and union leaders view cost-related and access-related changes as top priorities in the health-care system. The cost of health care is seen as the primary barrier to obtaining it.[25]

According to the survey, all groups view hospitalization and laboratory work and X rays done outside of hospitals and clinics to be too costly. A primary cause is new and more expensive equipment and treatments. Little is done to encourage price competition such as publishing of prices. Physicians do not agree that they can keep prices down with competition. They are the least willing of all groups to accept changes that are likely to adversely affect the financial incentives for their profession.

The public is willing to accept a wide range of cost-containment proposals because they think them necessary. These include outpatient or ambulatory surgery, alternative treatments for the chronically ill, increased cost sharing of health insurance premiums and increased deductibles, diagnosis-related cost caps on hospital and physicians' fees, required second opinion on nonemergency surgery, insurance rate incentives for preventive care, prepaid plans and preferred provider plans, and use of low-cost alternatives to physicians and hospital care.

Corporate executives view cost sharing, increased coverage for home care for the chronically ill, and use of nurse practitioners, midwives, and physicians' assistants as cost effective. All but physicians oppose a tax on employer-paid premiums. If health insurance benefits were folded into wages and salaries, the use rates by employees buying and paying for their own care could diminish. The American public opposes shifting costs from Medicare patients to other patients. Many people favor programs of health insurance for the unemployed. The conclusion is that the American public is well informed about health-care coverage and services.

Disincentives

Many of the policies and practices of the U.S. government and of private payers of hospital bills have been disincentives to cost management. Tax-free bonds for hospital construction, although threatened by the U.S. Congress and the HCFA, remain a disincentive. While hospitals vow the bonds are essential to keeping costs down, there is an argument for letting the health-care industry compete as other industries in the free-enterprise system. Tax-exempt bonds can fuel inflation by encouraging unnecessary building of new plants. They can also encourage growth of for-profit hospitals to compete with not-for-profit hospitals at the cost of quality as well as increased price of patient care. This trend is happening at an increased rate with for-profit hospital chains either buying the not-for-profit hospitals or taking over their management.

In the past, there has been a bias by insurance carriers in favor of inpatient care. Certain procedures would be paid for only if the patients were hospitalized. Although this disincentive has been largely reversed, it exists as a bias for physicians who get paid higher fees for some procedures when performed on an inpatient basis.

Until recently there was a ban on advertising, which was a disincentive to cost containment. Hospitals now advertise all services, although few publish their charges as a matter of policy. Some physicians advertise their services but never list their fees.

There are still multiple barriers to providers' entry into the health-care field. Political barriers are the most common disincentives. Certificate of need

laws, designed to control costs, actually control competition. In addition, hospitals work to prevent other hospitals from acquiring new services they provide rather than coming to cooperative agreements to share facilities and equipment.

A further disincentive to cost containment is the fact that decisions regarding patient care are made by providers with no financial risk to them. The risk is always to the patient and the third-party payer. This practice is changing with the advent of PPS and the threat of health-care reform. It is to the hospital's advantage to prevent complications leading to extended hospitalization. Unfortunately, the physician is only at risk for malpractice and so risk-management programs attempt to stem the tide of malpractice lawsuits.[26]

The Chrysler Experience

Chrysler cut its health bill in 1984 by $58 million, down from the projected $460 million in its budget. This action saved $300 for each employee and retiree. Chrysler did so by setting up a Health Care Committee of the Board of Directors in 1981. To get health-care costs under control, committee members went after the facts from the insurer, Blue Cross/Blue Shield of Michigan, and the United Auto Workers. They examined 67,000 hospital admissions, 30 months of records, catalogued all care for each Chrysler employee, and found unnecessary care, inefficiency, waste, and even abuse and fraud.

What did they do to correct it? They made the use of generic drugs mandatory, thereby saving $250,000 in the first partial year. Also, when employees and retirees could find overcharges, they gave them part of the refunds, calling this program "One Check Leads to Another."

In addition, Chrysler saved $2 million in 1984 by encouraging outpatient surgery. The company offered incentives to HMO enrollment and formed a dental HMO with fixed, prenegotiated prices. It had more than 17,000 members, saved $3 million in 1984, and was fought by the Michigan Dental Association.

Chrysler mounted a major health-promotion and disease-prevention effort to keep people out of the hospital and in good health. Chrysler's employees have been led to view hospitals as institutions of last resort, and have placed emphasis on health promotion and disease prevention.

Blue Cross now reviews admissions and length of stay. Admissions for nonsurgical low back pain were reduced 64 percent in 6 months. Applying similar standards, maternity stays in excess of 3 days were reduced 67 percent in 6 months. All hospitalizations are now prescreened; nonemergency, nonmaternity cases are reviewed by a second, independent medical opinion. "Of the $58 million saved, we believe that about $32 million is attributable to hospital costs, and about $22 million to fees and tests, largely associated with hospitalization. The remaining $4 million comes from the acceptance of dental HMOs, our move to generic drugs, and other cost-cutting activities."[27]

Future savings are projected in reduced HMO charges and reduced physician fees. Chrysler intends to make the suppliers of health care efficient. Even after savings, Chrysler spends $1.1 million per day for health care. This amounted to $530 per car sold in 1984 and was more than it paid to its 65,000 pensioners. It was four times what it paid to shareholders in dividends.

The following principles may be derived from the Chrysler experience:

1. Fee-for-service payments encourage physicians and dentists to keep prices high. A cap should be placed on them by insurers and users of their services. This limit can be accomplished by competition, advertising, and expanded use of HMOs, PPOs, PHOs, and other entities.

2. Charge and cost-plus hospital reimbursement should end. This trend is being accomplished by prospective payment for Medicare (although cost driven) and by competition and advertising in the industry. There is room for improvement by involving physicians in controlling excess use of tests and procedures.

3. Artificial monopolization of the practice of medicine and dentistry should end. This is occurring through the increase in numbers of more practitioners and specialists. However, physicians still control through referral patterns, one example being the alliance forged between cardiologists and heart surgeons.

4. There is a need for physicians and consumers to set predictable standards of malpractice. When they are not lived up to, the guilty must be disciplined. Enormous judgments against doctors and hospitals are forcing good ones out of the business. It is the bad ones who need to go. If they do, one seldom hears about them, indicating that there is a cover-up or no action being taken.

5. Government, corporate, and union health-care plans need to set their own standards, rules, and rates of reimbursement. They should never let providers write their own checks.

6. The decades of cozy intimacy between the Blues and commercial insurers, and doctor and hospital providers must end.

Business, industry, and consumers will continue to take action to contain health-care costs. The same technique can contain costs at other large industries where more is sometimes spent for health benefits than for raw materials.

Overinsurance

Although it could be labeled a disincentive to cost containment, overinsurance is certainly a cause of health-care costs. There is more and more coverage through group plans. People use that for which they believe they have already paid, a fact that is true in any form of insurance. For example, a car owner who has a broken windshield will file for the insurer to pay the cost of replacement if the premium will not rise. However, if a driver knows the premium will rise with more claims, that driver may be inclined to increase deductibles, reduce premiums, and risk personally paying small replacement costs such as for a windshield.

The same is true of health insurance. People want total coverage if premiums will be paid by the employer or someone else. They will even carry supplemental insurance without considering whether the benefit is equal to or greater than the risk. It can be advantageous to pay deductibles out of pocket, thereby lowering premiums.

Deductibles for health insurance decrease use of health services and subsequently contain costs. Business and industry officials are using these techniques of cost containment, knowing there is little risk to needed health-care services.

Higher Expectations of Patients

Patients with health insurance are like customers at a car wash who are paying for "the works." They are aware of health-care benefits and expect to get everything available. They want insurance that covers all health-care providers. They expect their insurance to cover children in college including graduate school. They expect the maximum in diagnostic tests and the latest in applied technological therapies and prescribed drugs. These higher expectations of patients inflate health-care costs.

New Services and Technologies

Each physician demands that hospitals buy "state-of-the-art" equipment. Physicians sell their patients on being admitted to such hospitals. Hospitals that don't buy the new machines and implement the new services do so at their own financial peril. Often companies selling equipment convince physicians that a new model has the edge over the old ones. Questions are seldom asked to prove the advantage of the newer and more expensive equipment. The same principle applies to supplies such as arterial catheters with computers attached and indwelling urinary catheters with thermometers attached. They cost much more than simple catheters and their value in improving care is questionable.

To contain the costs of technologies, physicians must be asked to justify purchase, write criteria for use, and be held accountable for such agreements. Most of the increased cost for technology cannot be recouped by charges in a prospective payment system. Technology can help reduce costs by the exercise of clinical judgment. Physicians can reduce the use of expensive technology such as the CAT scan and MRI, restricting it to elimination of the need for exploratory surgery and invasive tests.

Competition among private hospitals and HMOs for patients and physicians increases purchases of the latest technological equipment whether services are needed or not. "Boston's Massachusetts General Hospital recently opened a new obstetrical service, despite being within three miles of five well-established maternity programs with surplus beds."[28]

The United States has a surplus of 300,000 hospital beds and at least 5,000 surplus mammography machines.[29] Acute-care hospitals decreased to 5,261 in 1993. They still have an occupancy rate of only 64.6 percent and the average cost per patient day increased by $61 from $820 in 1992 to $881 in 1993.[30] Excess raises costs due to decreased use. Quality is lowered when not enough procedures are done to maintain personnel competence. More than one-third of California's hospitals are performing open heart surgery with dangerously low volumes, increased death rates, and increased costs.[31] These results are true of any transplant and complex surgical procedure performed at low volume.

Failure of Competitive Market Forces

In past years the health-care industry has had little or no competition, determining its own supply, demand, and prices. The consumer had no incentive to look for the lowest priced physician, hospital, drugstore, or any other provider of health-care service or goods. All a hospital needed to do was encourage a

group of physicians to use it and neither the patient nor third-party payer had much to say about prices. Much of this is changing, although the effect on costs is still questionable.

There is little evidence that competition will contain costs. They are being shifted to other pockets—home health care, ambulatory surgery centers, family medical centers, and others. The claim is that HMOs, HPOs, and PPOs will ultimately be effective in containing costs, but they simply become the new pockets that may or may not provide quality and necessary services.

A balance between a competitive and a cooperative market can be explored. Providers, consumers, and insurers would become partners in financing and delivering health care. Together they would decide what is necessary and what is an expensive option.

Health personnel must be effectively used to reduce costs. Competition among physicians does not drive down costs. Excess physicians create an excessive demand for health services. Specialty physicians order more procedures than family practice physicians and general practitioners. They also have longer encounters. Use of nurse practitioners and physicians' assistants reduces health-care costs.[32]

Increased use of emergency rooms increases health-care costs. They are frequently used by low-income people because they cannot pay private physicians and lose working time. High-income families use less expensive physicians' offices. This is a distributive problem that could be corrected by a health-care policy that provides vouchers to low-income families. Someone pays the higher costs through taxes or cost shifting.[33]

In Canada, monies have been redirected, although redirection to physicians' offices did not redirect patients away from emergency rooms. Canadians are reputed to have brought health-care costs under control by establishing hospital care as a basic human right, insuring everyone through one government plan, increasing the ratio of general practitioners to specialists, and reducing prescription drug prices. They have virtually eliminated the two-class system of health care and have reduced infant and maternal mortality rates.[34]

Government Programs

Even with the PPS, government programs increased costs of health care by imposing complex accounting and reporting procedures. In addition to the annual Medicare Cost Report, there is a PRO reporting system that requires full-time personnel to prepare and provide numerous documents. However, the administrative overhead of Medicaid is 5 percent, of private insurance an average of 13 percent. Medicare overhead was 2 percent in 1991.[35]

Sources of Pressure

The public is putting pressure on the health-care industry to contain costs. A uniform unit of service is needed to index the productivity of the industry and of individual hospitals. Also needed is a way to measure quality or outcome of individual hospitals and nursing care. For Medicare the outcome of measure is the DRG and a discharge from the hospital. Specific outcome standards are being developed by insurers, subsequently by providers. They must include quality standards.

Health-care costs are still accelerating as a result of inflation, regulation, technological advancements, public demands, excess capacity, malpractice lawsuits, regionalization, an aging and disabled population (35 million persons older than 65), changes in insurance coverage, and changing roles of hospitals. Consequently, charge structures, cost settlements, insurance premiums, and out-of-pocket payments are increasing. Pressure to restrain costs will come from:

- *Government payers*—Medicare and Medicaid are already in the forefront.
- *Government regulations*—Government activities will increase in areas of rate setting and review.
- *Other third-party payers*—Businesses and industries are encouraging them to assume an adversarial relationship with the health-care industry.[36]

Potential Patterns in Cost Management and Cost Benefits

Increased use of computers will assist administrators, including nurses, in the health-care industry in gathering information on the effectiveness of services. Computers will be used to control costs and to teach. Their advantages will be utilized and information-processing technology should be included in teaching curricula early in the program.

The cost-containment squeeze will force or encourage hospital mergers. By 1995 most major hospitals in San Antonio, Texas, belonged to one of four major groups. Mergers decrease duplication of services; for example, all women's and children's services can be combined in one hospital, and so on.

The cost squeeze will increase. Present reimbursement caps and DRGs are only the beginning. New methods will have to be devised to increase cost-effectiveness as jobs are merged and departments combined. There will be more family and, we hope, community involvement. The structure of the entire system will change as the industry vies to maintain a structural and functional identity and integrity. Continuing education will become more important and stronger links between academics and clinical practice will be formed.

Market Influences

We have entered a buyers' market in the health-care field, which is due to the shift of responsibility for decisions about cost to the consumer. All health-care decisions cannot be made on the basis of economics. There are multiple impacts: legal, economic, clinical, public relations, and others.

Competition hasn't really occurred until prices decrease. Use of hospitals has declined but the overall price of health care is still increasing.

The insurance industry is changing. There are higher deductibles and co-payments since fringe benefits have reached 40 percent of an employee's salary. Between 1979 and 1983, required employee-paid deductibles went from 14 percent to 32 percent.

Reputed benefits that have accrued from this high-cost health care include

- a 25 percent drop in cancer rates
- a 40 percent drop in death from stroke

- 72.1 years average life expectancy for males (projected to 74.5 by 2010)
- 78.9 years average life expectancy for females (projected to 81.3 by 2010)[37]

There should be some diagnostic restraint on the part of physicians. While appropriate tests are necessary to initiate and continue a plan of care, they should be ordered judiciously and with purposes fitted to diagnosis and therapeutic response. Trial-and-error use and overconcern for litigation should not be overriding forces for ordering tests. Physicians should consider expense when ordering tests and they should accept responsibility for making difficult decisions that will reduce costs. Computer systems to monitor physicians' practices are available and have proven to save considerable sums of money.

With a potential for 2.5 million persons over 85 years of age, 100-bed nursing homes would have to be built at a rate of one a day for 16 years to take care of them. Alternative systems must be found, such as tax credits for families who care for their aged relatives and a voucher system that allows them to shop for care. A means test is probably politically unacceptable.[38]

Approaches to Containing Health-Care Costs

Systematic Effort

The containment of health-care costs requires a systematic and coordinated effort. These facets of the problem must be understood before the problem is solved:

1. Health involves personal health services, education, housing, income, nutrition, environment, lifestyle, and training of providers. It is a total system requiring a total effort.
2. The weakness of the system must be acknowledged by all, by providers, insurers, and consumers alike. They must be acknowledged by the rich and by the poor, the educated and the illiterate, by government employees and private citizens.
3. Change must occur gradually and consistently with clear objectives. There is no simple solution to a problem that involves such vast national resources as 15 percent of the GNP, and which is projected to increase to 18 percent of the GNP by the year 2000.
4. The system must be dealt with as a whole. This is not occurring as competition is forcing divisiveness.
5. A comprehensive program can be administered by public and private sectors.
6. There are problems of organization, administration, and leadership at all levels.
7. Leaders from all sectors must work with, not against, each other. Otherwise the answer will be that the strongest will prevail. This begs the question of the nature of health care. Although it is not a legal right, the question of compassion must be addressed.
8. There must be a continuum of health care—ambulatory, institutional, and home.[39]

Health care is "big business," requiring careful coordination of its components to control costs. However, fragmentation of responsibility and duplication

of services are common. Poor leadership exists in health care because of frequent turnover in administration.

Physicians have had the greatest influence over provision and utilization of services. They alone can admit and discharge patients and order the use of diagnostic tests and therapies. They must be partners rather than antagonists.

Responsibility for health care is shifting to the state governments. The federal government will remain involved but will regulate the industry through directives related to Medicare and Medicaid. The private sector must find a way to work together with less reliance on the government.

There is some suggestion that group practice and a comprehensive, prepayment system can improve service and promote economy. In addition, a mission-oriented continuum of health care leading to a minimum of continued professional supervision of patients is needed. Health and social programs in other countries should be examined.[40]

Health-care reform is being successfully curbed by a well-organized medical-industrial complex of insurers, pharmaceutical companies, HMOs, medical trade associations, health-care providers, and similar groups. They fill the coffers of congressional campaigns, paying to influence legislative agendas and policy making. The insurance industry is a root cause of increased costs and decreased coverage.[41]

The insurance industry gives selective health security and safety to Americans with insurance and minimal to moderate health care needs. It increases costs.[42]

Efficiency

As one attempts to untangle the web of causes of high health-care costs, one is struck by the obvious inefficiency of the system. Resources are developed on a cumulative basis with few eliminations. These resources have not been controlled or used well. Planning and decision making have been sporadic and unconnected to providers, insurers and consumers operating independently among themselves and within their entity. They seldom planned for technical efficiency that would find the cheapest way of doing specific tasks. Nor did they plan for social efficiency to determine which group of tasks society wanted, given limits.

In nursing, the budget has often been developed by hospital administrators and spent by nurses and physicians. Information on profits and losses has been poor, while information on costs has ranged from meager to nonexistent.

More attention has been given to the activity of costing. This has been done for Medicare patients through the Medicare Cost Report and the DRG system. The same information can be used to determine the cost related to any patients as all fall within the 494 DRGs (with expansion to 652 proposed). Analysis of costs will provide the source for determining whether the unit cost of the services has been reduced. When it can be reduced and a safe level of care provided simultaneously, efficiency has increased.

Ten percent of the trillion-dollar health-care budget is eaten up by a bloated administrative bureaucracy. This bureaucracy could be reduced by a single-payer approach that would also reduce insurance companies' roles.[43]

The United States spends 40 percent more per capita on health care than any other nation but ranks twenty-first among the twenty-four largest industrial nations in infant mortality, and sixteenth worldwide in life expectancy.[44]

Twenty-four and eight-tenths percent of hospital budgets now go for billing and administration.[45] Canada, with universal coverage, has health-care costs around 10 percent of GNP, 11 percent of which is spent on billing and administration.[46] United States health care costs 15 percent of GNP with 24 percent of that spent on billing and administration.[47]

In 1991, $159.1 billion (21 percent of health-care spending) went for costs of health insurance overhead, hospital and nursing-home administration, and doctors' office overhead. The goal of insurers should be to spread costs of illness over a broad pool of people, healthy as well as sick.[48]

Improved Medical Practice

Medical malpractice has become a crisis. One approach to solving it has been to revise tort laws. In Illinois a "reform package included limits on attorneys' contingency fees, elimination of a special damages provision that prevents physician countersuits for malicious prosecution, establishment of pretrial screening panels, and standards for expert witnesses."[49] Opposition to malpractice tort reform comes mainly from trial lawyers. Since costs of medical malpractice are charged to the health-care system and passed on to patients, insurers, providers, and consumers should all work for tort reform that benefits society. Providers whose records for malpractice are bad should be put out of business or brought up to standards. In addition, a system that rewards the plaintiff who is at fault and causes payment by the person or entity with the best finances is in need of reform.

Tort reform in California and Indiana has not resulted in lower health-care costs. It has resulted in increased profit to insurers. States with the highest medical costs were more likely to be the states that have adopted tort reforms.[50]

The AMA claims that defensive medicine costs $15 to 30 billion per year. Between 66 and 80 percent of malpractice premiums are consumed by insurance overhead and legal costs.[51]

Medical negligence kills 80,000 persons per year and injures 150,000 to 300,000 more according to a 1991 study by Harvard Medical Practice Study Group in Cambridge, Massachusetts (study of 1984 hospital data). Only one in eight patients suffering from medical malpractice files a claim; only one in 19 ever sees compensation. The state or federal government disciplined 10,289 questionable doctors, and this is the tip of the iceberg. Still the AMA pushes for control of lawsuits. Insurance companies earned $1.41 billion in profits on medical malpractice premiums in 1991. More than 20 states have enacted legislation limiting physician accountability. Caps on damages hurt most those with the most severe injuries.[52] The real cause of liability for medical malpractice is medical malpractice.[53]

Controls

Corporate Controls

Top management, operating management, and personnel can all be involved in cost-management strategies. The strategies can be instituted with a cooperative arrangement between the business enterprise and providers. One of the first areas to look at is cost analysis and safety. There are safety alternatives to illness

and injury and the savings can be high when lost time and physical and emotional misery are converted to monetary terms.

Quick processing with analysis of claims can reduce costs, and can be done on both the consumer and provider reviews of claims. Risk analysis often results in self-insurance, particularly when it can be shown that health care costs a specified amount year to year.

Control can be initiated with the operational or cost-center manager who works directly with employees and can be rewarded for cost-management strategies that reduce claims and boost productivity.

All managers need accurate information from their computer systems. There should be a system to identify computer errors resulting in duplicate claims. In addition, claims audits should look at covered charges, acceptable charges, payments by other companies, and whether the service was provided.

Employees should be involved in cost-management strategies. If co-payments are involved, employees should be given educational support. Some benefits such as smoking control, weight control, outpatient surgery, home care, counseling, HMOs, and drug and alcohol rehabilitation can be cost effective. Refunds of unused premiums can be an incentive to employees to change their behavior. Such programs should involve employees in planning, implementing, and evaluating. Screening programs for early identification of disease can reduce disabilities and lost time. Rehabilitation of alcoholics can cost less than disability, as has been shown by industries that have reduced poor performance from 28 percent to 12 percent while increasing good performance from 22 percent to 58 percent, saved $419,200 from absenteeism, and had an 80 percent recovery rate.[54]

Supply Controls

Supply controls include the following measures:

1. Limit the available supply of health services, thus controlling total amount of spending and causing efficient utilization. Whatever services are available will be used.

2. Certificate of need (CON) programs have not been successful in cost containment to date. Standards of need have been established but they apply to new facilities only. Although new beds can be controlled, investment has shifted into other types of facilities and equipment. CONs are reputed to reduce competition, thereby increasing costs. They represent regulatory control aimed at restraint of entry.

3. Eliminate an excess of between 60,000 and 100,000 beds through hospital conversion and closure. This number increases daily as ambulatory facility services are built. Communities resist closures because of unemployment, loss of community prestige, and various social service reasons. Physicians resist closures because they believe closures reduce the quality of physicians' services.

4. Mandate hospital revenue ceilings instituted by the Economic Stabilization Program of 1971-1974 and other legislation to control the total revenues that a hospital could receive over a year. Although effective in controlling hospital

employee wage increases, these measures had little effect on overall hospital costs. This approach is one of price control.

5. Restrict the number of physicians who control approximately 70 percent of personal health-care expenditures. In 1977 a physician was estimated to generate an average expenditure of $370,000 per year. At an average increase of 8.37 percent per year in the Index of Medical Care Prices, this crudely translates to more than $1,204,400 in 1992. It may be easier to redistribute the supply geographically than to restrict it.[55]

Incentive Reimbursement Controls

Incentive reimbursement controls include the following measures:

1. Prospective institutional rate setting establishes the rates of third-party reimbursement with regard for actual costs. This is working. Emphasis has extended from determination of prices to development of new incentives to modify the decision-making and behavioral patterns within hospitals. Hospitals are doing this themselves with peer-review committees that look at standards related to numbers and kinds of diagnostic tests, lost charges, unnecessary admissions, and other items.

2. Reimbursement for physician services changes to a maximum allowable charge to the patient subject to modification only on the basis of negotiation with third-party payers. Total physicians' earnings are more indicative of controls than are prices. There are indications that when physicians' fees are controlled use of their services increases to maintain increased levels of earnings. The Canadian experience is that limits on physicians' fees slows the growth of their net earnings.[56] Red tape decreases physicians' participation in controlled programs. When reimbursements by Medicare are reduced, physicians bill patients the additional charges, or curtail services, or increase the number of patient visits.

3. Physician reimbursement cost-management proposals include higher rates for personal time than for diagnostic tests, salaries, blends of salaries and fee-for-service reimbursements, and some HMOs.

Market Reform Controls

Some of the market reform proposals are:

1. Consumer cost sharing—more deductibles, coinsurance, and co-payments.
2. Utilization review—services are evaluated to show compliance with professionally recognized standards of quality, medical necessity, and provision in an economical fashion. There is conflicting opinion as to whether such review has reduced use of services. There has been an attempt to educate physicians to be cost conscious and the review process is reputed to have reduced government costs for beneficiaries.
3. Promoting alternative modes of care—HMOs, extended-care facilities (did not save money in Canada), second consults, patient participation in utilization decisions, and education of physicians in health economics. Although prevention of illness and injury can reduce costs, it is only now coming into vogue, and only because employers are paying for it.

4. The private sector is working to reduce costs while advertising better value for money, better access to care, and better results than from comparable services.

Regulation

While still a potent cost-management strategy, regulation has given ground to competition. Public regulatory strategies include CONs, budget review, other general rate-setting programs, DRGs, RBRVS, and utilization review (UR) by PROs.

Public regulations contain certain values that should be retained: political accountability, public participation, and public information. Successful sojourns into both regulation and incentives should be retained and built upon. Nurse managers should be ready to participate through appointments to agencies and to control boards; through expert opinion expressed in publication, before legislative authority, and before the judiciary; through participation in programs to inform consumers about costs of alternative health plans; and through application of regulatory and incentive principles in the world of work. When health-care costs are contained, services can be expanded or premiums reduced. Nurse managers should be informed of the record of these activities by various health plans so as to keep employees informed.

Antitrust Laws

The learned professions, including physicians, are bound by antitrust laws. This was decided by the Supreme Court in the *Goldfarb v. Virginia State Bar* case.[57] Arguments notwithstanding, nursing is included and for this reason price-fixing is prohibited. Antitrust laws prohibit an entire profession or organization of institutions from setting minimum and maximum prices. In short, hospitals cannot conspire to fix prices, including those of nurses' salaries.

Nurses should have freedom to compete in the open marketplace. If all hospitals in an area agree to the maximum salaries they will pay nurses, competition is eliminated and choice of employers must be related to some other benefit. Nurses then no longer have freedom to determine their own prices. *Arizona v. Maricopa County Medical Society* and *Kartell v. Blue Shield of Massachusetts, Inc.*, are two relevant cases.[58]

Medicare and Medicaid reduce the effectiveness of antitrust laws because they pay the same price for each DRG, exceptions being outliers. However, providers have the option of competing for these prices through alternative delivery systems. Nurse administrators participate in the competition by developing alternative nursing delivery systems. Too much effort is spent in attempting to beat the system rather than modify it. Alternative delivery systems may invent new product lines of care.

Ohio Medicaid Approaches

Finding that health-care costs were increasing at the rate of $500,000 a day, 365 days a year, Ohio's governor Celeste decided to do something about it. He established the Governor's Commission on Health Care Costs in 1983, whose members recommended that Ohio:

- create standards that are consistent with those of the Medicare program,
- make changes in the way the state pays for Medicaid services,
- achieve appropriate use, quality control, and efficiency in the delivery of health-care services,
- expand alternative health-care delivery services, and
- refinance the children's portion of the General Relief Medical Program.

In this system, the primary care physician is chosen or assigned as "gate-keeper," screening everything. The system has as an objective containment of government spending on health care without shifting costs to the private sector.[59]

Competition

Competition is an idea whose time has come. It is the opinion of many that free market forces must control health-care costs.

The components of a competitive health-care market are:

- Consumer choice among multiple competing health insurance and health-care plans, with freedom to move from one plan to another through various forms of open enrollment
- Full consumer knowledge of the services to be purchased
- A fixed-dollar subsidy for all health-care plans by an employer or the government, through payments for insurance by an employer, for instance, or vouchers for Medicare or Medicaid
- Responsibility for cost sharing or savings saved by the consumer
- A supportive tax structure to ensure compliance with the fixed-dollar subsidy, with only the latter tax exempt
- Organization of providers into competing economic units, in order to provide minimally comprehensive services, thereby assuming ease of entry for all providers and competition at all levels of service
- Uniform rules to govern competing units so that competition would be through cost and level of services, not through collusive behavior

The benefits would include cost-efficiency and cost-effectiveness. Both consumers and providers would be at economic risk for loss of patients, and for cost-sharing requirements. Overall use of services would decrease, thereby decreasing health-care costs through decreased demands. The number of HMOs would increase. Reimbursement by insurance companies would be limited to amounts established by the most efficient providers. Private initiative and innovation would be stimulated.

In the competition model consumers become aware of available health services. This does motivate providers to aim to enroll low-risk/low-cost patients. Although both are beneficial, teaching and research do not fit into the competition model. Unproven technology is sometimes overused. Some providers think the competition model too commercial and too quantity driven.

Competition models do not lend themselves well to the public-health sector, which is oriented to cooperation and to populations and systems. Public-health clients tend to be uninsured, the poor, minorities, children, and the chronically ill. Public-health services have not been expected to generate profits. Competition could have advantages and serious disadvantages for the public-health sector. Competition for MediCal (Medicaid in California)

patients has forced hospitals to reduce rates to these patients by up to 40 percent.[60]

Exhibit 7.3 illustrates efforts to contain costs and to promote competition in health care.

Employer Coalitions

Employer coalitions are a relatively new strategy for cost containment. They are useful for:

- Studying and understanding the health-care delivery system.
- Impacting federal and state legislation by PRO. Most employers have contracts with PROs to monitor use of services.
- Exchange of cost-containment ideas.
- Assembling databases for evaluation of provider performance.

A coalition includes the public sector and provider organizations. The business community is becoming extremely aware of health-care costs, but so should the individual. Of prime importance are preadmission certification, concurrent review during hospital stay, and discharge planning.

Executives of business and industry have taken the lead in reducing health-care costs. A Harvard survey of 397 CEOs indicated that only 39 percent of their companies still paid the entire premium for major medical policies. Hospital occupancy rates fell from 78 percent in 1972 to 64.6 percent in 1993.[61]

Other efforts of business and industry include flexible compensation, PPOs, and audits of claims. All have reduced costs. Deductibles have been increased, employee contributions increased, and penalties for weekend admissions have been effected. Further methods include requiring second opinions, preventive care, wellness programs, and outpatient services. Even drivers' training can be a wellness program. Some groups are working to control malpractice claims. Fees would continue to be paid by providers but lawyers' fees would be limited. Only 18 percent of malpractice fees go to injured patients. It has been shown that insured persons have twice as many surgeries as the general public.[62]

Good cost-control programs are working for business and industry. Costs are down while quality remains high.

Consumer Awareness

In the competitive marketplace there is much focus upon awareness of the consumer. Consumers are offered a choice of multiple plans with full knowledge of what they will get and how it impacts their pocketbooks. Corporate money spent on health insurance decreases other employee benefits. Nurse administrators will have to prepare competitive marketing strategies such as tours of their facilities during which nurses describe the care options available. They will need to speak before consumer groups, offering presentations skillfully prepared with attractive visual aids that illustrate the service and the cost benefit. Kwon and others designed and used surveys to "uncover" the consumers' knowledge of health costs and their opinions regarding the Federal Trade Commission's ruling on advertising by physicians. The surveys of consumers of health-care services revealed the following facts:

EXHIBIT 7.3   Efforts to Contain and to Promote Competition in Health Care

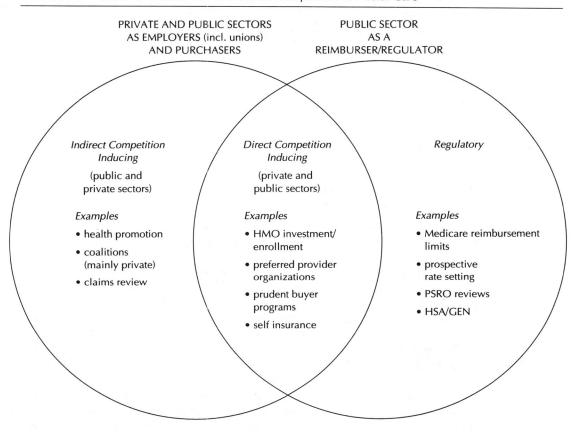

1. Most consumers are not informed of hospital costs and physicians' fees in advance but want to be.
2. Most consumers want cost information on health care available via the usual media.
3. Most providers do not agree that advertising will reduce health-care costs.
4. More consumers want to compare hospital costs and physicians' fees before making decisions.[63]

Second Opinions

A second opinion for surgery can avoid needless pain, anxiety, and time out of commission, thereby decreasing health-care costs. A 1983 study of employees of Owens-Illinois, Inc., showed that of 435 proposed operations, 76, or 17 percent, were opposed by a second physician.[64]

Developing New Provider Organizations

What will happen when hospitals are no longer the major source of health care? Most hospitals will survive but many will close (1,820 closed between 1972 and 1993). People are being kept out of hospitals. There are satellite outpatient surgical centers, mobile diagnostic laboratories, walk-in clinics, hospice care for the dying, home renal dialysis, and decreased insurance benefits with increased amounts paid by the insured. There is increased competition for all health-care services—nursing homes, clinics, medical equipment, and supplies. Hospitals and physicians are being forced to contain costs even when new equipment must be purchased as the old wears out.[65]

The consumer has replaced hospitals and physicians as the "driving force in a new health-care power hierarchy, giving rise to a radically different medical marketplace."[66] There are several major areas that offer ways to contain costs.

Provider Participation in Paid-in-Full Programs

Providers accept predetermined rates for covered services as payment-in-full. This prevents shifting of costs to other patients in the form of higher fees.

Improved Administrative Functions

There would be pre- and postpayment review of claims, coordination of benefits among payers, and shifting of profit or loss onto the provider. One format for billing would eliminate hundreds of different forms.

Alternative Delivery Systems

Patients are beginning to accept health-care plans that limit their freedom of choice. Some of them are:

- Health Maintenance Organizations (HMOs)
- Preferred Provider Organizations (PPOs)
- Health Care Cost Coalitions (HCCCs)
- Prudent buyer systems
- Health promotion and wellness programs
- Hospital Physician Organizations (HPOs)

Health Maintenance Organizations

Financing is done by fee-for-service, prospective payment, or capitation in which there is a predetermined payment per patient or per service.

Health Maintenance Organizations have the following characteristics:

- Utilization risks are shifted from payer to provider.
- Competition draws consumers to less costly services when there is a choice of plans.
- Use of preventive care and ambulatory facilities decreases hospital admission rates, lowering insurance costs by 10 to 40 percent.
- Use of primary care physicians at fixed salaries decreases use of expensive surgeons and specialists.

- They do not operate unneeded facilities such as hospitals, operating rooms, or radiation therapy units.
- Paperwork and overhead are reduced.

Pilot programs of HMOs treating patients insured by Medicare indicate hospitalization of this population could be decreased 30 percent. HMO membership increased from 9.1 million in 1980 to 37.2 million in 1991.

Hospitals that do not succeed in the growing competition will be faced with empty beds, unused ancillaries, decreasing reimbursement revenues, closings, and layoffs. Hospital administrators will learn not to respond to physicians at all costs. Many will employ physicians, give up beds and services, seek out special markets and relationships, adopt aggressive marketing strategies and techniques, and look outward. Hospitals will save management fees by managing their own HMOs.[67]

Wolfe indicates that HMOs do not decrease costs because they increase profits. Forty-five percent are owned by eight insurance companies. Their average profit from first quarter 1992 to first quarter 1993 was 40 percent.[68]

As HMOs expand, health costs increase. In California with 80 percent of employees covered by managed care, costs are 19 percent above the national average and rising more rapidly.[69]

Preferred Provider Organizations

A group of providers acts as health-care brokers providing services to a group of patients at reduced fees.

PPOs have the following characteristics:

- They contract with consumers through employers and insurers, and with providers including physicians, hospitals, and allied services.
- Services are discounted and there are no out-of-pocket expenses.
- Patients are limited to using the listed providers.
- They are intermediaries between payer and subscriber groups, furnishing marketing and administrative services.
- They set their own size, number of staff specialists, geographic availability, time limits for claims and payments, and other features.
- They place hospitals but not physicians at risk.

Arguments that the traditional physician-patient relationship will be destroyed are relatively inconsequential. These relationships will soon disappear anyway. Working people want efficiency and do not want to sit in physicians' offices waiting hours past their appointed time. Given adequate information they will make choices about their care, and they should. The old concept of withholding information is outmoded and dangerous. The objective of all competitive health-care plans is to provide good quality care as cheaply as possible.

Health Care Cost Coalitions

Organizations of employers, and sometimes unions, join to effectively bargain for better rates and parity with Medicare, Medicaid, and other insurers. They work to develop PPOs and utilization review programs.

Prudent Buyer Systems

Prudent buyer systems are characterized by joint purchasing arrangements, purchasing consortia composed of multiple providers, and competitive bidding for exclusive contracts.

Health Promotion and Wellness Programs

Increased education and awareness enable such programs to emphasize illness prevention. Programs are offered at work sites, in schools, at community centers, and at health-care facilities.

Hospital Physician Organizations

A relatively new entity, the objective of HPOs is to combine and reduce overhead. This can be done by sharing such services as billing.

Other Approaches

Research does not always produce cost savings but basic research often benefits society and should be supported both privately and publicly. For example, polio vaccine has eliminated expensive care of polio victims, and CAT scans eliminate invasive diagnostic procedures, thereby reducing the risk of complications and pain. Unfortunately, new procedures and equipment are sometimes used indiscriminately and result in third-party payers setting standards (limits) for reimbursement. Physicians will ultimately have to return to making difficult decisions about appropriate use of high technology.

Rubin offers the following as evidence that creative new approaches can and do control health-care costs:

- In Minneapolis, 78 percent of General Mills' employees belong to HMOs.
- DuPont offered its employees in Texas a choice of health plans: the original health plan, which has relatively low cost sharing for basic medical and hospital care and no catastrophic limit on out-of-pocket costs, or a new plan that couples more front-end cost sharing with catastrophic coverage. At the first offering, 47 percent of DuPont's employees elected the second more soundly structured plan.
- John Deere's utilization review program has reduced the company's utilization rate by about 30 percent over a 30-month period.
- Gimbel's and Bloomindale's have reduced their disability and hospitalization costs for hypertensive employees by 25 percent through a blood pressure control program.
- Kennecott Copper's employee assistance or mental health counseling program has a benefit-to-cost ratio of 6:1.[70]

In these instances costs were reduced by cost sharing, aggressive claims review, employer-sponsored health promotion programs, and choices of consumers who were given information and alternatives.

A Single-Payer System

Health care in the United States is treated as a commodity rather than a right. Medicare and Medicaid have increased access to care and improved morbidity

and mortality of both poor and elderly people. Approximately 35.7 million Americans, 14.2 percent of the civilian population, live in poverty; 21.8 percent of children live in poverty. Seniors spend 18.1 percent of income on health care not covered by Medicare. CBO states that a single-payer system offers the best prospects for cost control.[71]

In June 1991, the U.S. General Accounting Office (GAO) found that "(if) the United States were to shift to a system of universal coverage and a single payer, as in Canada, *the savings in administrative costs would be more than enough to offset the expense of universal coverage.*"[72]

"The Congressional Budget Office estimated that the Senate version of the American Health Security Act would save the nation $110 billion below the projected cost of the current system even *after* covering all the uninsured and dramatically improving coverage for the underinsured."[73]

A single-payer system would save $40 billion per year in insurance-industry profits and overhead.[74] It would save $117.7 billion on overall bureaucracy.[75] A National Health Program (NHP) would include

- a single-payer system
- fee-for-service private physicians
- a regional simple, binding fee schedule
- nonprofit HMOs which would receive capitated annual lump sums
- capital allocated separately to remove incentive for undertreatment or overtreatment
- a global budget for neighborhood health centers, clinics, and home-care agencies employing salaried providers
- pharmacists paid wholesale costs plus a reasonable dispensing fee for prescription drugs on the NHP formulary
- medical equipment covered similarly[76]

Private insurance and the profit motive increase the costs of health care. They put profits before patients or go under. Most single-payer systems are universal, effective, and popular. The United States needs a health-care philosophy and system "that is kind to patients, satisfying for caregivers, and financially conservative."[77]

Input into Public Policy

Cost management means that hospitals and health-care personnel cannot continue to do business as usual. The AHA, ANA, AMA, ADA, and other associations can take the lead to increase efficiency of the system or they will follow business, industry, and the consumer. What does this mean? For nurse administrators it means they will have to make hard decisions about personnel and material. With shrinking reimbursements from cuts in Medicare, Medicaid, decreased census, increased patient acuity, and closer scrutiny for admissions, there will be less revenue. Less revenue means fewer personnel and less material. Nurse administrators must tighten the purse strings.

As an example, suppose increased patient acuity dictates that another intensive care unit be opened. Revenues will increase only marginally, the difference being in amount generated by increased nursing hours. A decision is made not to increase permanent staffing. Nineteen FTEs are required to staff the projected ICU. There are 14 FTEs in a PRN pool. The nurse administrator decides

to transfer the permanent FTEs from the pool to the ICU. Temporaries will re-place permanent employees through attrition. Fringe benefits will be saved on the temporary employees.

While this kind of activity will solve a problem and increase efficiency, what happens to the approximately 40 million uninsured people? They include chil-dren born into poverty and older persons with only Social Security income. Predictions are that without preventive medical care their medical conditions worsen and ultimately use more scarce resources. Health-care professionals, sin-gularly and in organizations, must influence public policy. It will involve con-tacts with legislators on a local, state, and national level. It will mean contacts with administrators of government agencies. It will mean contacts with com-munity groups who can influence health-care policy. Even though there is no constitutional right to health care, health professionals cannot stand by while citizens suffer and die. Their contacts must be made in reasoned and logical terms without recourse to emotions.

This input into public policy is not in order to improve the financial status of the provider. That is to be done by improving efficiency and foregoing un-necessary use. The goal is to have an impact on the health-care needs of the indigent, the working poor and their children, and the needy elderly.

Nursing Approaches to Cost Management

Systems

A first step in nursing is to establish a systems approach to cost management. This will include a framework that delineates responsibility throughout the organizational entities and their functions. It begins with statements of mission, philosophy, and strategic objectives that specify cost management and a reason for existence of the organization and service. The system should serve as a con-duit for decentralization of these cost-management statements to cost-center levels, each unit or clinic having specific references to them in stating its mis-sion, philosophy, and objectives. Job descriptions and responsibility contracts should refer to them and they should be further developed into operational plans. Both responsibility contracts and operational plans are reviewed by supervisors and employees at intervals to maintain clear responsibility and accountability for cost management.

The key to a successful cost-management program is to educate and entrust responsibility to front-line managers who make the decisions that drive costs. Non–value-added costs should be identified and eliminated.[78] One of the ele-ments in achieving this is to have a course that incorporates the information and skills required for clinical and manager nurses to become continuing partners in the financial planning. Gregg and Britten describe such a course presented to staff development departments as the target population. Knowledgeable prac-titioners and administrators who share a common philosophy of caregiving and fiscal accountability can achieve a balance of quality care delivery and organi-zational economic stability.

The financial philosophy is reflected by the organizational design of the nursing department. Seldom is the staff nurse involved in planning the nursing

department's budget. Consequently, the practitioners in a nursing department lack comprehension of the financial framework that has an impact on the structure and design of their practice. This financial management course based on the practical realities of day-to-day practice can provide impetus for all practitioners to develop the skill and knowledge necessary for understanding and participating in the budgetary process.

Nursing executives and staff development educators experienced in budgeting can replicate this course with minimal preparation. This will result in increased contribution of the staff nurses and the nurse managers in partnership with the nurse executive and the organization.[79]

The conduit for cost containment and cost management can be the clinical nurse specialist (CNS). Gardner indicates that the CNS is in a key position to guide and influence decision making about cost savings. CNS activities include:

- Monitoring a patient's condition in such a way as to produce a cost advantage
- Balancing quality and cost
- Identifying variables that influence cost in a particular patient population and modifying them
- Learning to perform nursing work more efficiently to manage direct costs of nursing time multiplied by salary
- Organizing the work flow and eliminating small elements of downtime caused by actions such as running back and forth to obtain supplies or to communicate with other workers
- Implementing case management to expedite completion of tests, early discharge teaching, and coordination with other services
- Instituting prevention and self-care programs such as reduction of falls
- Managing indirect costs by having nonclinical tasks delegated to others
- Instituting use of acceptable substitutes for more costly items of supply and equipment
- Cancelling unneeded orders
- Rewarding nurses for cost savings[80]

A main element of an effective system is monitoring and controlling resources. There should be cost-containment objectives and operational plans to monitor planning, organizing, and directing. The system should periodically relate the mission and philosophy statements to the work of people, to the achievement of objectives, to the budgeting process, and to the effective use and control of supplies and equipment. Continuous feedback will indicate that output (of cost management) is being achieved.

Nursing Administration

Nursing being the largest department in most health-care institutions, it becomes the main focus for cost management. In the systems approach, there are processes to implement the mission, philosophy, and strategic objectives of cost management at the practicing clinical nurse level. As an example, the nurse administrator sets a responsibility objective for each head nurse to reduce use of supplies. Each head nurse finds that excess supplies are frequently brought to the patient's room. They can be found in bedside table drawers, on the bedside table, on the overbed table, at the sink, and even on the window sills. Each head nurse makes conservation of supplies a cost-containment target for orientation of new personnel and for responsibility contracts. It will be peer monitored.

Personnel are told the benefits of reduced use of supplies, which might include money for reference books, staff development, or even increased wages (pay-for-performance).

Nurse administrators must provide patient and family education to reduce costs. Patients and family should be told that supplies and services cost money and increase bills to patients and third-party payers. They can be told this as part of the admissions process. It can be emphasized in patient information booklets. Patients and family members can be asked, both at times of admission and discharge, for their suggestions to reduce waste.

Emphasis on efficiency, accountability, and productivity naturally addresses cost management. Nurse administrators should provide mechanisms for clinical nurses to accept concepts of safe care as opposed to quality care. With reduced inpatient censuses, increased patient acuity, increased outpatient services, and reduced elective services, nurse administrators must proactively restructure nursing services to establish and enforce professional standards that maintain job satisfaction within a cost-management environment. An effective system should be planned with input from all levels of nursing. It will result in new nursing organizations, with peer review as part of the directing and evaluating functions. This new system will create an organizational and functional structure to fully utilize nursing personnel time.

Implications for Nurse Administrators

While spending for inpatient hospital care and physician services that account for 90 percent of Medicare spending have increased at high rates, expenditures for home health services and outpatient services have grown faster than spending for other Medicare benefits. There has been an annual increase of 30 percent in home health care spending.[81] This has continued to increase as medical and health care services have shifted from inpatient to outpatient. In 1990 hospitals got 23 percent of revenues from outpatient services. This is predicted to be 50 percent by the year 2000. In 1990 52 percent of 22 million surgical procedures were done in outpatient settings. A 1990 study of BCBS of North Carolina showed surgery centers charged an average 47 percent less than hospitals for 21 common procedures.[82] No studies have been reported of the impact on home health care.

Because the prospective payment system places hospitals at risk, it places nurses at risk. They will have to examine how their nursing decisions account for clinical costs. They will have to examine alternative nursing prescriptions and decide which achieves the desired outcome with the least costs. Nurses will need to develop valid means for measuring their practice and its cost and revenues, or have it done by non-nurses.

It is essential that nurses know how to use computer technology. The world of medical care is one of computer-generated information and will become more so. Nurse leaders need to be strong and highly qualified in knowledge, skills, and research methods related to the cost containment and related efficiencies that are changing the nursing practice arena. Nurse managers and nurse executives need education and continuing education in financial management, health economics, computer technology skills, and management of resources.

Seed indicates that cost management can be improved by using cash flow reporting and forecasting to gauge the consequences of investment decisions. A computer-based model for forecasting and discounting cash flows for determining net present values of future cash flows is used by potential corporate acquirers, investment bankers, and valuation firms. With the present tempo of health-care mergers and acquisitions increasing, nurse managers can improve their value to the organization by learning the principles of life-cycle costing of products and projects, and of doing so with computer forecasting and simulation modeling.[83]

Hospital organizations are changing with horizontal integration into for-profit chain and multihospital systems. Vertical integration is taking the form of extension into manufacturing and distributing hospital supplies, home health care agencies, skilled nursing facilities, and clinics. The benefits of vertical integration include effective distribution of emergency care, hospital care, and home health care. Hospital discharges must be effected as soon as possible. If a patient requires it, he or she can be discharged to a nursing facility with the expense going to Medicare rather than the hospital.

As the costs of medical care transfer from inpatient hospital care to ambulatory care, nursing home care, or home health care, Medicare is considering putting limits on these services.

As part of the prospective payment system, a 15-member commission of physicians, nurses, health professionals, and hospital and business groups operates from the Office of Technology Assessment. They evaluate the DRG system at least every 4 years and make recommendations for revisions to the Secretary of Health and Human Services and to the U.S. Congress.

Although legitimate capital costs can be "passed through" under the PPS, they will be limited by what hospitals can afford in operational costs. Eventually, capital costs will be integrated into the DRG system. New technology will be evaluated by the commission before costs are reimbursed. This will require careful investigation before hospitals make technological investments. Hospitals will expand or reduce specialized services on the basis of volume and profitability.

Nurses need to be completely versed in all aspects of the PPS. Nurse executives will be on the front line of hospital administration, setting policy and implementing it. Clinical nurses need to learn economic principles and methods to implement them.

Nursing services are a subsystem of the hospital system. As a subsystem they are allocated portions of three kinds of resources in delivering services—human resources, technological resources, and financial resources. To maintain equilibrium, changes in financial resources are reflected by changes in human and technological resources.

Nurse administrators make an assessment of costs of nursing services to support budget requests and as a basis for rate setting, which will include variable and fixed costs. Variable costs are based on direct services provided to patients. They make use of a patient classification system and data on amount of nursing care hours per patient DRG and/or acuity to determine nursing hours per patient day for each level of care. Patient classifications are revised daily providing current figures for determination of direct costs of nursing to individual patients.

Fixed costs are based on indirect services including salaries of unit managers and secretaries. Fixed costs do not depend upon census or acuity mix. Fixed cost is determined by dividing total indirect costs by the bed capacity of the unit. Fixed costs plus variable costs equal total nursing-care costs.[84]

Cutting the Budget

One of the ways a budget can be cut is to decentralize the process. Experience has shown that practitioners and unit managers can set and reach goals of budget cutting. They do this by deciding what they want to preserve and then deciding what to cut.

Cost cutting actions that have worked include

- eliminating expendable positions
- substituting less expensive nursing positions
- taping nursing unit reports
- changing administrative coverage
- giving more autonomy to unit managers
- increasing management training for unit managers
- preprinting records
- reducing overtime by using per diem employees
- using flexible staffing
- using centralized staffing
- expanding use of computers
- expanding financial information[85]

Most budget cuts can be accomplished through the development of specific objectives. They are then developed into management plans that are carried to successful completion.

Decentralization and Increased Productivity

Nurses should have the responsibility for setting productivity standards and should share in the determination of what their productivity goals will be. Their goals may include additional patient care hours with fewer staff. Perhaps they will decide to use fewer supplies or to decrease cancellation of diagnostic tests and of surgical operations due to errors. There are many ways to increase productivity.

Nursing productivity can be increased by pulling nurses from non-nurse duties. Census can be graphed by day of the week to set staffing patterns and over a period of several years to show peaks and valleys. Vacations, educational travel, and other events can be scheduled around the valleys.

Incentive

Nurse managers must have an incentive. What they save can be used to buy needed items, even continuing education. It is important that they get their information printouts. Prospective nurse managers should be interviewed with the budget in mind. All nursing personnel should be educated about costs of supplies. Nurses can also be motivated to develop salable products to new markets, thereby increasing revenues, protecting jobs, and producing money for continuing services and developing new ones.

IV Teams

IV teams reduce patient problems and decrease patient length of stay. There is a greater need for this with DRGs.[86]

Staff Reduction

A 1980s ANA survey of 118 nursing department heads indicated that two-thirds of hospitals were shifting patterns in favor of RNs through attrition and more part-time employment.[87] Recent events have resulted in changes in the nursing care delivery systems to shift nonclinical work to non-nurses and to adjust the mix of RNs, LPNs, and nurse aides in the opposite direction.

Nursing staff expense is one of the largest items in the hospital budget. Matching staffing requirements with patient care requirements can improve care and control expenditures. This is done with a patient classification system. Patient care is calculated on the census and on acuteness of patient's condition. Basic schedules are related to normal workload with personnel being called in on the basis of specific criteria such as special qualifications. Workload variances are covered by reallocations of scheduled staff, who come from a float pool or have been cross-trained to work on several units.

There is a difference between orientation and cross-training. Orientation fits the employee into the hospital environment and to her or his position on a given unit. As the employee becomes familiar with the unit, that person will become more efficient with the assignments. Cross-training broadens the competency of persons already employed and familiar with the environment. It increases their value as human capital and produces a flexible workforce to meet demands. The cost of broadening their competence is much less than the cost of hiring extra help or contracting agency nurses.

At Highland Park Hospital, there was a good response to postings for cross-training. The response was so overwhelming it was difficult to match the many candidates to so few training positions. Applicants for cross-training received a letter informing them that staff members who had educational and clinical experience related to specialized areas were eligible for cross-training. They were to contact the head nurse if they were still interested. The head nurse made the final decision about who was qualified. The program worked very well and the head nurses were very pleased. The personnel were also pleased and enjoyed learning new skills while functioning as support staff.[88]

Staffing practices need to be evaluated on a continuing basis. They require very specific standards for quality control including performance appraisal.

Supplies

Cost-containment is altering the distribution of hospital supplies. Institutions are increasing standardization of supplies and placing more emphasis on costs.

To counter this, manufacturers are developing their own sales forces to sell their products, putting small suppliers or distributors out of business. Costs of

supplies can be reduced by centralized purchasing, requiring bids for products according to written specifications, and selecting the lowest bid that meets all specifications. This procedure has been required in some public institutions and the practice is now spreading to others.

While every single health-care product does not have to be evaluated, those that focus on needs, problems, issues, or concerns should be. The aims of product standardization include improved quality of patient care, cost management, evaluation of new products and equipment, and creation of an environment to objectively handle product requests.

Nurses are often primary users of supplies and equipment. They observe how others use them. It is important and credible to have users on product evaluation committees. The top 10 percent of patient-care items account for 70 percent of costs, the next 20 percent for 20 percent of costs, and the bottom 70 percent for 10 percent of costs. Supplies account for about 42 percent of all hospital budget dollars, making them an obvious area for cost control.[89]

Productivity increases when managers attend to the motivation, dignity, and greater personal participation of employees in designing and performing the work of the organization. Managers promote productivity by promoting partnerships and teamwork in which they and their employees create unity and harmony. Communication improves, innovators increase productivity, and managers help by doing self-assessment.

Nursing Education

Federal support of nursing education programs is not only being evaluated according to national needs and priorities, it is being reduced. Institutions of higher education are facing increased enrollment of nursing students. While enrollment increases, costs rise and government support decreases. Female students have almost total options for career fields and their intellectual talents propel them into medicine, dentistry, law, engineering, business management, and computer science. More people view nursing as a source of jobs, even for second careers.

Nurse administrators in both education and service are identifying new program goals. They are changing curricula to meet supply demands for ambulatory care nurses skilled in health assessment, health maintenance, and disease prevention. They are evaluating new job opportunities when getting students ready to function in the health-care system. If they are to compete in other fields, nurse leaders will have to upgrade salaries and redefine roles. Professional nursing skills will become a costly commodity fueled by competition from other career fields. This change will require that nurse administrators become more skilled in cost analysis as they relate the personnel resource to the job performed.

All of these changes will be accomplished by closer evaluation of nursing programs and nursing faculty. If they are not addressed by nurse administrators in education and service, the quantitative characteristics of nursing students will decline including entrance test scores and course grades. There will be continued efforts by hospital administrators to increase use of LPNs and technical nurses. Professional nurses will be expensive practitioners to be used in direct patient care and as resources to other personnel.

Clinical Practice

Clinical practice is being influenced within this changing system. It is also influencing the system. Nurses are establishing practice standards for use of equipment and supplies. This will be done through their participation in product evaluation. They can test the use of products and determine whether the cheaper one is safe and effective. This was vividly evident in a situation when the cheapest bid for an intercath was accepted. But the intercath was not cost effective—more were wasted than used. The second highest bid was then used with effective results. By this time the item could be rebid and the original supplier with the superior product brought the price down below the others. Patience and perseverance of clinical nurses effectively reduced supply costs for intercaths. This can be done with numerous items of supply and equipment and reinforces the Deming theory of staying with suppliers.

Responsibility Accounting

An activity that has as its object the cutting of costs is responsibility accounting. It purports to make nurses responsible for financial resources used in patient care. Descriptions of the activities of a responsibility center indicate it to be similar to a cost center or a profit center. Information from a responsibility accounting system is used in making decisions and evaluating the outcomes. This information is used by nurse managers "to evaluate resource volume and cost per unit of resource input, units of output, and input/output relationships, that is, productivity ratios."[90]

There must be standards by which accounting reports are compared. Variances indicate performance of responsibility accounting, favorable variances indicating reduced costs or increased productivity. Standards are set through the planning process. A standard can be an activity such as identifying all non-nursing functions on a unit and reducing staffing by one RN while increasing non-nurse staffing by one clerk. The difference in salaries is a cost savings. Other specific standards can relate to goals for reducing supply usage, using alternative brands of supplies, modifying procedures, shifting tasks, and others. Application of the standard must be under the control of the responsible and accountable person.

A responsibility accounting system can be effective down to the practicing nurse level. It must be an organized system attended to by hospital administration. Practicing nurses must be educated in financial management for their participation to be effective.

The following questions can be used to evaluate a responsibility accounting system:

1. What commitment has the administration made to a responsibility accounting program?
2. Have comprehensive standards been set?
3. Is the information relevant and useful?
4. Has the information been made available to the user in time to favorably cut expenditures?
5. Does the benefit or money saved exceed the cost of the activity?
6. Do people understand the program, the standards, and the process?

7. Does the information collected make a difference in the decisions to be made?
8. Does the information mean what it is purported to mean?
9. Can the cost savings be verified by comparing inputs and outputs?
10. Can the impact of the program be verified?
11. Can the results of the program be compared with similar information about other units or the same unit during another time period?
12. Is the system free of bias?
13. Has feedback been provided?
14. Does feedback confirm the expectations?[91]

Functional Value Analysis

Cost reduction can be achieved through a process called functional value analysis. The first step in the process is to describe all of the end functions of nursing care. Once this has been accomplished a cost is identified for each end function. Using brainstorming sessions, nurse managers look at other methods of achieving the end functions. Goals for reducing costs are set and each is evaluated in terms of both savings and risks. Finally, staff members with extensive knowledge of the functions and costs are asked to challenge the proposals. Proposals that pass the test are implemented and evaluated at the end of 6 months.[92]

Other Nursing Approaches

Nurse managers may consider nursing utilization review (NUR). This approach has frequently been applied to hospital use and physician management of patient care. The concept of functional value analysis could be used by nurse managers to develop UR standards for nursing.

Product line management should be studied by nurse managers to determine which nursing products can be developed as product lines. Product line management is a process under which products are defined, priced, marketed, and sold. The goal of product line management is to secure a competitive edge in the marketplace. An orthopedic product line management at St. Joseph Medical Center in Albuquerque, New Mexico, was developed and sold the following:

- 50-bed adult orthopedic nursing care unit (unit was downsized from 61 to 50 beds to meet the market demands for private rooms)
- Traction service—marketed and sold to inpatients, outpatients, and other facilities through physicians, nurses, and managers
- Orthotic services—contracted as a convenience service
- Orthopedic education services—to patients, families, staff, physicians, and community (some are gratis; some charged)
- Orthopedic technician services—marketed and sold same as traction service; expanded to service traction in place[93]

There are many potential nursing product lines such as pricing services for medications. Nurses price medications and provide clients with options. There are great variations in such prices; see Exhibit 7.4. The same product line services could be offered for durable medical equipment and medical supplies. A product line could be developed for handling health insurance claims, for

EXHIBIT 7.4   Medication Price List

		BARNEY'S	DRUG E.	ECONOMY	REVCO	PHAR MOR
LASIX 40 mg 30 tabs	B	6.84	4.27	8.07	5.74	3.60
	G	4.89	3.00	5.58	3.74	1.99
AMOXIL 250 mg 30 CP	B	8.89	4.04	10.77	9.18	5.69
	G	8.89	x	8.72	6.77	x
PROVERA 10 mg 10 TB	B	7.89	2.69	8.93	7.46	5.99
	G	5.25	2.22	7.07	4.13	1.99
BENADRYL 50 mg #30	B	8.29	6.67	8.57	7.18	6.39
	G	4.89	2.90	5.10	3.74	1.99
VALIUM 5 mg #50	B	22.89	19.78	25.99	20.99	17.50
	G	7.89	3.23	10.72	8.67	2.49

	LASIX		AMOXIL		PROVERA		BENADRYL		VALIUM	
HARRIS	B	3.92	B	6.17	B	4.75	B	4.42	B	20.23
WHOLESALERS COSTS	G	.32	G	6.17	G	2.00	G	.54	G	.91

Note: (B = brand, G = generic)

negotiating provider prices, and many others. Product lines should be set up with input from the clinical nurse staff. Specific goals are established and a sound management (business) plan developed. The objective is increased productivity as an element of cost management.

Education programs to inform consumers so they can reduce health-care costs include these points:

- Making sure providers accept "customary" fees
- Auditing hospital and other provider bills
- Increasing deductibles on health insurance (decreasing monthly payment by $30 would increase deductibles by $360 a year)
- Buying group rate insurance
- Accepting assignment of specific physicians and hospitals
- Joining HMOs
- Setting aside tax-deductible medical annuity
- Accepting "pre-certification"
- Comparing insurance companies
- Seeing physician early
- Asking physician to prescribe double dose per tablet of medication, then breaking tablet in half
- Using generics
- Looking for drug discounts; mail order
- Asking for free medication
- Using clinics[94]

Insurers often reduce bills. Customers' co-payments should be based on actual insurer payment, not on amount billed. For example:

Provider Bills	Insurer Accepts
$50,000	$35,000 (70 percent of amount billed) as full payment

A customer who has 20 percent co-payment should pay 20 percent of $35,000 ($7,000) not 20 percent of $50,000 ($10,000). The customer needs to be sure

co-payment is written in the policy for amount paid, not amount billed.[95] This is another service nurses can sell or teach their clients.

Problems of Cost Management

Problems are emerging from cost-management methods now in effect. They include capital shortages, because it is no longer possible simply to buy equipment or build new plants and services and have the cost automatically charged to the consumers and insurers. Insurers look at the effectiveness of the new service and set standards for reimbursement. Nurse administrators must be involved in capital investment. They should get information on standards for reimbursement for services before making decisions. This becomes more important as we head toward billing for nursing services.

Capital equipment is currently a passthrough for DRG reimbursement but will be absorbed in the individual DRG price. Government entities are attempting to restrict use of tax-free bonds by the health-care industry. These developments will potentially decrease technological advancement as fewer dollars become available for research and development.

There will be adaptations in the development of regionalized programs. Because of competition, hospitals can elect to form groups or to effect takeovers. Few hospitals will want a patient or case mix that increases intensity of care. They will not be able to afford to develop large or sophisticated services. New businesses are being formed to contract with community hospitals through joint ventures. These include treatment centers, psychiatric services, and many others.

There will be fewer dollars for modernization and maintenance of facilities particularly in not-for-profit and public hospitals. For-profit groups will have the competitive edge. While revenue-producing activities have been projected to receive priority over community services and education, these activities are receiving attention as marketing strategies.

Cost management is used as the pressure to contain pay levels and staffing levels and to reduce services and schedules.

Nurse administrators must pursue strategies for survival within the public and political areas, making sure they are represented and involved in planning, regulations, and reimbursement mechanisms. Shared services can be another strategy for cost containment and survival. Whether hospitals will pursue this strategy is uncertain. While there have been a number of mergers, many seem to be totally involved in competitive strategies. Nurse administrators can lead in this area, particularly with regard to clinical nurse specialists, staff development, and nursing research.

New corporations are being formed to pursue revenue-producing services. Services that are increasing are HMOs, nursing homes, and ambulatory services. Hospitals are becoming more involved in hotel, restaurant, and other profit-making services. Fund-raising is another strategy. The ultimate cost-management strategy is to decrease consumer demand for services by increasing health promotion. Health (illness) technology must be used more sparingly. Nurse administrators must make sure nursing is well represented in all of these events.

In the area of human resources, decreased hospital usage results in workforce reductions, wage and hiring freezes, reduced employee work hours, staff

cuts by attrition, increased productivity, and increased part-time and contract employees.

Few personnel shortages exist except in some rural areas. Employers are encouraged to upgrade clinical competencies of personnel through training, continuing education, and credentialing. Personnel who can work in more than one clinical area will be in high demand.

Because of the problems related to the need for cost management, nurse administrators will arrange incentives and start rewarding for constraint. Rearrangement will provide for measurement by the health of people, not for the amount of services provided. They will seek input and support of private corporations outside of the health-care industry. Health-care cost management is a problem of our society, not just the health-care industry.

Needs versus Frills

A system is needed that ensures access to necessary health care for all who are in "need," but retains frills for those who can afford them. There is no "free lunch." Everybody is becoming more aware of rising costs. Employers, insurance carriers, organized labor, consumers, and government must quit placing blame and start working together. Employers can design plans to:

1. Involve employees in premium and cost sharing. It will include deductibles and co-payments. Incentives can be designed to compensate for these increased costs to employees. They will include use of generic drugs, health maintenance programs, and lists of choices that are now part of charges to third-party payers but can be charged to the employee or patient. In the latter instance, patients do not buy the items unless they want them. All of these actions can reduce the cost of health insurance.
2. Encourage effective utilization of system. There are more than 100 surgical procedures that will only be reimbursed as outpatient ones. Third-party payers now encourage use of second opinions, home health care, and medical recovery in nursing homes.
3. Promote alternative systems and practices, including HMOs, PPOs, and wellness centers.
4. Promote employee education in shopping for services and understanding coverages.

Summary

The rising bill for health care requires that all categories of professional nurses be involved in cost management. They will be challenged to make rational and economic choices that relate to use of personnel, supplies and equipment, and services. Professional nurses are at risk if they do not learn the processes related to the economics of health care. They include cost-benefit analysis, economics of scale, productivity research, normative economics, responsibility accounting, and functional value analysis.

Health providers and consumers are all devoting increased interest to control rising health-care costs. Nurses must not only be aware of developments,

they must be involved in policy decisions and proposed solutions. This includes providing information to consumers to make them informed users of the system.

Disincentives to health-care cost containment are tax-free bonds, lack of advertising, certificate of need laws, overinsurance, and shifting of risks to consumers. In the latter instance, hospitals have been placed at some risk by the prospective payment system but physicians absorb few, if any, risks.

Approaches to cost containment need to be systematic and cooperative, involving public and private sectors, consumers and providers. Controls will include those initiated at the corporate level, supply controls, and laws and regulations. Competition will continue to evolve, eventually bringing health care into the marketplace of the free-enterprise system. Nurses will teach consumers how to shop for health care, strategies related to insurance, health maintenance, and provider selection including HMOs, PPOs, HCCCs, HPOs, and prudent buyer systems.

Nurse administrators will soon be in the forefront of cost management and reform. They need to be fully informed on developments, and highly skilled in applications. When they are charged with cutting the budget, they must prepare themselves to convince hospital administrators that nursing services are the best bargain in health care and will continue to be so when professional nurses are retained in nursing through well-planned and administered career development programs.

Experiential Exercises

1. Obtain the budget records of a cost center, preferably the one where you work. These records include budgets for personnel, supplies and equipment, capital equipment, and monthly reports of revenues and expenditures. Working with a peer group identify areas for cost management and write goals to cover them. You would need the cooperation of the cost-center manager beforehand. Present your goals to the cost-center manager with specific recommendations for achieving them including pay-for-performance incentives. Your final product should be a complete business plan.

2. Evaluate the mission, philosophy, values, vision, and objectives of a cost center. How do they support the notion of cost management? If they do not, prepare statements to include this important management concept and present them to the cost-center manager. You may also do this exercise with your peers.

3. Work with a group of your peers to explore the issue of health-care coverage. Conclude whether your group would support or oppose universal coverage from evidence gained during the exercise. Outline a strategy to support your position.

Notes

1. E. Ubell. "What It Will Take to Fix Health Care." *Parade Magazine* (Jan. 3, 1993):16-18; E. Ubell. "When Is a Caesarian Really Necessary?" *Parade Magazine* (Oct. 25, 1992):26, 28; R. A. Knox. "Many Caesarian Births Are Unnecessary, Group Claims." *The Augusta Chronicle* (Feb. 2, 1989):2B; J. Anderson and D. Robinson. "Isn't It Time

to Clean Up Medicare?" *Parade Magazine* (Nov. 8, 1992):8, 10; M. Beck. "Rationing Health Care." *Newsweek* (June 27, 1994):30-31, 34-35; J. B. Quinn. "Taking Back Their Health Care." *Newsweek* (June 27, 1994):36.

2. L. F. Samson. "Economic Trends in Health Care." *Nursing Dynamics* (Sep. 1993): 5-8, 10.

3. D. S. Salkener and A. L. Sorkin. "Economics, Health Economics and Health Administration" *The Journal of Health Administration Education* (Mar. 1983):228.

4. J. Buchan. "Cost-Effective Caring." *Int. Nurse Rev.* 39, 4 (1992):117-120.

5. L. L. Hicks and K. E. Bales. "Why Health Economics?" *Nursing Economics* (May-June 1984):125-180; D. S. Salkener and A. L. Sorkin, op. cit., 236-237, 247-249.

6. L. F. Samson, op. cit.

7. J. C. Morley. "The Cleveland Health Care Experiment." *The Wall Street Journal* (Feb. 10, 1992):A18.

8. R. Winslow. "How Local Business Got Together to Cut Memphis Health Costs." *The Wall Street Journal* (Feb. 4, 1992):1, A6.

9. J. Lindauer. *Economics: A Modern View* (Philadelphia: W. B. Saunders, 1977):16.

10. C. McCarthy as told to T. Lowry, C. Valle-Rogers, and J. Berker-Daily. "Under Fire: When Crime Hits Home." *Ladies Home Journal* (July 1994):82, 84-86, 88; J. Canham-Clyne, S. Woolhandler, and D. Himmelstein. *The Rational Option for a National Health Program* (Stony Creek, Conn.: Pamphleteer's Press, 1995):16.

11. J. Buchan, op. cit.

12. C. F. Chang. "Towards a Better Understanding of Health Care Economics." *Medical Group Management* (Mar.-Apr. 1981):48-52.

13. "Alabama Exceeds Goal for Number of Medical Doctors." *Report of State Health Planning Agency* (May 27, 1985).

14. U.S. Bureau of the Census. *Statistical Abstract of the United States 1995* (Washington, DC: 1995).

15. R. B. Spitzer. "Legislation & New Regulations." *Nursing Management* (Feb. 1983):20.

16. Ibid.

17. D. Fox. "Experts Debate the Costly Game of Health." *San Antonio Express-News* (June 2, 1994):3C, 5C.

18. D. Cassak. "$9.5 Billion Bonanza." *Surgical Business* (Jan. 1980):25-29, 37.

19. L. F. Samson, op. cit.

20. Retirement Systems of Alabama. "The Tyranny of America's Old." *Advisor* (Feb. 1992):1-2 (Compiled from *Fortune Magazine*).

21. C. F. Chang, op. cit., 48-49.

22. Ibid., 49.

23. S. M. Wolfe, Ed. "$1.06 Trillion for Health in 1994, $1.20 Trillion by 1995, $2 Trillion by 2000." *Public Citizen Health Research Group Health Letter* (Feb. 1994):1-2.

24. H. Koontz and C. O'Donnell. *Essentials of Management* (New York: McGraw-Hill, 1974):92-94.

25. "Options for Controlling Costs: A Survey of the American Public and Selected Professionals in the Health Care Field." *North Carolina Medical Journal* (Apr. 1984): 258-260.

26. E. P. Ehlinger. "Implications for the Competition Model." *Nursing Outlook* (Nov.-Dec. 1982):518-521.

27. J. A. Califano, Jr. "Chrysler's Health Care Cost Containment: The First Results." Remarks made before the Health Insurance Association of America, Kansas City, Mo. (Apr. 29, 1985):8-9.

28. J. Canham-Clyne, S. Woolhandler, and D. Himmelstein, op. cit., 23.

29. Ibid., 23; M. L. Brown, L. G. Kessler, and F. G. Reuter. "Is the Supply of Mammography Machines Outstripping Need and Demand? An Economic Analysis." *Annals of Internal Medicine* 113(1990):547; D. Himmelstein and S. Woolhandler. *The National*

Health Program Chartbook (Cambridge: Center for National Health Program Studies (Harvard Medical School, 1992):79.

30. U.S. Bureau of the Census, op. cit.
31. J. Canham-Clyne, S. Woolhandler, and D. Himmelstein, op. cit., 65.
32. T. C. Tillock. "Cost Containment in the Health Care Industry." *Aging and Leisure Living* (Feb. 1981):5-15.
33. Ibid., 8-9.
34. Ibid., 10-13.
35. J. Canham-Clyne, S. Woolhandler, and D. Himmelstein, op. cit., 30, 44.
36. D. H. Hitt and M. P. Harristhal. "Financing Health Care in the 1980s." *Hospitals* (Jan. 1, 1980):71-74.
37. J. Mortimer, C. C. Hampton, B. Campbell, R. E. Thompson, and P. Francise. "Controlling Health Care Costs: Five Industry Spokesmen Express Their Opinions." *Cost Containment Newsletter* (Dec. 1984):3-6; U.S. Bureau of the Census, op. cit.
38. Ibid., 3-6.
39. A. W. Snoke. "What Good Is Legislation or Planning—If We Can't Make It Work? The Need for a Comprehensive Approach to Health and Welfare." *American Journal of Public Health* (Sep. 1982):1028-1033; J. Canham-Clyne, S. Woolhandler, and D. Himmelstein, op. cit., 60.
40. A. W. Snoke, op. cit.
41. J. Canham-Clyne, S. Woolhandler, and D. Himmelstein, op. cit., 13-15.
42. Ibid., 91.
43. Ibid., 11-12.
44. Ibid., 18.
45. S. Woolhandler, D. Himmelstein, and J. Lewontin. "Administrative Costs in U.S. Hospitals." *New England Journal of Medicine* 329(1993):400-403.
46. D. Himmelstein and S. Woolhandler, op. cit., 79.
47. S. Woolhandler, D. Himmelstein, and J. Lewontin, op. cit.
48. J. Canham-Clyne, S. Woolhandler, and D. Himmelstein, op. cit., 43-50.
49. "AMA Urges Action in Three Medical Liability Areas." *Medical Staff News* (July 1985):1.
50. P. H. Corboy. "Medical Malpractice Insurance and Defensive Medicine: The Myth of Tort Reform 'Savings.'" *National Forum* (Summer 1993):33-36; J. Canham-Clyne, S. Woolhandler, and D. Himmelstein, op. cit., 60.
51. J. Canham-Clyne, S. Woolhandler, and D. Himmelstein, op. cit., 58.
52. M. Dye. "Silent Danger of Medical Malpractice: Third Leading Cause of Preventable Deaths in U.S." *Public Citizen* (May-June 1994):10-13, 21.
53. Ibid.
54. K. Per Larson. "Taking Action to Contain Health Care Costs: Part I." *Personnel Journal* (Aug. 1980):640-645.
55. I. E. Raskin, R. M. Coffey, and P. J. Farley. "Controlling Health Care Costs: An Evaluation of Strategies." *Evaluation and Program Planning* (Jan. 1980):1-14; U.S. Department of Commerce, op. cit.
56. I. E. Raskin, et al., op. cit., 1-14.
57. D. L. Shapiro. "Cost Containment in the Health Care Field and Antitrust Laws." *American Journal of Law and Medicine* (Apr. 1982):425.
58. Ibid., 432-433.
59. E. Burkland and S. Porter. "What Government Is Doing to Cut Health Care Costs." *The Ohio State Medical Journal* (Dec. 1983):919-921.
60. R. E. Schlenker and N. H. Shanks. "The Private Sector and Competition in Health Care Markets." *Journal of Health Politics, Policy, and Law* (Fall 1983):598-606.
61. J. N. Horchler. "CEOs Take the Cure." *Industry Week* (July 22, 1985):27-28; U.S. Bureau of the Census, op. cit.
62. J. N. Horchler, op. cit., 30.

63. Ik-Whon Kwon, R. T. Overman, and J. H. Kim. "Consumer Information on Health Care Costs." *Missouri Medicine* (Jan. 1980):31-32.
64. "A Second Opinion." *Advisor* (May 1985):1.
65. R. B. Spitzer, op. cit., 13-21; J. G. O'Leary. "Can Nursing Survive the Cost Containment Crunch? *RN* (Mar. 1983):85-88.
66. Alabama Hospital Association. "Environmental Assessment of the Alabama Hospital Industry." (May 1985):1
67. P. L. Grimaldi. "HMOs and Medicare." *Nursing Management* (Apr. 1985):16, 18, 20.
68. S. M. Wolfe, op. cit.
69. J. Canham-Clyne, S. Woolhandler, and D. Himmelstein, op. cit., 400.
70. R. J. Rubin. "How We Finance Care." *Issues in Health Care* (Jan. 1983):64-67.
71. J. Canham-Clyne, S. Woolhandler, and D. Himmelstein, op. cit., 34-41.
72. Ibid., 24.
73. Ibid.
74. Ibid., 23.
75. Ibid., 46.
76. Ibid., 80.
77. J. P. Callan, W. N. Tredup, and R. S. Wissinger. "Elgin Sweeper Company's Journey Toward Cost Management." *Management Accounting* (July 1991):24-27.
78. A. C. Gregg and S. M. Britten. "Budgeting from Bedside to Boardroom: A Staff Development Course." *Journal of Nursing Staff Development* (Nov.-Dec. 1989):277-284.
79. Ibid.
80. D. Gardner. "The CNS as a Cost Manager." *Clinical Nurse Specialist* 6(2)1992:112-115.
81. R. McPhillips, "The New Era in Nursing: A Time of Challenge and Change," Paper presented to the Southern Council on Collegiate Education in Nursing, Atlanta, Ga. (Oct. 31, 1984).
82. "More Outpatient Services Beef Up Hospital Revenue." San *Antonio Express-News* (Feb. 21, 1993):5K.
83. A. H. Seed, III. "Improving Cost Management Accounting" (Feb. 1990):27-30.
84. H. Lombard. "What Can Nursing Do to Control Costs?" *The American Nurse* (June 1980):11-13.
85. J. Trofino. "Managing the Budget Crunch." *Nursing Management* (Oct. 1984):42-47.
86. M. Larkin. "The Need for I.V. Teams Is Stronger Than Ever." *NITA* (Mar.-Apr. 1983): 82-83.
87. "National News." *Trim* (June 21, 1985):3.
88. R. F. Lyons. "Cross-Training: A Richer Staff for Leaner Budgets." *Nursing Management* (Jan. 1992):43-44.
89. T. C. Smith. "Materials Management: A Model for Product Review." *Nursing Management* (Mar. 1985):51-52, 54.
90. J. H. Kersey, Jr. "Responsibility Accounting: Making Decisions Efficiently." *Nursing Management* (May 1985):14.
91. Ibid., 14-16.
92. F. M. Hoffman. "Functional Value Analysis." *The Journal of Nursing Administration* (Dec. 1984):25-28.
93. C. E. Maye. "Product Line Management." *Orthopedic Nursing* (Jan.-Feb. 1991):56-61.
94. "How to Save on Health Care." *San Antonio Express-News* (Nov. 8, 1993):11B.
95. S. M. Wolfe, Ed. "Hospitalization Costs: What Is Customary and Reasonable?" *Public Citizen Health Research Group Health Letter* (Apr. 1994):7.

References

Allen, D. "The Search for Greater Efficiency." *Nursing Mirror* (Feb. 9, 1983):44-46.

Althaus, J. N., N. M. Hardyk, P. B. Pierce, and M. S. Rodgers. "Decentralized Budgeting: Holding the Purse Strings, Part 2." *Journal of Nursing Administration* (June 1982): 34-38.

Cassak, D. "The Hospital Supply Market in the 80s: A Study." *Surgical Business* (Jan. 1980):44-46.

Davis, E. "Does Money Make a Difference?" *Nursing Times* (Sep. 28, 1983):35-36.

Eusebio, E., K. Louisignau, M. Horber-Scheuter, and J. Jorlett. "Product Selection in the Hospital: Controlling Cost." *Nursing Management* (Mar. 1985):44-46.

Gackenbach, J. G. "Understanding the Attempts to Contain Health Care Costs." *Journal of the American Optometric Association* (July 1984):529-532.

Glassman, A. "Employer Strategies for Health Care Planning." *Alaska Medicine* (Apr.-May-June 1984):36-40.

"Good Housekeeping at Wythenshawe." *Nursing Times* (July 28, 1982):1269-1272.

Goldman, H. H. "Determining a Fair Price for Inpatient Psychiatric Care." *Hospital and Community Psychiatry* (Feb. 1991):139-140.

Hoffman, F. M. "The Capital Budget." *AORN Journal* (Oct. 1986):604-610.

McAlvanah, M. "Fiscal Planning: The Capital Budget." *Pediatric Nursing* 15(1)1989:70.

McMahon, J. A. "Inflation, Hospitals, and the Soaring Costs of Health Care." *College of American Pathologists* (Apr. 1980):192-194.

Norby, R. B., J. W. Cody, C. A. Anderson, J. K. Brown, S. Williams, H. Weber, J. Pooler, and M. V. Baby. "Cost Containment." *Oncology Nursing Forum* (Summer 1980):27-34.

Ontario Hospital Association. "Cost Containment in the Nursing Department." *Dimensions in Health Care* (Mar. 1981):34.

Pelfrey, S. "Cost Categories Behavior Patterns & Breakdown Analysis." *Journal of Nursing Administration* 20(12)1990:10-14.

Peddecord, R. M. "Health Care Competition in the 1980s: Its Potential Impact." *Radiology Management* (Feb. 1983):9-14.

Polakoff, P. L. "Do PPOs Answer a Need, or Create a New Set of Problems?" *Occupational Health and Safety* (Jan. 1984):69-70.

"Pre-Admission Testing Benefits Patient, Physician and Hospital." *The Quarterly* (Winter 1984-85.

Quinn, C. C. "Health Regulation and Market Forces." *Nursing Economics* (May-June 1984):204-209.

Rayner, G. "U.S. Health Care: Assessing the Evidence." *Health and Social Service Journal* (Apr. 26, 1984):502-503.

Sheetz, M. "Can Indirect Cost Funding Be Improved?" *News and Features* (Nov. 1992): 3234-3235.

Sheridan, D. R., J. E. Bronsein, and D. D. Walker. "Using Registry Nurses: Coping with Cost and Quality Issues." *Journal of Nursing Administration* (Oct. 1982):20-34.

Weiner, S. M. "On Public Values and Private Regulation: Some Reflections on Cost Containment Strategies." *Health and Society* (Feb. 1981):269-296.

"Who's Holding the Purse Strings?" *Nursing Times* (May 26, 1982):870-871.

Yeater, D. C. "Are You Keeping Up with Health Care Cost Containment Strategies?" *Occupational Health Nursing* (Apr. 1984):193-198.

8

Business Plan for Developing a Health-Care Management Service

Lynn Burgamy, M.S.N., R.N.
Pat Christenson, Ph.D., R.N.
Susan R. Colgrove, Ph.D., R.N., F.N.P., C.S.
Deborah Natvig, Ph.D., R.N.
Kay Russell, M.S., R.N., C.N.A.

Some organizations do not develop separate goals and objectives. Instead, they develop objectives and from the objectives develop management or business plans. In actual practice, organizational objectives are often goals labelled *objectives*. As they are developed into operational plans, specific goals and objectives are written for each major activity.

The goal is to plan, to assess progress toward goals and objectives at all levels, and to provide feedback to all levels of management. Efficiency is also a goal; all levels of management should guard against unnecessary time spent in meetings. At the same time organizing changes are occurring, controlling activities are in operation and activities are being evaluated.

Planning New Ventures

In an era of competitiveness, each nurse manager can be called on to develop ideas for new ventures, be they nursing products or services. For example, continuing education courses can be packaged, marketed, and presented within the organization or taken on the road. Hospitals have moved into home

health care, durable medical goods, wellness and fitness programs, and many other ventures. The basic rule for undertaking new ventures is to do sound planning.

Any new venture should have a marketing plan. The nurse manager should consult marketing department personnel and develop a marketing plan that will:

- Define problems and opportunities that may confront the new enterprise and product.
- Define the competitive position of the product and set objectives to meet anticipated problems and opportunities.
- Detail work steps, schedules, assignment of responsibilities, budgets, and other elements of implementation.
- Describe the monitoring (control) plan.[1]

The marketing plan should be separate from a primary operational plan. This plan includes gathering and analysis of data related to the product or service as it already exists in the area. If the product is continuing education, who will the customers be? They could be nurse managers, nurse educators, RNs, or LPNs. What is the competition in the market area? Is it local or imported from educational institutions and for-profit companies? Who will pay for the course—employers or individuals?

In addition, the marketing plan includes gathering and analyzing data to pinpoint possible strengths and weaknesses, problems, and opportunities. It identifies strategies for taking competitive advantages. Each opportunity, problem, strength, and weakness should be addressed by definitive objectives developed into operational plans for advertising, product development, and even personal selling.

Before any new venture is launched, a control plan is made. This plan includes measures of performance such as numbers or amounts of products or services to be sold within specific time frames. Managers are assigned responsibility for comparing expected results with actual results and for making corrections in all elements of the plan and its implementation. This plan can be monitored based on the marketing and operational plans with checklists.[2] Exhibit 8.1 illustrates an operational plan for development of an intermediate cardiac rehabilitation program.

Nursing service planning supports the mission and objectives of the institution. For this reason the nurse administrator needs to know the plans and programs of the health facility administrator and of other departments where personnel contribute to the joint effort of providing health-care services. The nurse administrator should be a voting member of all important committees of the institution and should give input into the planning done by these committees. This includes committees dealing with budgets, planning, credentialing, auditing, utilization, infection control, patient-care improvement, library, and all other areas concerned in any way with nursing service, nursing activities, or nursing personnel.

The nurse administrator who participates in institutional committee work achieves an overall view of hospital problems and activities and is in a position to interpret problems, policies, and plans of the hospital to nursing personnel. He or she can also interpret nursing needs and problems to hospital personnel of other departments. This planning integrates the nursing-care program into the total program of the health-care institution.

EXHIBIT 8.1 Division of Nursing—Cardiac Rehabilitation Program

Strategic Objective

The patient is provided with an effective patient and patient-family teaching program, which will include guidance and assistance in the use of medical center resources and community agencies that can contribute support to the patient's total needs.

Operational Objectives	Actions	Target Dates and Persons Responsible	Accomplishments
Determine cardiologist's perception of the program: goals, resources to be used, breadth of services to be provided, etc.	1. Prepare an agenda for meeting with cardiologist.	Do by April 1 19xx. S and P	The following agenda was developed: • Need for new services. • What will it be? • What will it cost? • What will be charged? • Who will pay? • Where will it be done? • Who will do it? • How many patients? • What equipment and supplies are needed?
	2. Make appointment with cardiologist.	May 3 19xx at 11 A.M. in Dr. C's office; S and P	May 3 19xx. Had a meeting with Dr. C, the cardiologist. The purpose of this program is to rehabilitate patients following open-heart surgery, angioplasty, and post-MI. It is the intermediate phase between acute care and when they enter "bounce back." The following decisions evolved from the meeting: 1. We will undertake this program on a limited basis; there is no other such service available. 2. The service will include physical exercises, monitoring, progress report by patient, counseling as indicated. 3. Only patients with insurance or with ability to pay will be accepted. 4. It will be done in PT on Mon., Wed., and Fri. from 7 to 9 A.M. 5. Equipment and supplies will be in-house. 6. The CV clinical nurse specialist will be the project director.
Meet with the CV clinical nurse specialist and plan the program.	3. Make appointment with nurse D to plan the program.	May 4 19xx at 8 A.M. S and P with D	Plan: 1. D will coordinate with PT director. 2. P will figure cost of program by the hour and set charges with accounting office.

(Continued)

EXHIBIT 8.1   Division of Nursing—Cardiac Rehabilitation Program *(Continued)*

Operational Objectives	Actions	Target Dates and Persons Responsible	Accomplishments
			3. D will borrow equipment to run the program until the next capital budget. 4. Accomplish this by May 12 19xx.
Have plan completed by May 31, 19xx.	4. Set up a control chart to identify when each phase of project will be completed.	May 12 19xx; P.	May 10 19xx: Done. Posted.
	5. Write policy and procedure for the program. Include admission and discharge procedures and emergency plan.	May 31 19xx; D.	May 29 19xx; Draft presented; minor changes needed. May 31 19xx: Done.
	6. Obtain equipment and supplies.	May 31 19xx; D.	May 17 19xx: Done.
	7. Coordinate with PT director.	May 12 19xx; D.	May 17 19xx: Done.
	8. Meet with cardiologist when all of this is done.	June 1 19xx; P, S, and D.	Met with cardiologist June 2 19xx. Dr. C is happy with plan and will be ready to start on July 1 19xx.
Provide for third-party reimbursement.	9. Discuss with insurance companies.	June 15 19xx; P.	June 15 19xx: Insurance reps will visit the program and make decision. Appointment made.
Develop marketing plan.	10. Prepare detailed marketing plan.		Marketing plan is already in operation with announcements mailed to all area cardiologists.
Develop evaluation plan.	11. Prepare evaluation plan.	June 30 19xx; P and D.	D has a good evaluation plan.
	12. Implement program.	July 1 19xx; D.	July 1 19xx: Had our first patient today. Cardiologist was there as required by insurance companies. All went well.
	13. Evaluate the program weekly until stabilized.	D, beginning July 8 19xx.	

Business Plans

Business plans are detailed descriptions of the process for launching a new product or product line, project, unit, or service. Business plans meet many of the standards for strategic planning as they are projected over an extended time period of months or years. Their purpose is to provide sources of information

for investors, decision makers within and external to the organization, motivation, and measurement of performance.[3] They are the blueprints for ventures.

There are 10 key elements of a business plan as described by Johnson and others.

1. Introduction—nature, goals, objectives, and desired outcomes of the proposed business
2. Description of the business—goals, nature, and history of the sponsoring institution, nature and history of the product, and industry trends
3. Market and competition analysis—including target audience, pricing, promotion, placement, and positioning—based on data from solid market research
4. Product development—product description, resources, time frames for development, and quality control plan
5. Operational plan—location, facilities, labor force, and equipment
6. Marketing plan—mission, marketing research, measurable goals, strategies, and a staffing and financial plan
7. Organizational plan—organizational chart and job descriptions
8. Developmental schedule
9. Financial plan
10. Executive summary[4]

Business plans are often categorized as strategic plans. Many of the key elements are the same, however a business plan is more detailed than a strategic plan. Actually, a business plan is developed for each new venture emerging from a strategic plan.

This chapter discusses each of the key elements of the business plan for a hypothetical health-care management service. Exhibits showing documents are grouped at the end of the chapter as appendices to the business plan.

Mission

The mission of Health Care Management Service (HCMS) is to assist consumers in gaining access to appropriate care within the fragmented health-care delivery system. By maintaining individuals in their own surroundings as long as appropriate, HCMS will help prevent inappropriate and unnecessary hospitalizations and long-term residential care.

Philosophy

The HCMS of the greater Augusta area is a privately owned for-profit corporation. It takes a case-management approach to health care, providing a single entry point into the health-care system for adults 50 years of age and older.

The HCMS accepts the American Nurses' Association's statement regarding rights of clients as basic tenets for their case-management services.

The client shall have:

- The right to be given a fair and comprehensive assessment of his or her health, functional, psychological, and cognitive ability.
- The right to have access to needed health and social services.

- The right to be treated with respect and dignity.
- The right to self-determination, including the opportunity to participate in developing one's plan for services.
- The right to privacy and confidentiality.
- The right to know the cost of services prior to rendering of services, especially in cases where the client will be responsible for payment.
- The right to be notified of any changes of services, termination of service, or discharge from the program.
- The right to withdraw from the case-management program at any time the person is dissatisfied with the case-management service being given.
- The right to a grievance procedure in the event that the client feels his or her rights have been violated or perceives discrimination or inappropriate treatment.[5]

Description of the Business

The Health Care Management Service (HCMS) of the greater Augusta area is a privately owned for-profit corporation jointly owned by the Autumn Retirement Village and three private investors. The joint venture is designed to increase business, provide efficiency in operations, and allow economies of scale so that health-related services are provided in an effective way. The Autumn Retirement Village owns 49% of the business while the other three investors own equal parts of the remaining 51% (17% each).

The HCMS is a case-management system that will focus on health promotion and maintenance activities of individuals 50 years of age or older. The agency will serve as a single entry point into the health-care system by providing and coordinating services related to identified health, financial, and legal services relevant to the aging population. Services include health assessments, financial management, assistance with insurance and Medicare, home care services, services to maintain independent living, health-related legal services, counseling, rehabilitative services, and social services. Referral services will also be available to health agencies providing services not provided by HCMS. These services will be provided at the health club or, if necessary, in the individual's home.

The HCMS centers around a health club that will provide a focal point for social activities and interaction among the members. Case-management activities currently provided to the residents of the Autumn Retirement Village will be taken over by HCMS. In addition, case-management services and the health club will be available to individuals living outside the retirement village. The health club will provide scheduled leisure-time activities and will be available to members for private meetings and group functions. The projected date to begin operations is January 2.

The target population for HCMS is private-pay individuals aged 50 and over. Membership in the health club will include use of the clubhouse facilities, reduced rates on fee-for-service products, and discounts at several health-related businesses. Nonmembers will be charged for use of the clubhouse and will pay regular rates for services provided.

The HCMS will be the only service organization providing comprehensive health-related services to the target population. Marketing research revealed a positive response from individuals polled regarding their desire to purchase both memberships and fee-for-service options.

The Autumn Retirement Village was established in 1972. It is a continuous-care retirement community that offers living arrangements including two-bedroom cottages, duplexes, one- and two-bedroom apartments, a congregate living center, and a 102-bed health-care center that is dually licensed for skilled and intermediate nursing care. The other partners in the corporation are educated and experienced in the area of health-care administration with emphasis on gerontology, health promotion, and home care. They are well connected with the other Augusta-area health-care service providers.

The success of the Health Care Management Service is contingent upon the staff's and management's commitment to attain clear and measurable goals. The long-term goals and short-term objectives for the HCMS include:

1. LONG-RANGE GOAL: Identify and/or develop a collaborative network of health and social services capable of responding effectively to the needs of individuals 50 years of age and older

   Objectives
   (1) To maintain a comprehensive portfolio of written referral service agreements with existing providers of social and health services within the geographical boundaries of the agency
   (2) In those instances where appropriate service providers do not exist or choose not to participate, to recruit appropriate professionals and develop the components for provision of needed services

2. LONG-RANGE GOAL: Provide the services to make each client's life healthier, more socially connected, and more manageable, thus enhancing the individual's self-esteem and ability to cope with health-related situations

   Objectives
   (1) To prioritize the needs of the client to maintain the highest level of independence possible, to slow the transition into dependency, or to accept the inability of regaining a high level of health
   (2) To re-evaluate the need for continued service within 1 month after the first five needs have been met

3. LONG-RANGE GOAL: Assist individuals in obtaining appropriate health care for the most economical price

   Objectives
   (1) To maintain an up-to-date register of fees charged by providers of health and social services in the greater Augusta area
   (2) To develop written agreements for group rates (discounts) when possible
   (3) To monitor the quality of services and give each provider a written evaluation of its services at least once a year
   (4) To advise clients regarding financial reimbursement systems and assist them in obtaining reimbursement as necessary

4. LONG-RANGE GOAL: Increase the accessibility of health and social services needed by individuals 50 years of age and older

   Objectives
   (1) To develop written agreements with current transportation services to provide services to the target population, establishing rates and schedules that promote independent use
   (2) To purchase and obtain specialized vehicles necessary to transport individuals with special needs

5. LONG-RANGE GOAL: Assist individuals 50 years of age and older in reaching their highest level of health through health education programs

Objectives

(1) To increase public awareness of health, social, and financial services available to individuals 50 years of age and older

(2) To increase the level of awareness of clients and their families regarding the management of their health care

Market and Competition

Customers

The HCMS will provide services to private-pay individuals aged 50 years and older. Services will also be provided to younger individuals with chronic illnesses. All persons in this target group living in the greater Augusta area are eligible for services.

Market Size and Trends

The percentage of individuals aged 55 and older is projected to increase by 22 percent over the next 5 years, thus indicating an escalating need for the comprehensive services to be provided by HCMS.

Competitors

No other businesses in the greater Augusta area provide the comprehensive services of HCMS. Other agencies, including the Area Agency on Aging, offer some of the services offered by HCMS. There are three agencies in the direct vicinity that may provide competition to HCMS.

1. Healthmaster Home Health Care of Georgia provides home health care to private-pay individuals in Columbia and Richmond counties. Services include nursing, physical therapy, occupational therapy, speech therapy, social services, home health aides, personal care aides, homemaker aides, and private sitters.

2. Humana Hospital Senior Association provides discounts on private-room costs, insurance specialist to fill out Medicare and Medicaid forms, support groups, trips at reduced rates, and an exercise group that meets three times weekly. The association is run by an RN. Cost = $15.00 per year.

3. The YMCA provides exercise rooms, swimming pool, running track, handball courts, gymnasium, and team sports. It is currently overcrowded, noisy, and heavily used by families with young children and young executives.

Potential Market Share

The HCMS has the potential to capture the entire market for coordinated health-care management. The Market Development Analysis shows the following Strengths, Weaknesses, Opportunities, and Trends (SWOT).

Strengths

- Rapid increase in the number of individuals aged 55 and older in the greater Augusta area.
- Complexity of the health-care system frequently requires professional assistance to navigate successfully.
- Case management may help provide more cost-efficient care.
- Case management may result in increased quality of health care.
- Wealth and diversity of nursing expertise of owners.
- Extremely marketable.
- High growth potential.
- High profitability potential.
- May provide government incentives through cost containment.

Weaknesses

- Limited capital budget, necessitating loans for start-up.
- Concept is new and may not be readily accepted initially.
- Not all services are reimbursable through insurance.

Opportunities

- No direct competitors in the area.
- Expanding elderly population has more discretionary income.

Trends

- Agencies offering competing services may market more vigorously once competition begins.
- Government regulations are stringent and rapidly changing. It may be difficult to respond in a timely manner.
- Potential lack of cooperation among physicians who may perceive erosion of power base.

Operational Plan

The starting date for the project is January 2 with a starting date for the opening of HCMS 1 year later. One year will allow time to remodel the building, acquire and train staff, and promote the business. The official opening will be a major part of the marketing strategy. The health-club facility will be open from 6:30 A.M. to 11 P.M. Professional services provided by social workers and nurses will be available from 8 A.M. to 5 P.M. Monday through Friday, in the evenings, and on Saturdays by appointment. Lawyers and accountants will be available by appointment during regular office hours Monday through Friday, in the evenings, or on Saturday mornings. Home care services will be available 7 days per week, 24 hours per day through prearranged contractual agreements.

Location of the Business

The HCMS will purchase a 15,000 square foot building located in Columbia County for $750,000. Although the building is zoned for commercial use, the

facility is in a nonindustrial area with several professional and medical plazas nearby. The facility is centrally located and easily accessible via highways I-20, Washington Road, and the Bobby Jones Expressway. The surrounding buildings and businesses are attractive and the market value has increased by 46% over the past 3 years. HCMS will utilize all portions of the building except for seven offices, which will be available on a rental basis. The rental space could be remodeled to accommodate a medical suite or be used as individual offices for organizations such as the American Cancer Society, the American Lung Association, or the Boy Scouts of America.

Building and Equipment

The major capital expense will be the purchase of the building and necessary remodeling. Other major expenditures will include the exercise and health training equipment for the health club, equipment for an examination room, lounge furniture for the health club, appliances and dishes for the kitchenette, and office furnishings for five offices. Financing will be obtained through a commercial lender. A down payment of $250,000 will be required, half of which will be raised through contributions from community groups, businesses, and individuals. The remaining $125,000 will be received through matching funds from the Papp Foundation, which offers philanthropic support to worthwhile, community-centered projects.

Personnel

The key to success will be the managing and coordinating of HCMS. Individuals with backgrounds in nursing administration with an emphasis on family health, gerontology, and rehabilitation will serve as the product line specialists. These individuals will plan and implement programs in their particular areas and serve as consultants to one another. Specific responsibilities are discussed in the Management and Personnel Plan. Administrative and clerical support will be the responsibility of the office manager.

Marketing and Distribution Plan

Attempts will be made to market services to both health-care providers and consumers. Providers may be able to participate by offering group rates or special discounts for referrals. Consumers will be provided cost-effective coordinated health-care services.

Objectives to Attract Providers

1. Build acceptance of service concept.
2. Increase referrals from physicians and other health-care and social service providers.
3. Offer educational seminars open to the greater Augusta medical community.

Objectives to Attract Clients

1. Gain support of community leaders and politicians.
2. Focus on population aged 50 years and older.

3. Build acceptance of service among consumers.
4. Inform consumers of benefits of service by
   * using multimedia advertising.
   * placing an advertisement in the telephone directory's yellow pages.
   * placing brochures in physicians' offices and throughout the community.
   * arranging speaking engagements at all local organizations (Kiwanis, Rotary, Women's Clubs, AARP).
   * submitting press releases to local television news channels and newspapers.
   * advertising in local newspapers.

To increase future business, HCMS will expand through the addition of new services. Projected additions in the next 2 years are a 30 ft. × 60 ft. indoor pool and adaptive and health-related equipment either on a rental or purchase basis from a shop located adjacent to the health club.

Management and Personnel Organizational Plan

The organizational chart for HCMS is presented in Appendices 1A and 1B [Exhibits 8.2 and 8.3].

The director will have ultimate responsibility for the operation of HCMS. All aspects of the business will be coordinated by this individual who will serve as liaison to the Board of Trustees. Initially two product line specialists will be hired with the intent of adding the third when financially feasible. First-year financial projections indicate that this may be possible in 24 to 36 months. Each product line specialist (Advanced Practice Nurse [APN]) will be a resource person concerning aspects of her or his specialty to clients, physicians, community groups, and other health and social service providers. The APN will have responsibility for line management of her or his assigned department. The office manager will be responsible to provide clerical and administrative support to the HCMS staff. This individual will also coordinate all bookkeeping functions and serve as an assistant to the director in financial coordination of HCMS. Full position descriptions of the director, the product line specialists, and the office manager will be found in Appendix 2 [Exhibit 8.4].

Board of Trustees

HCMS is a small business corporation as defined in Section 1244(cc)(2) of the Internal Revenue Code of 1954. The stock will be owned by the Autumn Retirement Center (49%), and three principal stockholders (17% each) who will also serve on the Board of Trustees and as consultants to the business. The Autumn Retirement Center will have two representatives on the Board of Trustees.

The chief function of the board will be to approve strategic plans, programs, and organizational policies and procedures. The board will ensure quality services, represent the organization's interests to the community, and monitor the organizational efficiency and effectiveness. The following compose the board of trustees:

1. A. B. Smith has a Ph.D. in nursing with a specialty in nursing administration. She was successful in restructuring the discharge planning process at

Perly Gates Rehabilitation Hospital. She is a well-known speaker and sought-after consultant in rehabilitation programs.

2. J. L. Jones has a Ph.D. in nursing with a specialty in gerontology. She has taught gerontological aspects of health care at the University of Georgia and is responsible for the federal grant to the Georgia Department of Aging and Rehabilitation to establish homemaker service programs throughout Georgia.

3. Nancy Brown has a Ph.D. in nursing with a specialty in health promotion. She has been involved in establishing well-health programs throughout the southeastern United States. She currently is on faculty at the Medical College of Georgia.

Two additional members of the board (yet to be determined) will represent the Autumn Retirement Village. Brief position descriptions for the director of HCMS, the product line specialists, and the office manager may be reviewed in Appendix 2 [Exhibit 8.4].

Development Schedule

Careful planning and coordination of HCMS is mandatory. A planning year will permit time for the physical plant to be readied, the equipment obtained, and the staff hired and trained. The opening of HCMS will be a main focus of a marketing and advertising campaign that will be carefully timed and coordinated with community leaders so it does not interfere with or serve as competition to other service organizations. The three private investors on the Board of Trustees will be responsible for coordinating and carrying out the marketing strategy and campaign.

Quality Assurance Plan

The Quality Assurance (QA) methods to be used by HCMS are based on the critical path model of the New England Center for Case Management in Massachusetts. The advantages of this model include

- a standardized way to identify patterns of care
- an outcome-directed methodology
- the ability to focus staff on "what day it is in the client's case"
- incorporation of regular review procedures

As the client enters HCMS, he or she will be assigned a case manager who will initiate the critical path with the client and family. At that time a plan of care will be established from the results of the assessments and consultations. Activities, treatments, medicines, teaching, and discharge planning will be planned on a time frame based on client's needs. The CareMap® (Appendix 3A [Exhibit 8.5]) records the type of service(s), the length of anticipated service(s), the client problem/nursing diagnosis, the goals, and outcomes. The CareMap® and the critical path (Appendix 3B [Exhibit 8.6]) are individualized and then plotted to reflect the time frame for each service. Time frames range from 1 visit

to 3 weeks for each plan. All CareMaps® and critical paths must be renewed after a maximum of 3 weeks or after the assigned time, whichever comes first. This 3-week limit reflects the overall objective of HCMS's evaluation plan, which is to evaluate overall performance every month.

If the client's care varies from the preset time frame, the variance is recorded, its cause identified, and appropriate action taken and recorded on the form labeled Variance from Critical Path (Appendix 3C [Exhibit 8.7]). At the time of the monthly overall performance evaluation of HCMS, an Aggregate Variance Analysis Report (Appendix 3D [Exhibit 8.8]) is compiled to list all the variances from the critical paths for all clients that month. These cases are reviewed by the staff and the board and recommendations are made to decrease variance in subsequent reporting periods.

An additional quality improvement (QI) survey will be taken. Every 6 months all clients of HCMS will be sent a Client Satisfaction Assessment (CSA) questionnaire (Appendix 3E [Exhibit 8.9]). This tool is designed to elicit the opinions of the clients specifically in regard to whether their needs were met, whether the staff was courteous, and whether managers were responsive to their needs. Clients will be asked to respond to a series of questions on all HCMS services that they used during the previous 6 months. The responses to the CSA will be tabulated and used to evaluate the overall performance of HCMS.

Financial Analysis

The HCMS is a corporation developed as a joint venture of the Autumn Retirement Village and three private investors. The Autumn Retirement Village owns 49% of the business and the remaining 51% is equally divided among the other investors. A loan of $800,000 will be secured through a commercial lender by the Autumn Retirement Village after a $250,000 down payment is obtained by the private investors. One-half of the down payment will be raised through contributions from community groups, businesses, and individuals. The remaining $125,000 will be received as matching funds from the Papp Foundation.

The Autumn Retirement Village currently provides some case-management services for its clients. Once HCMS is established, all case management will be coordinated through HCMS.

Autumn Retirement Village clients will receive membership at reduced rates ($300 per year) and will not be required to pay the introductory fee.

Memberships will be sold to community members aged 50 years and older for $480 per year. A first-year introductory fee of $200 will also be assessed.

Companies and businesses will also have the opportunity to purchase memberships for their employees aged 50 and older. An introductory fee of $100 plus one half of the membership fee will be paid to HCMS by the company. The employee will pay the remaining $20 per month. Prices are comparable to prices of service providers in other cities the size of Augusta and are competitive with those services provided by other agencies. Research indicates that 5% of the charges will not be collected.

At start-up the occupational, physical, and speech therapists will spend their time assessing needs and establishing baselines for Autumn Retirement Village residents and other new members. This should be completed by the end of the

first quarter, at which time they will provide therapy to nonmembers on a fee-for-service basis. Baseline assessments will be provided to members at no cost.

The direct and indirect expenses specific to HCMS are projected in Appendices 4A and 4B, and are summarized in Appendix 4C. An itemized list of expenses for equipment and furnishings is presented in Appendix 4D. [See Exhibits 8.10 through 8.13.]

The financial analysis to determine revenues for the first 3 months (Appendix 5A [Exhibit 8.14]) and the first year (Appendix 5B [Exhibit 8.15]) are presented along with income statements for the same time frames (Appendices 6A and 6B [Exhibits 8.16 and 8.17]). The income statements reflect a loss of $37,407 during the first 3 months, but it is projected to decrease to $18,891 by the end of the first year. Break-even analysis reveals that monthly revenues must increase from current projections of $87,548 to $92,363 per month. The formulas to determine the break-even point are presented in Appendix 7 [Exhibit 8.18].

Plans to increase revenue include selling more corporate and community memberships, expanding home health services, and expanding rehabilitation services. An additional product-line specialist (APN with expertise in psychiatric nursing) will be added during the second or third year if necessary increases in revenues are realized.

Summary

This advanced business plan is a prototype for entrepreneurial nurses who are certified in advanced practice nursing. It is a blueprint for the development of nursing services in a climate of competition in the health-care industry.

Experiential Exercise

Form a group and do a nominal group process exercise to identify areas for developing advanced practice nurse businesses. Decide on a business and write a complete business plan.

Notes

1. D. W. Nylen. "Making Your Business Plan an Action Plan." *Business* (Oct.-Dec. 1985):12-16.
2. E. K. Singleton and F. C. Nail. "Guidelines for Establishing a New Service." *Journal of Nursing Administration* (Oct. 1985):22-26.
3. K. W. Vestal. "Writing a Business Plan." *Nursing Economics* (May-June 1988):121-124.
4. J. E. Johnson. "Developing an Effective Business Plan." *Nursing Economics* (May-June 1990):152-154; J. E. Johnson, D. G. Sparks, and C. Humphreys. "Writing a Winning Business Plan." *Journal of Nursing Administration* (Oct. 1988):15-19.
5. American Nurses' Association. *Nursing Case Management* (Washington, DC: ANA, 1988):7-8.

EXHIBIT 8.2   Appendix 1A

Table of Organization—Year 1

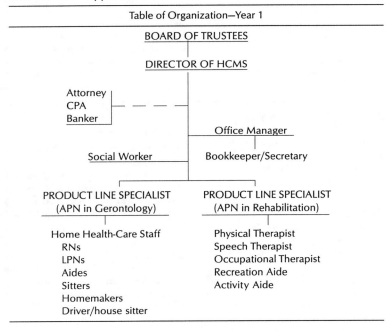

EXHIBIT 8.3   Appendix 1B

Table of Organization—Year 2 or 3

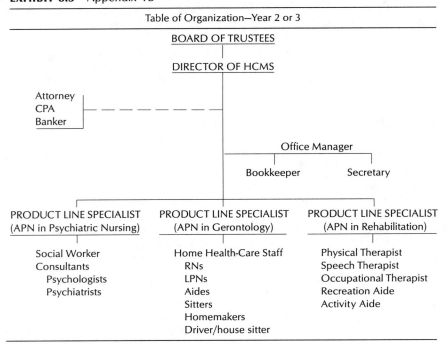

EXHIBIT 8.4   Appendix 2

Position Descriptions

Director of HCMS

Qualifications:
Master's degree in nursing administration
Licensed as a registered nurse in Georgia

Job Functions:
Responsible for developing mission and philosophy statements, determining goals and objectives, developing standards of practice, interpreting and ensuring compliance
with policies and procedures, serving as advisor and consultant as needed, submitting HCMS budget plans and
program development to the board of trustees.

Supervises: Product line specialists, office manager

Reports to: Board of Trustees

Product Line Specialists

Psychiatric Nurse Practitioner (Asst. Director) (to be added
after 24 to 36 months. Responsibilities will be taken by
the administrator of HCMS until the position is filled.)

Qualifications:
Master's degree in nursing with speciality in psychiatric/
mental health with emphasis on family health concerns
Licensed as a registered nurse in Georgia
Licensed as an advanced practice nurse in Georgia
Certified as an advanced practice nurse

Job Functions:
1. Coordinates all psychiatric and psychological-related
matters for the agency including but not limited to family and caregiver counseling, and support groups
2. In the absence of the director provides overall supervision and management of HCMS
3. Primary liaison with consultant psychologists and psychiatrists
4. Responsible for coordinating services with other social
service agencies

Supervises: Social worker, consultant psychologists, consultant psychiatrists

Reports to: Director of HCMS

Gerontological Nurse Practitioner

Qualifications:
Master's in advanced practice nursing with a specialty in
gerontology with background in home health care
Licensed as a registered nurse in Georgia
Licensed as an advanced practice nurse in Georgia
Certified as an advanced practice nurse

Job Functions
1. Coordinates and supervises home health-care program
including homemaker services
2. Performs physical assessments and conducts health
screening clinics
3. Conducts family and patient assessments in regard to
skills for daily living, support structure, and alternative
living arrangements
4. Assists in the acquisition of medical and rehabilitation
equipment

5. Provides nutritional counseling
6. Provides medication management services
7. Coordinates nursing home placement
8. Coordinates house and apartment sitters
9. Coordinates nonmedical transportation

Supervises: Home health-care nurses, aides, sitters, home-
makers, and drivers

Reports to: Director of HCMS

Rehabilitation Nurse Practitioner

Qualifications:
Master's degree in advanced practice nursing with spe-
cialty in rehabilitation and health promotion
Licensed as a registered nurse in Georgia
Licensed as an advanced practice nurse in Georgia
Certified as an advanced practice nurse

Job Functions:
1. Coordinates all rehabilitation functions within the agency
2. Overall responsibility for leisure-time and therapeutic
activities occurring in the health club
3. Responsible for acquisition, sale, and rental of rehabilitation equipment

Supervises: All rehabilitation staff (O.T., P.T., speech therapist, and activity aide) and health club activity aide

Reports to: Director of HCMS

Office Manager

Qualifications:
Associate's degree in business
Skills in office management, bookkeeping, word process-
ing, and transcribing dictation

Job Functions:
1. Assists the director in preparing and maintaining financial and material resources for HCMS operations
2. Coordinates schedules and manpower resources
3. Runs the office!

Supervises: Secretary/billing clerk

Other Personnel

Driver/transporter/house sitter
Billing clerk with insurance background
Secretary
RNs
LPNs
Aides
Sitters
Social worker (MSW)
Physical therapist
Occupational therapist
Speech therapist
Recreation aide

Consultants on Contract (available for referral)
Attorney
CPA for retirement planning and financial counseling

EXHIBIT 8.5   Appendix 3A

CareMap®

Name _____
Service type _____
Length of anticipated service _____

Client Problem/Nursing Diagnosis	Goal	Outcome

Visit(s) per day/week
1.

2.

3.

EXHIBIT 8.6   Appendix 3B

Critical Path

Client _____   Type of service _____
Case manager _____   Doctor _____
Date of review _____   Expected time needed
Reviewed by _____   (in visits, days, or weeks) _____

Date:

Day/week/visit

Time period (circle):   1.   2.   3.
Consultations: _ →
Activities (specify): _ →
Treatments (specify): _ →
Meds (specify): _ →
Discharge planning: _ →
Teaching: _ →
Evaluation (as soon as activity ends for this case type): _ →

Admission date _____ Discharge date _____
Renew activity (check one) _____ yes _____ no

Typical times: <u>Plan must be renewed after 3 weeks.</u>
Nursing 1 visit–3 weeks
Social work 1 visit–3 days
P.T./O.T. 1 visit–3 weeks
Health counseling 1 visit–3 days
Rehabilitation 1 visit–3 weeks
Legal/insurance counseling 1 visit

Source: Adapted from a New England Center for Case Management critical path. Used with permission.

EXHIBIT 8.7   Appendix 3C

Variance from Critical Path

Client's name _____

	Variation	Cause	Action Taken
Date Service Used			

Source: The Center for Case Management, South Natick, Massachusetts. Reprinted with permission.

EXHIBIT 8.8   Appendix 3D

Aggregate Variance Analysis Report

Date: _____

Case type: _____

DRG(s): _____

Period included in aggregate analysis: _____

Number of cases: _____

Variance Identified

System

Variance	No. Cases	Cause	Action Taken	Results

Practitioner

Variance	No. Cases	Cause	Action Taken	Results

Patient

Variance	No. Cases	Cause	Action Taken	Results

Submitted by _____

Source: Copyright © 1989, The Center for Case Management, South Natick, Massachusetts. Reprinted with permission.

EXHIBIT 8.9   Appendix 3E

Client Satisfaction Assessment

In order to continue to provide high-quality services to our clients, we need your input. We value your opinion of the comprehensive services we provide. Please answer the following questions by circling the answer that best fits your response.

Of the services listed, please indicate the ones your have used in the past 6 months and answer the questions related to those services.

	Yes	No	Does Not Apply
1. Home health nursing service	1	2	3
Nursing personnel met my needs	1	2	3
Nursing staff were courteous	1	2	3
2. Social workers	1	2	3
Social workers met my needs	1	2	3
Social workers were courteous	1	2	3
3. Physical therapy	1	2	3
Staff met my needs	1	2	3
Staff were courteous	1	2	3
4. Occupational therapy	1	2	3
Staff met my needs	1	2	3
Staff were courteous	1	2	3
5. Health counseling	1	2	3
Staff met my needs	1	2	3
Staff were courteous	1	2	3
6. Rehabilitation	1	2	3
Staff met my needs	1	2	3
Staff were courteous	1	2	3
7. Financial counseling	1	2	3
Staff met my needs	1	2	3
Staff were courteous	1	2	3
8. Legal/insurance counseling	1	2	3
Staff met my needs	1	2	3
Staff were courteous	1	2	3
9. Health club	1	2	3
Staff met my needs	1	2	3
Staff were courteous	1	2	3
10. Transportation	1	2	3
Staff met my needs	1	2	3
Staff were courteous	1	2	3
11. I have had my questions answered adequately by staff members.	1	2	3
12. Management staff have been responsive to my needs.	1	2	3

13. Please feel free to make any additional comments you feel will be helpful to deliver better care to our clients. Thank you for your help with this survey.

EXHIBIT 8.10   Appendix 4A

Projected HCMS Direct Expense		
	Annual	Start-Up
Salaries		
APN-1	$ 36,000	$ 9,000
APN-2	36,000	9,000
MSW	24,000	6,000
Driver/house sitter	15,000	3,750
PT (10 hr/wk @ $40/hr)	20,800	5,200
OT (10 hr/wk @ $35/hr)	18,200	4,550
SpT (10 hr/wk @ $35/hr)	18,200	4,550
Rec Aide	18,000	4,500
Total	$186,200	$46,550
Benefits (25% salaries)	46,550	11,638
Total Salaries & Benefits	$232,750	$58,188

Hourly Wages				
Class.	Rate/Hr.	Hrs. billed		
RN	$20	50/week	$ 48,000	$ 12,000
LPN	14	50/week	33,600	8,400
NA	7	400/week	134,400	33,600
Sitter	5	800/week	192,000	48,000
Total Hourly Wages			$408,000	$102,000
Total Salaries, Wages, & Benefits			$640,750	$160,188

Direct Equipment		
Van (Rent–$600, Maint.–$125, Gas–$210 = $935/mo)	$ 11,220	$ 2,805
Car (Rent–$300, Maint.–$65, Gas–$100 = $465/mo)	5,580	1,395
Total Direct Equipment	$ 16,800	$ 4,200
Total Direct Expenses	$657,550	$164,388

EXHIBIT 8.11   Appendix 4B

Projected HCMS Indirect Expense		
	Annual	Start-Up
Administrative Support		
Director	$ 40,800	$10,200
Office Manager	24,000	6,000
Bookkeeper/Secretary	18,000	4,500
Advertising ($1,000/mo plus $3,000 additional for start-up)	15,000	4,000
Telephone	1,800	450
Water	1,056	264
Electricity	7,200	1,800
Office supplies	1,200	300
Garbage	1,440	360
Copy machine	1,200	300
Cleaning	5,200	1,300
Other services	8,400	700
Total	$125,296	$30,174
Renovation Expense	$25,000	$25,000
Equipment/Furnishings		
Health club	$48,865	$12,216
Exam room	8,430	2,108
Offices	18,484	4,621
Lounge	12,200	3,050
Kitchen	3,850	963
Total	$91,829	$22,958
Depreciation (5 yrs useful life)	$18,366	$4,592

Interest Costs

Total projected funds	$1,050,000	
Amt borrowed	800,000	
Interest rate 11%		
Amortization—20 yrs 5-year fixed rate		
Payment	$99,084	$24,771

EXHIBIT 8.12   Appendix 4C

Projected HCMS Expense Summary		
	Annual	Start-Up
Direct		
Salaries, Wages, & Benefits	$ 640,750	$160,188
Equipment	16,800	4,200
Indirect		
Administrative support	125,296	30,174
Renovation	25,000	25,000
Equipment & furnishings	91,829	22,958
Depreciation	18,366	4,592
Interest	99,084	24,771
Total	$1,017,125	$271,883

EXHIBIT 8.13 Appendix 4D

Itemized Equipment/Furnishing Expenses	
Health Club	
Circuit weight training system—8 stations	$15,000
Exercise bikes—Aerobo-cycle (2 @ $2,000)	4,000
Treadmill	4,500
Handweights (small dumbbells)	595
Rack for hand weights	425
Scale	295
Mirrors	1500
Clocks (2 @ $25)	50
Whirlpool	10,000
Sauna/steam room	10,000
Sound system	2,500
Total	$48,865
Examination Room	
Examining table	$7,375
Sphygmomanometers (2 @ $37)	74
Opthalmoscope/otoscope	150
Scales	295
Gooseneck lamp	75
Examiner's stool	67
Chair	98
Reflex hammer	21
General supplies (tongue blades, cotton swabs, etc.)	150
Biological testing kit (neurological testing)	125
Total	$8,430
Offices (5)	
Desks (5 @ $241.60)	$ 1,208
Desk chairs (5 @ $188.25)	941
Extra chairs (10 @ $109.50)	1,095
File cabinets (8 @ $201.86)	1,615
Clocks (5 @ $25)	125
Pictures/wall decorations	1000
Computer system (5 PCs @ $2500)	12,500
Total	$18,484
Lounge	
Game tables—6	$ 1,200
Matching chairs—24	3,000
TV with remote—1	500
Conference table—1	850
Chairs—10	1,250
End tables—4	1,000
Settees—4	3,400
Wall decorations	1,000
Total	$12,200
Kitchen	
Refrigerator	$1,000
Stove	750
Dishwasher	500
Microwave	350
Trash compactor	350
Sinks with garbage disposal	300
Dishes	200
Silverware	200
Cooking Equipment	200
Total	$3,850

EXHIBIT 8.14 Appendix 5A

			Financial Analysis Determining Revenues—Start-up			
	1	2	3	4	5	6
Memberships						
Community Member	150	$ 48,000	$ 45,600	$ 9,000	$36,600	$ 2,400
A.R.V. Member	100	7,500	7,125	6,000	1,125	375
Commercial Member	75	16,500	16,050	4,500	11,550	450
Services						
Client consult	90	9,000	8,550	4,500	4,050	450
Blood tests	125	1,250	1,190	625	565	60
Home visit	1300 hr/wk	152,400	144,780	101,600	43,180	7,620
Transportation	180	1,800	1,800	2,400	(600)	0
House sitting	7	700	665	350	315	35
Finance mgmt.	90	4,500	4,275	2,250	2,025	225
Office Rental	7	6,782	6,441	5,945	496	341
Totals		$248,432	$236,476	$137,170	$99,306	$11,956

Key:
1 Volume
2 Total Charges
3 Paid to HCMS
4 HCMS cost of service [Membership @ $20/mo., home health visits @ 66% of charge, all others @ 50% of charge]
5 Profit (loss) [Column 3 less Column 4]
6 HCMS write-off [Column 2 less Column 3]

Membership rates:
   Community Membership—$200 introductory fee plus $40/mo. ($480/yr.)
   Autumn Retirement Village Membership—No introductory fee, $25/mo.
   Commercial Membership—$100 introductory fee paid by employer. $40/mo fee paid 50% by company and 50% by
      employee.

EXHIBIT 8.15 Appendix 5B

	Financial Analysis Determining Revenues—Year 1					
	1	2	3	4	5	6
Memberships						
Community Member	300	$ 168,000	$159,600	$ 89,000	$ 70,600	$ 8,400
A.R.V. Member	150	41,250	39,188	33,000	6,188	2,062
Commercial Member	150	69,000	65,550	27,000	38,550	3,450
Services						
Patient consult	450	45,000	42,750	22,500	20,250	2,250
Blood tests	250	2,500	2,375	1,250	1,125	125
Home visit	1300 hr/wk	609,600	579,120	406,400	172,720	30,480
Transportation	1080	10,800	10,400	16,200	(5,800)	400
House sitting	32	3,200	3,040	1,600	1,440	160
Finance mgmt.	45	27,000	25,650	13,500	12,150	1,350
Office Rental	7	27,128	25,772	23,780	1,992	1,356
Nonmember Services						
Building rental	4	1,000	1,000	200	800	0
Client consult	18	2,700	2,565	1,350	1,215	135
Speech therapy	273	16,380	15,561	9,550	6,011	819
Occup. therapy	78	4,680	4,446	2,730	1,716	234
Physical therapy	78	5,460	5,187	3,120	2,067	273
Finance mgmt.	225	16,875	16,032	8,438	7,594	843
Totals		$1,050,573	$998,236	$659,618	$338,618	$53,337

Key
1   Volume
2   Total charges
3   Paid to HCMS
4   HCMS cost of service [Membership @ $20/mo., home health visits @ 66% of charge, all others @ 50% of charge]
5   Profit (loss) [Column 3 less Column 4]
6   HCMS write-off [Column 2 less Column 3]

Membership Rates
   Community Membership—$200 introductory fee plus $40/mo. ($480/yr.)
   Autumn Retirement Village Membership—No introductory fee, $25/mo.
   Commercial Membership—$100 introductory fee paid by employer. $40/mo fee paid 50% by company and 50% by
      employee.

Figures reflect 50 community memberships added each quarter, 50 A.R.V. memberships added in the 2d quarter, and 75
commercial memberships added in the 3d quarter.

EXHIBIT 8.16 Appendix 6A

Income Statement—Start-Up		
Revenue		
Gross Revenue	$248,432	
Allowance for bad debts	(11,956)	
Net revenue		$236,476
Expenses		
Direct Expense		
Salaries & benefits	160,188	
Equipment	4,200	
	$164,388	
Indirect Expense		
Administration	30,174	
Renovation	25,000	
Equipment/furnishings	22,958	
Depreciation	4,592	
Interest	24,771	
	$107,495	
Total Expense		$271,883
Gain (Loss)		$ (35,407)

EXHIBIT 8.17 Appendix 6B

Income Statement—Year 1		
Revenue		
Gross Revenue	$1,050,573	
Allowance for bad debts	(52,337)	
Net revenue		$998,236
Expenses		
Direct Expense		
Salaries & benefits	640,750	
Equipment	16,800	
	$657,550	
Indirect Expense		
Administration	125,296	
Renovation	25,000	
Equipment/furnishings	91,829	
Depreciation	18,366	
Interest	99,084	
	$359,575	
Total Expense		$1,017,125
Gain (Loss)		$ (18,889)

EXHIBIT 8.18 Appendix 7

Break-Even Analysis	
Gross Income	$87,548
less: allowances for bad debts	(4,362)
Adjusted monthly gross income	83,186
less: Direct Costs	(54,796)
Gross Profits	28,390
less: Fixed Costs	(29,965)
Net profit (loss)	(1,575)
Fixed monthly costs	29,965
Adjusted monthly gross income	83,186
Average direct costs/month	54,796
Margin (billing less direct costs)	28,390

Formula: $\dfrac{\text{Fixed Costs}}{\text{Margin}}$ = % of billing needed to break even

$\dfrac{\$29,965}{\$28,390}$ = 105.5

$\begin{array}{r}\$87,548 \\ \times\ 1.055 \\ \hline \$92,363 \end{array}$ Amount needed in revenue each month to break even

9

Personal Financial Management for Nurses

Russell C. Swansburg, Ph.D., R.N.
Philip W. Swansburg, M.S.N., R.N.
Richard J. Swansburg, B.S.N., M.S.C.I.S., R.N.

Planning for Financial Security

All nurses have concerns for their personal financial security. This includes both present and future. It may be more acute for the average clinical nurse than for the average nurse manager or administrator. It becomes less acute as income increases but only because one has more income to budget. In today's employment climate temporary and part-time workers are on the increase making it essential that they plan for their own financial security in their retirement.

The Personal Budget

Financial management begins with the personal budget, a plan that balances income, or revenue, with expenses. Personal budgets are important to a person's lifestyle. They are the object by which one decides upon what to spend one's money. Included are such decisions as whether to spend less money on living quarters in order to have more money to travel; whether to save money for retirement or spend it on a car; whether to contribute to charity or buy a waterbed. All of these are personal choices related to personal values. It is important for any nurse to have a budget so as to stay relatively debt free. This does not mean one should not have debts, but rather that one should be able to meet the commitments of the indebtedness.

EXHIBIT 9.1   Format for Personal Budget

Budget for 19___

	monthly	yearly
Income		
Bonuses	$ ____.__	$ ____.__
Dividends	$ ____.__	$ ____.__
Honorariums	$ ____.__	$ ____.__
Insurance benefits	$ ____.__	$ ____.__
Interest	$ ____.__	$ ____.__
Pensions	$ ____.__	$ ____.__
Royalties	$ ____.__	$ ____.__
Salary or wages	$ ____.__	$ ____.__
Tips	$ ____.__	$ ____.__
Other	$ ____.__	$ ____.__
Total Income	$ ____.__	$ ____.__
Expenses		
Cable TV	$ ____.__	$ ____.__
Car payment	$ ____.__	$ ____.__
Car servicing	$ ____.__	$ ____.__
Charge accounts	$ ____.__	$ ____.__
Charity	$ ____.__	$ ____.__
Child care	$ ____.__	$ ____.__
Clothes	$ ____.__	$ ____.__
Electricity	$ ____.__	$ ____.__
Food (including eating out)	$ ____.__	$ ____.__
Furniture	$ ____.__	$ ____.__
Garbage collection	$ ____.__	$ ____.__
Gas	$ ____.__	$ ____.__
Gasoline for car	$ ____.__	$ ____.__
Insurance, life	$ ____.__	$ ____.__
Insurance, medical	$ ____.__	$ ____.__
Insurance, house	$ ____.__	$ ____.__
Insurance, car	$ ____.__	$ ____.__
Rent or house payment	$ ____.__	$ ____.__
Repairs and improvements on house	$ ____.__	$ ____.__
Savings and investments	$ ____.__	$ ____.__
Taxes, property, license tags	$ ____.__	$ ____.__
Telephone	$ ____.__	$ ____.__
Toiletries	$ ____.__	$ ____.__
Other	$ ____.__	$ ____.__
Total Expenses	$ ____.__	$ ____.__

Income should always be greater than expenses.

Income less expenses equals "disposable" funds
$ _____ – $ _____ = $ _____.__

Liquid assets should equal monthly expenses times the number of months
a person wants to plan to cover financially.

Exhibit 9.1 is a format for a personal budget, which can be followed on a monthly basis. A good plan is to keep a personal budget book with a page for each month of the year. As bills are paid, the amounts can be checked off. If you are running shy of money you can decide where to cut expenses. If you have extra cash you can decide how to spend it. A personal budget book is also a source of data for preparing personal income tax returns.

Hints for Adjusting the Personal Budget

1. Make your money work for you. Do not prepay bills too far in advance. When you do you are giving banks, businesses, and others your money to use. Pay a mortgage payment two or three days before it is due. The date stamp on the envelope is the proof you paid the bill on time. The same holds true for charge accounts. Insist advance payments be applied to principal to reduce interest charge.

2. Avoid late payments; they exact a penalty in money that could be spent on something you want.

3. Pay charge accounts on time and in full when possible. Otherwise you will pay exorbitant interest rates, sometimes as much as 20% and seldom less than 14%.

4. If you want to borrow money, do so through a credit union or a bank. Such places frequently use savings accounts or bonds as collateral for a loan at lower interest rates. Shop around. Some retailers allow you to charge items for 90 days without interest. Or they set up installment accounts at lower interest rates than regular charge accounts, especially for large purchases such as furniture.

Liquidity

Liquidity is being able to convert assets into cash in a short time and to take care of an emergency. Sources of quick cash are savings accounts, corporate, discount, and zero coupon bonds, cash loans on life insurance policies, certificates of deposit, money market funds, government securities, Government National Mortgage Association (GNMA), common stocks, preferred stocks, utility stocks, convertible securities, mutual funds, unit investment trusts, stock options, stock warrants, real estate investment trusts, and precious metals.

Liquidity is a personal choice, usually something about which people are concerned. What happens if one is ill or injured for periods not covered by income? What happens if one is fired or demoted and cannot work for any reason? People make a personal choice about the degree of their liquidity. They may plan for income to cover from 1 month to 1 year. They set aside savings, in multiple forms, to cover personal living expenses for a specified period of time. They do this in vehicles that are relatively safe, quickly available, and that will earn the most interest.

Tax-Sheltered Annuities

If you are a teacher, professor, or other employee of a public institution such as a nonprofit hospital or home health agency, you may be able to take advantage of a special tax-sheltered retirement/savings plan called a tax-sheltered annuity (TSA). You should check with your personnel office because this plan will reduce your current federal income taxes and provide a source of savings for your retirement.

A tax-sheltered annuity is a plan whereby your employer pays part of your earned income directly into a savings account with a company with which you

contract. This reduces income tax currently being paid because the participant has federal income tax deferred during years of highest income and pays it in retirement years when income will usually be lower. TSAs also supplement other retirement income.

Facts about Tax-Sheltered Annuities

1. "403(b)" annuities are available to employees of teaching institutions, hospitals, churches, and home-health service organizations.

2. Elective salary reduction contributions are limited to $9,500 per year since the Tax Reform Act of 1986. In some states, contributions to pension plans are included as part of the tax-exempt annuity.

3. Whereas these funds could be withdrawn without income tax penalty, they now have a 10% tax on distributions. The tax does not apply if

- you are then 59½ or older, or
- you separate from the service of your employer at any age and then begin annuity income, for life or a period equal to your life expectancy (or the joint lives or life expectancies of you and your beneficiaries), or
- the distribution is made following your separation from service, after attaining age 55, under the "early retirement" provisions of your employer's pension or Tax Deferred Annuity (TDA) plan, or
- you have unreimbursed medical expenses that exceed 7½% of your adjusted gross income, or
- the distribution is attributable to your being disabled, or
- the distribution is a death benefit, or
- the distribution is made to an alternate payee because of a "qualified domestic relations order" granted by a court.

4. At this time distributions must begin no later than April 1 of the calendar year following the year in which the individual attains the age of 70½ in most instances. Each policyholder should determine the distribution requirements of this new law.

5. After August 1, 1986, already taxed contributions were included as a tax-free portion of each monthly payment until the investment in the contract is recovered. The question of already taxed contributions should be raised with any annuitant's retirement plan(s) now because some state retirement plans include them.

6. The new tax law includes other changes such as a 15% "excise" tax on the amount in excess of distributions above $112,500 a year (adjusted for inflation).

7. Contributions are made through payroll deduction and are taken from before-taxed earnings. Thus they lower the amount of earnings on which current income tax is paid.

8. Tax-sheltered annuities are still an excellent tax shelter to reduce income tax while working. They also provide excellent pension income.

9. Some plans charge commissions and administration or management fees at the front end and on an annual basis. Others do not. Choose one that does

not. An example is USAA Life Insurance Company (USAA Building, San Antonio, TX 78288; Tel. 1-800-531-8000; San Antonio only 498–8000). They charge no commission, pay a high rate of interest, are safe and portable, and the withdrawal, surrender charge is only $150.00 the first year, $50.00 the second year, and $25.00 each year thereafter. The charge can never exceed 7% of the value of your account. See Exhibit 9.2.

10. There is usually a minimum contribution but in some instances it is as low as $25.

11. An employer will sometimes match a percentage of an employee's salary. They can require that this be done with a specific plan. If an employer matches 3% of a salary of $50,000, the employee earns $1,500 a year extra in tax-sheltered income, making the earned salary $51,500 a year. The matched salary is included as part of the total earned income that can be sheltered. Some employers match part of a person's total salary, others part of a specified amount.

12. Tax-sheltered annuities are handled through personnel programs. Usually there are several plans to choose from.

13. TSA loans are available with a fixed annuity. The loan will use a collateral assignment arrangement for the accumulated value in your TSA contract. TSA loans usually are for minimum amounts, last a maximum of 5 years, require monthly payments, may be repaid early without penalty, and are not taxable distributions.

14. 401(k) plans are available at many companies. These plans allow workers to voluntarily contribute pretax earnings to a tax-deferred retirement savings account that can grow. Many employers match employees' contributions, making 401(k)s an almost unbeatable deal. The maximum amount that can be put into a 401(k) plan is approximately $9,500 per year (employee + employer contributions). For 1995 it is $9,240, for 1996 $9,500. The contributions are usually tax-deferred; the interest is tax-deferred until withdrawn. Employees should know:

- 401(k) plans are portable.
- Employers should make contributions promptly.
- By law the employer is required to distribute a plan: who is covered; eligibility requirements; vesting arrangements; amount employee may contribute; matching policy of employer; and details of benefits payouts.
- Plan termination requires vestment.
- The account can be rolled over into an IRA.
- The employee can borrow up to the lesser of 50% or $50,000 of the vested account balance.
- Employee can manage his or her account of more than $3,500.
- 401(k) accounts are protected against bankruptcy.[1]

Individual Retirement Accounts

There is some similarity between individual retirement accounts (IRAs) and tax-sheltered annuities. IRAs are personal retirement plans. They were originally

EXHIBIT 9.2   What to Look for When Selecting a Company for Tax-Sheltered Annuities

1. What are the front-end loading charges?
2. Are there annual maintenance charges in the contract?
3. What are the withdrawal and/or surrender charges/values?
4. How are surrender values calculated?
5. May payments be periodically increased, decreased, stopped, or started without having to rewrite the policy or be assessed penalties?
6. If payments are discontinued, does the policy continue to earn the current rate of interest paid by the company or only the guaranteed interest rate?
7. What is the guaranteed rate of interest?
8. What is the current rate of interest?
9. Is the current rate of interest paid on the full contract balance or is the interest rate banded where money continues to earn only the interest rate in effect at the time of payment?
10. When is interest credited to the contract balance? Annually? Quarterly? Monthly? Daily?
11. May the contract be transferred to another employer in the event you change employers?

created to supplement other retirement plans including Social Security. Under the 1986 Tax Reform Act individuals may continue to contribute to an IRA; however, it will not be fully tax-deductible if they are covered by a qualified retirement plan or a TSA pension plan and earn more than $40,000 a year for a married couple or more than $25,000 a year if single. If they are not covered by a pension plan, employees may make tax-deductible contributions to an IRA on a sliding scale up to $2,000 a year for salary ranges between $25,000 and $35,000 if single and between $40,000 and $50,000 if married. Anyone can continue to put after-tax money into an IRA and the interest will accumulate without being taxed until withdrawn. An individual retirement account has a maximum contribution of $2,000 per year and must not exceed 100% of income earned in that year.

There is a federal penalty of 10% for withdrawing money from IRAs before age 59½. Exemptions are death or disability. Federal income tax is paid on interest earned on IRAs at the time the interest is withdrawn. As with TSAs, some companies charge administrative fees. There are minimum contributions to an IRA, which are set by the company.

A married couple can each have an IRA. If both people work, each can have up to $2,000 in an IRA. If only one spouse works, the total is $2,250 with each IRA split but no more than $2,000 in any one IRA per year.

More than 37 million Americans have IRAs. They have them as retirement planning investments and as tax-savings strategies. Investments in IRAs include mutual funds, bank products, stocks, real estate partnerships, and government securities. The only exceptions are collectibles and gold bullion. Tax laws probably diminish participation in IRAs when they do not provide an income tax deduction to people.

A retired person with self-employed income who is not making contributions to any retirement plan may be eligible for a tax-deferred IRA.

IRA Tips

1. Make an IRA investment early in the tax year to earn maximum interest. It can be made any time before April 15 of the next year and still qualify for federal income tax deduction for eligible persons.

2. Choose an investment with the highest rate of interest. The amount of risk increases the rate of interest. A young person may want to take a higher risk at a higher rate of interest while the older person may want a lower risk at a lower interest rate. Bank or life insurance investments are less risky than high-growth mutual funds but pay lower interest rates.
3. IRAs, like TSAs, can be held in multiple accounts. They can be moved by a procedure called "rollover." There are many options and a person can select a variety of them and have multiple accounts.
4. IRAs must be related to earned income. Retired pay does not qualify a person.
5. Distributions to IRA holders *must* begin at age 70½ years.
6. If you are not comfortable with a particular IRA investment vehicle, do not buy it. You should do what is best for your security, stability, and peace of mind.
7. Investment advice is available free from sellers. Get advice from more than one and as many as possible.
8. Manage your IRA if you have the time, knowledge, and desire to do so. Otherwise, choose a reputable agent to do it for you.
9. Decide the minimum distribution you wish to receive between ages 59½ and 70½, the period of no federal penalties to mandatory distribution. At age 70½, you may take payout in

   - a lump sum (be careful of tax penalty),
   - an annuity purchase,
   - equal payments over fixed-life term, or
   - yearly recalculation based on life expectancy.

IRAs can be invested in any one of the following vehicles.

Annuity

An annuity is a long-term savings or investment plan. It combines high-interest earnings and tax-deferral on those earnings until a person is ready to draw on those funds. Ideally, this happens at a time when that person is in a lower tax bracket. The contract provides periodic payments for a specific length of time—a specific number of years or the lifetime of the owner.

Certificate of Deposit

Certificates of Deposit (CDs) are documents issued by banks for receipt of money. Dollar amounts, maturities, and interest rates are flexible. Withdrawal of the principal before maturity incurs a penalty. Interest is compounded monthly, quarterly, or at maturity, and credited to the account.

Limited Partnership

A limited partnership is one that has one or more partners whose potential liability is limited to the investments in the business. It must also have one or more general partners who have limited personal liability for the debts of the partnership. Limited partnerships frequently involve real estate transactions. They have higher risks than do most annuities, CDs, or money markets.

Money Market

Money market vehicles are instruments that reach maturity in 1 year or sooner. They include government issues (T-bills or Treasury bills), certificates of deposit, short-term notes issued by businesses or governmental agencies, and others. Money market investments are made through bank money market accounts or money market funds.

Bank Money Market Accounts

Bank money market accounts include checking accounts such as Super NOW accounts and money market deposit (savings) accounts. Interest rates are competitive with the money market rates. They can include check-writing privileges, are insured, and usually require a deposit of $1,000 to open.

Money Market Funds

Insurance and other investment companies pool money of small investors to purchase money market instruments. They pay interest and the rates change frequently. They generally match money market interest rates.

Mutual Funds

Mutual funds are investment companies that pool the savings of a large number of investors and invest these savings in securities such as stocks, bonds, and short-term money instruments. Thus small investors can share the advantages of large investors through broad diversification and economies of scale that lower costs of professional management including transaction costs and custodian fees.

Portfolio

A collection of investments is a portfolio. Some persons have large portfolios that they manage themselves. Others choose reputable financial managers.

Securities

Bonds, stocks, mortgages, and other written instruments of investment are termed *securities*.

Stocks

Stocks are the certificates of ownership in a corporation.

Retirement

To calculate the amount you need to save to retire in style, use Exhibit 9.3.

EXHIBIT 9.3   Your Retirement Budget

No matter how far off retirement is, consider these items: Will your mortgage be paid off? What kind of life and health insurance will you need? Do you have any special medical or lifestyle considerations? Some people put travel, gourmet dining, or other high-cost leisure activities on their priority lists.

Financial planners traditionally suggest you will need 70 to 80 percent of pre-retirement income after you retire to live comfortably and to meet expenses. Their assumptions are that by retirement most debts will be paid, children will be independent, income taxes will be lower and certain work-related expenses will become unnecessary. But your situation may be quite different. Many people are waiting until their 30s to have children, meaning college tuition costs may come just as they prepare to retire. Others may foresee a need to provide financial help to aging parents.

Whatever your obligations, you may not be willing to live on this reduced amount. If you are within 5 to 10 years of retirement, you can approximate future expenses fairly accurately. You will have a good feel for what will be a satisfactory level of pre-retirement income.

Retirement represents a dramatic change of lifestyle for most people, and many aren't prepared for the change. Before you make financial plans, consider what you want your retirement to be like. You have many choices; no single retirement style is right for everyone. You might want to travel, go back to school, or devote more time to hobbies. You might decide to work part-time or devote yourself to volunteer work. Be sure to consider all aspects of your ideal retirement lifestyle, not just the financial concerns.

Retirement Income and Expenses

Preparing a budget is essential to developing a comprehensive financial plan. Using the previous discussion on income sources and expenses, complete the "Projected Retirement Budget." The budget work sheet will determine if your anticipated resources are likely to meet your future income needs.

To factor inflation into the picture, multiply current income and expenses that are likely to rise by the appropriate "inflation multiple" for each year you would like to project. Between 1983 and 1992, the average annual inflation rate was 3.81 percent. Between 1988 and 1992,

inflation averaged 4.3 percent. Depending on the current economic climate, you may wish to choose a different inflation rate for your projections.

To complete the work sheet:

1. Fill in your current income from all sources applicable to your situation.
2. Enter your current expenses, using the chart as a guide.
3. Subtract expenses from income. This is your annual budget surplus or shortfall.
4. Now estimate your income and expenses for each retirement scenario listed. Choose any year of retirement for which you can reasonably project. To use the inflation chart, find the number of years for which you would like to project. Then, multiply the appropriate figure by your current expense.

Example: A given expense is currently $900 a year. Assuming an average annual inflation rate of 5% each year, you would need $1,466.01 ($900 x 1.6289) to meet that expense 10 years from now.

The Effect of Inflation

Year	Your Age	Multiple		
		3%	5%	7%
1	_____	1.0300	1.0500	1.0700
2	_____	1.0609	1.1025	1.1449
3	_____	1.0927	1.1576	1.2250
4	_____	1.1255	1.2155	1.3108
5	_____	1.1593	1.2763	1.4026
6	_____	1.1941	1.3401	1.5007
7	_____	1.2299	1.4071	1.6058
8	_____	1.2668	1.4775	1.7182
9	_____	1.3048	1.5513	1.8385
10	_____	1.3439	1.6289	1.9672
12	_____	1.4258	1.7959	2.2522
14	_____	1.5126	1.9799	2.5785
15	_____	1.5580	2.0789	2.7590
16	_____	1.6047	2.1829	2.9522
18	_____	1.7024	2.4066	3.3799
20	_____	1.8061	2.6533	3.8697
25	_____	2.0938	3.3864	5.4274
30	_____	2.4273	4.3219	7.6123

(Continued)

Home Ownership

Owning a home is a part of financial management for many Americans. Most nurses will not be able to buy a home outright and will need to obtain a mortgage. The home-buying market in 1986 became one of advantage to the buyer. Interest rates decreased from 12% and higher to around 9.5% and even lower. Following an increase, they decreased again in 1993–1994.

EXHIBIT 9.3   Your Retirement Budget *(Continued)*

| | | Projected Retirement Budget | | |

Your age _____

	Current	Retirement Self & Spouse (Year ____)	Retirement Self Alone (Year ____)	Retirement Spouse Alone (Year ____)
Income				
Pensions				
Corporate	_____	_____	_____	_____
Government	_____	_____	_____	_____
IRAs	_____	_____	_____	_____
Self-Employment: SEP	_____	_____	_____	_____
IRA/Keogh Plans	_____	_____	_____	_____
Social Security	_____	_____	_____	_____
Investments/Savings				
Annuity Installments	_____	_____	_____	_____
Rental Income	_____	_____	_____	_____
Bond Interest	_____	_____	_____	_____
Stock Dividends	_____	_____	_____	_____
Mutual Fund Dividends	_____	_____	_____	_____
Money Market Accounts	_____	_____	_____	_____
Life Insurance Cash Value	_____	_____	_____	_____
Total Income	_____	_____	_____	_____

Your age _____

	Current	Retirement Self & Spouse (Year ____)	Retirement Self Alone (Year ____)	Retirement Spouse Alone (Year ____)
Expenses				
Mortgage/Rent	_____	_____	_____	_____
Real Estate Taxes/Homeowner's Insurance	_____	_____	_____	_____
Income Taxes	_____	_____	_____	_____
Contributions to Savings	_____	_____	_____	_____
Home Maintenance/Improvements/Furnishings	_____	_____	_____	_____
Utilities	_____	_____	_____	_____
Food	_____	_____	_____	_____
Clothing/Dry Cleaning	_____	_____	_____	_____
Medical Expenses/Health Insurance	_____	_____	_____	_____
Life Insurance	_____	_____	_____	_____
Car Payments/Insurance/Gas/Repairs	_____	_____	_____	_____
Charitable Contributions	_____	_____	_____	_____
Gifts	_____	_____	_____	_____
Travel/Entertainment	_____	_____	_____	_____
Education	_____	_____	_____	_____
Loans/Credit Cards (Interest)	_____	_____	_____	_____
Other	_____	_____	_____	_____
Social Security Taxes	_____	_____	_____	_____
Total Expenses	_____	_____	_____	_____
ANNUAL SURPLUS/SHORTFALL (annual income – annual expenses)	_____	_____	_____	_____

(Continued)

EXHIBIT 9.3   Your Retirement Budget *(Continued)*

Making up the shortfall

Projecting a budget with the previous work sheet gives you an idea of how well your resources match current and anticipated expenses. If you computed an annual shortfall, the charts below are designed to help you develop a systematic savings plan to cover it.

Use the following charts to calculate how much you would need to have in savings in order to withdraw $100 a month over a given number of years. The first chart assumes the account balance is reduced to zero after the period specified; the second chart shows the amount you need to maintain your principal.

Reducing Your Balance to Zero

Example: To withdraw $500 a month from savings for 20 years from an investment earning 7 percent interest, you would need an initial balance of $64,490 (5 × 12,898).

Years of Withdrawals	Average Annual Return		
	5%	7%	9%
5	$ 5,299	$ 5,051	$ 4,825
10	$ 9,428	$ 8,613	$ 7,937
15	$12,646	$11,126	$ 9,962
20	$15,153	$12,898	$11,293
25	$17,106	$14,149	$12,176
30	$18,628	$15,031	$12,776

Note: Chart figures do not include the effect of inflation or income taxes on investment earnings.

It is far wiser to plan your investments so that you maintain your principal. To calculate how much you would need in savings, simply divide the interest rate you expect to earn on your money into the amount of your annual withdrawal.

Maintaining Your Principal

Example: To withdraw $100 a month at the interest rates shown in the first chart, you would need:

Amount Needed in Savings

At 5% interest: $\dfrac{100 \times 12}{.05}$ = $24,000

At 7% interest: $\dfrac{100 \times 12}{.07}$ = $17,143

At 9% interest: $\dfrac{100 \times 12}{.09}$ = $13,333

Accumulating a Nest Egg:

The chart below shows how much you will need to save each year for each $1,000 you would like to accumulate at various interest rates.

Annual Savings to Reach Goal of $1,000

Example: To accumulate $100,000 in 20 years, assuming a 9 percent rate of interest compounded annually, you would need to save $1,954 each year (100 × $19.54).

Years to Retirement	Average Annual Return		
	5%	7%	9%
5	$180.98	$173.89	$167.09
10	$ 79.51	$ 72.38	$ 65.82
15	$ 46.34	$ 39.80	$ 34.06
20	$ 30.24	$ 24.39	$ 19.54
25	$ 20.95	$ 15.81	$ 11.81
30	$ 15.05	$ 10.59	$ 7.34

Note: Chart figures do not include the effect of inflation or income taxes on investment earnings.

Source: From "Financial Guide for Retirement." Copyright © 1990. The USAA Educational Foundation, San Antonio, Texas. Reprinted with permission.

There are several factors to consider when buying a home. These include whether to have a fixed-rate mortgage or an adjustable-rate mortgage, and the costs of a down payment, closing, monthly payments, taxes, and insurance. Most mortgages are for 30 years, although they can be for any number of years, depending on the amount of the down payment and the method of financing. If for less than 30 years, the payments will be somewhat higher but the amount of interest will be lower.

Fixed-Rate Mortgages

Fixed-rate mortgages have the same interest rate during their lifetime. The buyer knows exactly what the monthly payments will be for the life of the loan. When

interest rates were high and fluctuating, neither buyer nor lender wanted fixed-rate mortgages. The buyer wanted lower rates while the lender wanted to get as much interest as possible for a 30-year loan.

Two problems with fixed-rate loans can be due-on-sale clauses and prepayment penalties. Due-on-sale clauses prevent another buyer from assuming the home loan. Prepayment penalties require a sum of money be paid the lender if the loan is paid in full before due.

Some fixed-rate loans can be tied to increasing monthly payments if the buyer desires. The increases are in principal payments while the interest rate remains fixed. In these instances the loan is repaid quicker and the total interest paid is decreased. However, the borrower must be able to meet the increased payments.

Adjustable-Rate Mortgages

Adjustable-rate mortgages (ARMs) provide for the rates to be negotiated and adjusted at intervals. The intervals are agreed upon in the contract. Thus the buyer takes advantage of lowered rates and the lender of higher rates of interest. A borrower should insist on a cap on the interest rate that will keep the payment within payment capacity.

As a rule of thumb, a mortgage payment, including adjustments for taxes and insurance, should not exceed 25 to 28% of monthly income. Thus a person earning $2,000 a month should keep the mortgage payment between $500 and $560. If other debt is considerable, then even this amount should be reduced. In a real estate market where interest rates are 9.5%, a home that costs $48,000 to $50,000 will result in a monthly payment of around $500.

There are other types of mortgages. Graduated-payment mortgages require low payments initially and higher payments in later years. They support the concept of increased earnings by buyers as they grow older. Rising interest rates coupled with rising mortgage payments can create financial problems.

Balloon mortgages result in early monthly payments with a large final payment. Although interest rates are fixed, payments on the principal may not be. The difficulties with other than fixed-rate loans should be fully understood by any buyer-borrower when buying a home with a mortgage.

Closing Costs

There are many costs to the buyer on closing a home loan. These costs can be from $2,500 to $5,000 on a $50,000 loan depending on the source. Closing costs can be paid in cash or can be added to the mortgage principal.

During 1986 and 1993, when interest rates dropped, many homeowners refinanced their houses to take advantage of lower interest rates and thereby bring down their monthly payments. VA and FHA interest rates decreased to 9.5% and lower, which was lower than current market interest rates. This resulted in higher discount points, sometimes as high as 6% of the face value of the loan. A buyer could sometimes fix the discount points at the time of loan application, thereby risking that the rate would increase rather than decrease.

Other closing costs include

1. Loan origination fee to cover costs of processing the loan—limited to 1% on VA and FHA loans but can be much higher on conventional loans
2. Appraisal fee, usually around $100 to $150
3. Credit report fee of approximately $30
4. Hazard insurance premiums of $350-plus depending on the appraisal value of the home or the loan amount
5. Property taxes varying from a few hundred dollars to thousands of dollars depending on location and value of home
6. Funding fee of 1% on VA mortgages
7. Realtor's fee of 3 to 10%
8. Title insurance to guarantee clear title to the property, the fee for which can be hundreds of dollars
9. Escrow fees to an account to pay taxes and homeowner's insurance
10. Survey fees
11. Termite and other inspections
12. Recording deeds
13. Attorney's fees
14. Home warranty fees
15. Recording fees

Down Payments

Down payments range from 0 to 10% of the price of the home. VA home loans require no down payment. FHA loans require a 5% down payment. Conventional loans can range from 5 to 10%, although creative financing can be arranged through some sellers and lenders. Usually, the down payment must be made with a cashier's check. Personal checks are not acceptable.

Homeowner's Insurance

A homeowner's insurance policy includes coverage for dwelling, personal property, and liability. When you purchase this you will need to know and supply the following information:

- Correct name of the policyholder, as it appears on the deed
- Complete address and legal description of the property
- Whether the property is inside or outside the city limits or fire district
- Distance (in feet) to the nearest fire hydrant and distance (in miles) to the nearest fire department
- Year of construction (for homes more than 30 years old, additional information about wiring, plumbing, heating systems, and recent improvements to the property)
- What the house and roof are built of (frame, brick veneer, asbestos siding, or the like)
- Number of square feet of living space and number and types of rooms
- Premises alarm systems, if any, including type, name of manufacturer, and whether it is approved by Underwriters Laboratory (UL)
- Replacement and market value of the dwelling only (without the land) and the amounts of insurance you want
- Amount of the loan, name and address of the lender, and loan number
- Name and address of the person or company handling the closing
- Date to be effective

The homeowner's policy should start on the closing date of the loan. It is due at this time. Ideally, it should cover the replacement cost of the house but is usually required to be equal to the loan amount. Minimum liability insurance can be $100,000 but insurance companies frequently recommend limits of $300,000.

If a home is in a flood hazard area, flood insurance is required. Rates for flood insurance are set by the federal government but must be prepaid.

Borrower Precautions

When buying a home, a person should take the following precautions:

- Have an assumable clause in the loan to guarantee freedom of selling. This protects the interest rate and increases the selling options.
- Avoid prepayment penalties.
- Know rate changes—amounts, dates, and procedures.
- Know changes that may or will occur in the amount of the monthly payment.
- Know payment cap.
- Know interest cap.
- Know the highest monthly payment that can occur.
- Know whether negative amortization can occur and what it will mean.
- Negotiate the best deal possible including payment of any or all closing costs by the seller.

Wills

A will ensures that a person's property goes to the desired person or charity. Otherwise a person's property is distributed by state laws and courts. In the latter instances property is usually divided among surviving spouse and children. If there are no surviving spouse or children, the estate goes to parents, then brothers and sisters, and then to other blood relatives. If there are no blood relatives, property can pass to the state.

Although you can draw up your own will, doing so can create legal problems. The best approach is to have a lawyer do it. It can be cheaply done in a legal clinic or you can call several attorneys and inquire about fees.

All wills are subject to probate laws. They are expensive and time consuming. Any asset owned entirely by an individual is subject to probate. To avoid probate you should have property held jointly or in trust and should name the desired beneficiary on all insurance policies. You can give away assets of $10,000 per year tax free. A husband and wife can give assets of $10,000 each to any number of persons.

If you own a business, want special care for a loved one, want to disinherit someone, or want to set up a trust, you should consult a lawyer. Up to $600,000 can pass to a spouse tax-free if a marital deduction is specified in a will.

Wills contain the following information:

- Identity of the person making the will.
- Statement that the document is a will and revokes all previous wills.
- Name of executor or executrix of estate. This should be a person who agrees to do the job of inventorying assets, paying debts, selling property, and other work.

- Statement directing prompt payment of debts.
- Provision for distribution of assets.
- Provision for guardian of minor children.
- Provision for trust funds.
- A named trustee for any trust fund.
- Provision for gifts to charity or individuals.
- Witnessed and notarized signatures (usually of two uninterested adults).

Give a copy of the will to the executor or executrix. If locked in a safe deposit box, it can be sealed up for some time.

A will should be reviewed periodically and a new one written if changes are desired. To prepare for making your will, use Exhibit 9.4, Estimating Your Net Worth.

Life Insurance

A question often asked is, "How much life insurance do I need?" One answer is that a person should have enough life insurance so that the beneficiary can invest the death benefit and maintain a lifestyle by spending only the interest generated.

Employers often provide some free life insurance and incremental amounts at minimum costs. When buying additional life insurance, buy the maximum coverage at the minimal cost. As income increases, policies that pay dividends and accumulate cash reserves can be purchased. One problem with these policies is that the insurance company has the use of the money to invest at profitable rates. It is a good idea to look at loan rates for cash reserves of insurance policies. Older rates are often 4.5 to 6%. The policy owner can borrow the cash at this rate and invest it in CDs, bonds, or other liquid assets that make a profit. Also, be sure that interest earned is considerably more than interest paid. The tax-deduction benefit ended in 1987.

Insurance plans include annual renewable term, whole life, universal life, group life and health plans, and income replacement plans, among others. Use Exhibit 9.5, as a work sheet to determine your life insurance needs.

Pension Plans

Many employers have pension plans that supplement Social Security income. Some employees frequently participate in pension plans in which they contribute only part of the payment, the employer contributing equal or greater amounts. An employee should know all about any pension plan including vestment, age of retirement, amount of retirement, amount of retirement income, survivor benefits, and other information. This information must be provided to participating employees, but they do not always read it.

Vestment

An employee is vested in a pension plan after a specified period of time, usually 5 to 10 years. *Vestment* means the employee owns all assets of his or her

EXHIBIT 9.4   Estimating Your Net Worth

Assets

Cash in bank

Checking account	$_____
Savings account	_____
Other accounts	_____

Investments

Bonds	_____
Cash value of retirement plans (e.g., company pension, IRA, TSA)	_____
Mutual funds	_____
Stocks	_____

Life insurance	_____

Personal property

Auto and other vehicles	_____
Home furnishings	_____
Jewelry, clothes, silver, china, furs, art, sporting goods, etc.	_____

Real estate

Business	_____
Home (full market value)	_____
House trailer (or RV)	_____
Rental	_____
Vacation home	_____
Other (lots, etc.)	_____
Miscellaneous (e.g., business interests)	_____

Total	$_____

Liabilities

Loans

Auto and other vehicles	$_____
Life insurance	_____
Personal	_____

Mortgages

Business	_____
Home	_____
House trailer (or RV)	_____
Vacation home	_____
Rental	_____
Other (lots, etc.)	_____

Other indebtedness

Medical (physician, dentist, etc.)	_____
Stores (credit card and charge account balances)	_____
Miscellaneous (e.g., funeral and probate costs, inheritance taxes)	_____

Total	$_____
Total assets	_____
minus Total liabilities	========
Net worth	$_____

retirement account including amounts contributed by the employer. If the employee resigns or is fired after having become vested, the retirement account belongs entirely to the employee. Usually, the employer's contribution cannot be withdrawn at this time; however it can be paid at the age specified in the contract. The employee's portion of the retirement account can be withdrawn at any time, the only penalty being taxes if the contribution were tax

EXHIBIT 9.5   How Much Life Insurance Do You Need?

	YOUR ESTIMATES	SAMPLE ESTIMATES
1. **Annual income objective**	$_____	$ 30,000
2. **Minus other sources of annual income**		
Surviving spouse's salary	$_____	$18,000
Investment earnings	_____	820
Social Security	_____	4,000
Pensions	_____	0
Miscellaneous (rental income, etc.)	_____	0
Total income	_____	22,820
3. **Annual income shortfall**		
(Subtract total of item 2 from item 1)	_____	7,180
4. **Amount of death benefit needed** **to get annual income in item 3**		
(Divide amount in item 3 by either .06 or .04)	_____	119,667
5. **Expenses**		
Funeral expenses	_____	
Cost of last hospital stay/illness	_____	
Estate probate costs	_____	10,200
Federal estate taxes	_____	
State inheritance taxes	_____	
Mortgage balance	_____	0
Education fund	_____	44,232
Emergency fund	_____	6,480
Other outstanding debts	_____	5,000
Total expenses	_____	65,912
6. **Preliminary insurance needs**		
(Add total of items 4 and 5)	_____	185,579
7. **Existing liquid assets/other insurance**		
Group life insurance through employer	_____	36,000
Personal life insurance coverages	_____	0
Lump-sum pension payable at death	_____	36,200
Cash and savings	_____	3,300
Securities	_____	5,000
IRA and Keogh plans	_____	0
Employer savings plan (401(k))	_____	0
Other liquid assets	_____	8,000
Total assets/insurance	_____	88,500
8. **Total life insurance needed**		
(Subtract total item 7 from item 6)	_____	97,079

Source: From "Understanding Life Insurance." Copyright © 1996. The USAA Educational Foundation, San Antonio, Texas. Reprinted with permission.

sheltered when paid into the account. A young person may want to withdraw the account to earn higher interest rates on investments over an extended period of time.

Simplified Employee Pension IRA

Simplified employee pension IRAs (SEP-IRAs) are available for owners of small businesses looking for an inexpensive-to-maintain retirement plan for employees.

Start-up costs are minimal and there is no complicated paperwork. All payments are considered a tax-deductible business expense. They are tax deferred for the employee. Maximum contributions are the lesser of $22,500 or 15% of income per year.

Keogh Plans

Keogh Plans are retirement plans for self-employed persons. They can put up to $30,000 per year, or 20% of net income (25% less the contribution itself), into a Keogh Plan. These plans are available from banks, investment companies, and insurance companies. They are tax-deferred retirement plans. Administrative fees usually cost several hundred dollars each year.

Mutual Funds

When investing in mutual funds, be sure to understand their objectives and look at their performance over the last several years. There are some characteristics to consider:

1. Is the fund no-load? No-load funds have no fees for putting money into them. Other funds charge a fee each time a deposit is made.
2. Does the fund preserve capital? You do not want to lose any of your invested money.
3. How liquid are the fund shares? Can they be turned into cash in a short period of time?

There are mutual funds that have no sales charge or redemption fees, which are true "no-load" funds. Some funds allow you to redeem your shares on demand. While a young investor may want mutual funds with a high risk tolerance, long holding period, low liquidity needs, and low income requirements, the retirement-aged investor wants low risk income, a holding period, high liquidity, and high income requirements.

Reputable mutual fund companies attempt to reduce the market risk by diversifying, by selecting highly rated securities, and by continuous monitoring of each holding. Their net asset value per share (NAV/PS) is listed in the business or financial section of most daily newspapers including *The Wall Street Journal*.

Dividends

A buyer of mutual funds should determine when dividends are paid. Some are paid quarterly in cash or in additional shares, whichever is desired. Capital gains are distributed annually. You can receive a monthly or quarterly check for a fixed amount if your investment is a certain amount (usually $10,000 or more).

Check Writing

Some mutual funds have check-writing privileges. The amount of the check is limited and there may be a small service charge.

Most tax-exempt securities fall into categories of general obligation or revenue bonds. General obligation bonds are backed by the authority of a government body such as the state, city, or county to tax its inhabitants. Revenue bonds are backed by income generated by the project they finance. Such projects include hospital, housing, pollution control, and industrial development.

Financial Management Tips

Checking and Savings Accounts

Most people keep money in noninterest-bearing checking accounts and low-interest savings accounts. They should go to credit unions, banks, savings and loan companies, and brokerage firms for information on the kinds of accounts that pay the highest interest and allow check-writing privileges.

Series G Savings Bonds

Series G Savings bonds issued between May 1941 and April 1952 will cease to pay interest after 40 years. Interest not reported will be taxed as income when they are cashed in. If these bonds are 40 years old, they should be cashed in or exchanged for Series HH bonds.

Tax-Free Income

While tax-free bonds reduce income taxes for some people, they do not always equal the advantages of high–interest-bearing taxable bonds. If tax-free bonds pay 7% interest but taxed bonds pay 10% with a net of 8% after taxes are paid, the financial advantage is with the taxable bonds. An account or investment manager can give you appropriate information.

Municipal or other tax-free bonds do not provide for growth during inflation. They make sense for the investor who is only concerned with tax-free income.

Employer Benefit Plans

Employees should examine their employers' benefit plans carefully. Each plan should be evaluated separately. Matching contributions to savings plans, stock accumulation plans, supplemental group term life insurance, and long-term disability coverage can each have a financial advantage to any employee.

Dependent Working Children

A parent who pays more than 50% of a working child's support can claim that child as a dependent. The child must be under age 19 or a full-time student, and unmarried. Scholarships received by the full-time student are not counted in making this determination.

Lump-Sum Distributions

Persons under 70½ years of age who receive lump-sum distributions upon retirement or termination should investigate treating it as a 5-year forward-averaging item or rolling it over into an IRA. Otherwise, they will pay income tax on the total sum in 1 year.

Home-Improvement Costs

It is important to keep track of all home-improvement costs because they can be added to the cost of the house when bought. The taxable profit will be the difference between the selling price and the sum of all home-improvement costs added to the original price paid for the house.

Itemizing Tax Deductions

Keeping accurate expense records is always useful. To gain the advantages of itemizing tax deductions, you should have proof of all expenses. In fact, the Internal Revenue Service requires that you be able to document itemized deductions.

Highly appreciated capital assets can sometimes be donated to charity and be deducted at full market value. Thus both taxpayer and charity benefit fully.

When giving annual gifts to friends or relatives, donors should consider giving appreciated securities. They have not been previously taxed as have other assets. Thus the donor avoids taxes and the recipient may be in a tax bracket that makes capital gains tax significant.

Donate all used goods to a charity and get a receipt. The amounts can be tax deductions.

Child-care credits are available for children under 15 years of age. Keep an account of all child-care expenses and have an income tax accountant determine which are deductible. This can save as much as $1,440 in 1 year.

Tax Withholding

Although it is exciting to get a tax refund, it is not good financial management. The government is using your money. Use form W-4 worksheet to determine your payroll deduction amount. Keep it at a minimum underpayment or overpayment and invest your money.

Summary

Prudent professional nurses plan their financial security. This planning begins with keeping a personal budget, and that includes provision for liquidity in times of emergency. Any tax-sheltered savings available to the individual should be considered for savings including a tax-sheltered annuity, an annuity, an IRA, or tax-sheltered bonds.

Home ownership is one of the major benefits available to the average nurse. Interest can be deducted on income tax returns and equity builds as mortgage payments are made. Care should be taken when changing the type of mortgage.

Every professional nurse should have a will to ensure that personal and real property goes to the desired individual. When buying life insurance, one should get the widest coverage for the cheapest price. Also seek employment with a company that has a pension plan and check all conditions of investment. Setting up a Keogh Plan or SEP-IRA for retirement is another alternative.

The best advice for the professional nurse: Make your money work for you!

Experiential Exercises

1. Prepare a personal budget using the format of Exhibit 9.1.
2. Determine from your employer the availability of TSAs and matching contributions. Decide whether you want to participate and act by contracting with the company providing the best benefits. Use Exhibit 9.2 to help make your decision. This exercise may be done as an individual or as a group.
3. Make a plan for your retirement income. Use the format of Exhibit 9.3.
4. Use Exhibit 9.4 to determine your net worth.
5. Use Exhibit 9.5 as a method of determining your life insurance needs.

Note

1. T. P. Pare. "Everything You Ever Wanted to Know About 401(k)s (But Were Afraid to Ask)." *Fortune* (Dec. 25, 1995):176-178, 180; R. S. Teitelbaum. "Getting the Most from Your 401(k)." *Fortune* (Dec. 25, 1995):183-184.

References

"A Will of Your Own." *AIDE Magazine* (Spring 1986):17-19.

Bamford et al., Consumer Reports Books Staff, and Jeff Blyskal, Eds. *Complete Guide to Managing Your Money* (Yonkers, NY: Consumer Reports, 1989).

Bromberg, B. S. "Significance of the Tax Reform Act of 1984 for Professionals." *Review of Taxation of Individuals* (Winter 1985):98-102.

Corrigan, A., and P. Kaufman. *How to Use Credit and Credit Cards* (Stamford, Conn.: Longmeadow Press, 1985).

Eisenberg. R. "Rating Your Firm's Retirement Plans/Premium Company Plans." *Money* (Nov. 1984):185-197.

Harris, H. "Creating a Budget." *Money* (Oct. 1983):71-76.

Hira, L. S. "Rollovers to IRAs and Tax Planning for IRA Distributions after TEFRA." *Tax Adviser* (May 1984):280-286.

"How Much Life Insurance Is Enough?" *AIDE Magazine* (Winter 1986):18.

"How to Choose the Right IRA for You." *AIDE Magazine* (Winter 1985):12-16.

"How to Take a Personal Audit that Tells You What You're Really Worth." *Professional Report* (Dec. 1980):13-15.

"Investing Now in Your IRA." *AIDE Magazine* (Winter 1986):22.

Johnson, R. H. "Spend It Only After You've Saved It, Johnson Says." *National Underwriter* (June 25, 1984):64-65.

Koehler, D. "Financial Planning; Key Considerations for Success." *Bank Marketing* (June 1984):19-30.

"Making Sense of Today's Home Mortgages." *AIDE Magazine* (Spring 1985):9-16.

Morton, L. "Money-Making Ideas for 401(k) Plans." *Insurance Sales* (Dec. 1984):20-26.

"The New Tax Act and Its Effect on TIAA-CREF Participants." *The Participant* (Jan. 1987):1-4.

Quinn, J. B. *Making the Most of Your Money* (New York: Simon and Schuster Trade, 1991).

Sheets, J. G. "Financial Planning with Life Insurance." *Wealthbuilding* (July 1983):16-17, 20-21, 33.

Sheets, J. G. "How Much Is Your Life Worth? *Wealthbuilding* (May 1984):14-15.

Weinstein, G. W. "Taking Charge of Your Finances." *Parade Magazine* (Feb. 1, 1987):12a-j.

"Your Budget and Your Life." *Wealthbuilding* (Nov.-Dec. 1984):32-36.

Index